Critical Care Nursing

Critical Care Nursing
Learning from Practice

Edited by

Suzanne Bench

*Florence Nightingale School of Nursing and Midwifery,
King's College, London*

and

Kate Brown

*Florence Nightingale School of Nursing and Midwifery,
King's College, London*

WILEY-BLACKWELL

A John Wiley & Sons, Ltd., Publication

This edition first published 2011. © 2011 by Blackwell Publishing Ltd

Blackwell Publishing was acquired by John Wiley & Sons in February 2007. Blackwell's publishing program has been merged with Wiley's global Scientific, Technical and Medical business to form Wiley-Blackwell.

Registered office: John Wiley & Sons Ltd, The Atrium, Southern Gate, Chichester,
West Sussex, PO19 8SQ, UK

Editorial offices: 9600 Garsington Road, Oxford, OX4 2DQ, UK
2121 State Avenue, Ames, Iowa 50014-8300, USA

For details of our global editorial offices, for customer services and for information about how to apply for permission to reuse the copyright material in this book please see our website at www.wiley.com/wiley-blackwell.

Library of Congress Cataloging-in-Publication Data

Critical care nursing : learning from practice / edited by Suzanne Bench and Kate Brown.
   p. ; cm.
  Includes bibliographical references and index.
  ISBN 978-1-4051-6995-0 (pbk. : alk. paper)
  1. Intensive care nursing–Case studies.   I. Bench, Suzanne.   II. Brown, Kate, MSc.
  [DNLM: 1. Critical Illness–nursing–Case Reports.   2. Critical Care–methods–Case Reports.
3. Critical Care–organization & administration–Case Reports.   WY 154]
  RT120.I5C763 2011
  616.02'8–dc22

                                                                     2010040962

A catalogue record for this book is available from the British Library.

This book is published in the following electronic formats: ePDF 9781444393088 ePub 9781444393095

Set in 10/12.5 pt Times by Aptara® Inc., New Delhi, India
Printed and bound in Malaysia by Vivar Printing Sdn Bhd

1   2011

Contents

Contributor list

Suzanne Bench, MSc, PGDipHE, BSc (Hons), RGN, ENB 100
Lecturer in Critical Care Nursing
Florence Nightingale School of Nursing
    and Midwifery
King's College
London

Kate Brown, MSc, PGDipHE, BA (Hons), RGN, ENB AO9
Lecturer in Critical Care Nursing
Florence Nightingale School of Nursing
    and Midwifery
King's College
London

Maureen Coombs, MBE, PhD, RN
Consultant Nurse
Critical Care
Southampton University Hospitals Trust
Southampton

Ruth Cork, BSc, PGDipHPE, RGN, ENB 100
Senior Sister
Staff Development and Training
Intensive Care
East Surrey Hospital
Redhill, Surrey

Cheryl Crocker, PhD, MSc, PGDipHE, BA, RNT, RN
Consultant Nurse
Critical Care
Nottingham University Hospital
Nottingham

Annette Davies, MSc, BSc (Hons), PGCAP, RN, ENB 134, ENB 100
Lecturer/Practitioner
Renal Critical Care
Renal Unit
King's College Hospital
London

Helen Dickie, BA, RGN, ENB 100, ENB 998
Renal Sister
Critical Care
Guy's and St Thomas' NHS Foundation
    Trust
London

Danielle Fullwood, BNurs (Hons), RGN, ENB 100
Lecturer/Practitioner
Liver Intensive Care
King's College Hospital
London

Julie Hamilton, MSc, BNurs, RGN, ENB 100
Practice Development Lead
Perioperative, Critical Care and Pain
   Division
Guy's and St Thomas' NHS Foundation
   Trust
London

Sinead Mehigan, PhD, PGDE, BSc (Hons), RN
Head of Department of Initial and Acute
   Nursing Practice
School of Health and Social Sciences
Middlesex University
London

Claire Merriman, MSc, PGDipHPE, BSc (Hons), RGN, ENB 148, ENB 998
Head of Professional Practice Skills
School of Health and Social Care
Oxford Brookes University
Oxford

Tina Moore, MSc, BSc, PGCEA, RN
Senior Lecturer in Acute and Critical Care
   Nursing
School of Health and Social Sciences
Middlesex University
London

Suzanne Sargent, MSc, PGCE (TLHE), BSc (Hons), RN, ENB 100
Lecturer/Practitioner
Liver Intensive Care
King's College Hospital
London

Deborah Slade, MSc, PGCertHPE, BSc (Hons), RGN, ENB 100, ENB 148
Senior Lecturer
Faculty of Health and Life Sciences
Oxford Brookes University
Oxford

Sue Whaley, BSc (Hons), PGCAP, RGN, ENB 199
Lecturer/Practitioner
Emergency Department
Guy's and St Thomas' NHS Foundation
   Trust
London

Preface

Nurses need to continually examine their own practice skills and knowledge in order to provide expert care for the critically ill patient. The content of the book is not intended as a comprehensive critical care text but rather aims to explore some of the common challenges faced by critical care practitioners. Each chapter focuses on a patient in practice, critically examining the knowledge and skills required to attain greater expertise. It provides opportunities for readers to reflect on their own experiences enabling professional growth and development. The book also promotes inter-professional collaboration, whilst valuing the unique position of the critical care nurse. Evidence-based practice is an essential goal within healthcare, and to reflect this, a relevant research paper has been included for each case study. This will enable the reader to examine the quality of available evidence and evaluate their own practice in light of this.

Critical care is an expanding area of healthcare, with an acknowledged requirement for practitioners to develop their skills in managing critically ill patients in a range of locations (DH 2000). As technology and research continue to advance, this book will support practitioners in meeting the challenges of the future.

We hope you find it enjoyable to read and a useful resource in supporting the delivery of high-quality critical care nursing practice.

Suzanne Bench
Kate Brown

Acknowledgements

We would like to express our gratitude to each of the chapter authors for their expertise, hard work and patience during the development of this book. We would also like to thank the following people for taking the time to review chapter content and for their insightful and valuable comments: Helen Dickie, Dr. Carol Ball, Mary Pennell, Chris Hill, Sandra Fairley, Doreen Patsika, Margaret Kirkby. We are also very grateful to all those who kindly gave permission to use their tables, figures, illustrations, pictures and photographs within the text.

Finally, we wish to thank our families, colleagues and friends for their unwavering encouragement and support in the preparation of this book.

Chapter 1

The patient with acute lung injury (ALI)

Julie Hamilton

Introduction

Acute respiratory distress syndrome (ARDS) is the severest form of acute lung injury (ALI) and presents one of the greatest challenges to health professionals within critical care. This scenario focuses on the knowledge and skills necessary to manage the complex needs of a patient with ARDS.

Patient scenario

Lee Kuan Yew, a 68-year-old gentleman who weighs 75 kg, was admitted to the intensive care unit (ICU) following intubation in the Accident and Emergency (A&E) department for acute respiratory failure. He had been unwell for four days with shortness of breath, pleuritic pain, fever and rigours and presented to the A&E with tachypnoea, followed by dyspnoea and progressive hypoxaemia and hypercarbia. Physical examination revealed focal findings of consolidation. His past medical history was unremarkable, but he smoked 30 cigarettes per day for the past 40 years. Three days following his admission to the ICU, Lee Kuan Yew remains sedated, intubated and mechanically ventilated. Assessment findings can be seen in Table 1.1.

Reader activities

Having read this scenario, consider the following:

- How do Lee Kuan Yew's symptoms suggest that he has an ALI?
- Consider the possible causes of Mr Kuan Yew's lung injury. Outline the factors that make him at risk for the development of ALI.
- What stage of ALI do you think Mr Kuan Yew is in? Explain this using relevant pathophysiology.
- Analyse the blood gas presented. Consider the possible causes of Mr Kuan Yew's altered results.

Critical Care Nursing: Learning from Practice, 1st edition. Edited by Suzanne Bench and Kate Brown.
© 2011 Blackwell Publishing Ltd.

- Do you agree with the current ventilation strategy? How would you manage Mr Kuan Yew's respiratory function?
- What therapies other than conventional ventilation can be utilised in the management of ARDS?

Table 1.1   Assessment findings.

Ventilator settings	• Ventilated on synchronised intermittent mandatory ventilation–volume control (SIMV-VC) • 50% oxygen (FiO$_2$ 0.5) • PEEP 5 cmH$_2$O • Preset tidal volume (Vt) 600 mL • Respiratory rate set at 14 bpm (no spontaneous effort) • Peak airway pressure (PAP) 31 cmH$_2$O • Inspiratory:expiratory ratio 1:2
Clinical findings	• Bilateral air entry with coarse crackles throughout • Frothy pink sputum obtained on endotracheal suctioning • Bilateral infiltrates on chest X-ray
Arterial blood gases	• pH 7.34 • PaCO$_2$ 6.5 kPa • PaO$_2$ 10.8 kPa • HCO$_3$$^-$ (standard) 20 mmol/L • Base excess −3 • PaO$_2$/FiO$_2$ 21.6 kPa • SpO$_2$ 92%
Haemodynamic data	• Heart rate (HR) 115 bpm (sinus) • Mean arterial blood pressure (MABP) 59 mmHg • Central venous pressure (CVP) 9 mmHg • Tympanic temperature 38.7°C • Feels peripherally warm to touch • 500 mL colloid administered over last 24 hours • Urine output 40 mL/h • Nasogastric feeding in progress at 80 mL/h
Laboratory results:	Sodium 137 mmol/l Potassium 4.5 mmol/L Lactate 2.8 mmol/L Glucose 8.2 mmol/L Haemoglobin (Hb) 10.5 g/L Raised white cell count (WCC) and C-reactive protein (CRP) level

Definitions of acute lung injury (ALI) and acute respiratory distress syndrome (ARDS)

Adult respiratory distress syndrome was first described by Ashbaugh et al. in 1967 as a clinical syndrome different from other types of acute respiratory failure, with clinical characteristics of tachypnoea, hypoxaemia resistant to supplemental oxygen, diffuse alveolar infiltrates and decreased pulmonary compliance (Ashbaugh et al. 1967).

Since its initial description in 1967, the criteria for defining ALI/ARDS have changed several times. In 1988 Murray and colleagues proposed a definition which described

Table 1.2 American–European Consensus Conference Definitions of ALI/ARDS.

	Onset	Chest X-ray	Left-ventricular pressure	PaO$_2$/FiO$_2$
ALI	Acute onset	Bilateral infiltrates on chest X-ray	No clinical evidence of left-atrial hypertension or PAOP <18 mmHg	<40 kPa
ARDS	Acute onset	Bilateral infiltrates on chest X-ray	No clinical evidence of left-atrial hypertension or PAOP <18 mmHg	26.6 kPa

Source: From Bernard et al. (1994).

whether the syndrome was in an acute or chronic phase, the physiological severity of pulmonary injury and the disorder associated with the development of the lung injury (Murray et al. 1988). In 1994, recognising that the study of ALI and ARDS was still hindered by the lack of a simple, uniform definition, the North American–European Consensus Conference (NAECC) published further revised definitions (Bernard et al. 1994) (see Table 1.2).

From the NAECC definition it can be deduced that Mr Kuan Yew has ARDS. He has developed acute respiratory failure requiring ventilation; he is hypoxaemic with a PaO$_2$/FiO$_2$ ratio of 21.6 kPa and has bilateral infiltrates on chest x-ray (see Figure 1.1).

Mr Kuan Yew does not have a pulmonary artery catheter *in situ* to enable determination of the pulmonary artery occlusion pressure (PAOP); however, he has no history of cardiac disease and clinically shows no signs of left-atrial hypertension such as a raised central venous pressure (CVP), although the latter can be normal in left-atrial hypertension. Mr Kuan Yew is also demonstrating symptoms of severe sepsis (see Chapter 4 for further information on sepsis), a common co-existing condition.

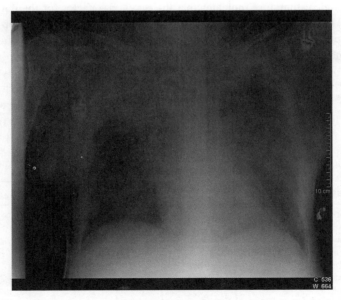

Figure 1.1 Chest X-ray. (X-ray courtesy of Dr Duncan Wyncoll, Consultant Intensivist, Guy's and St Thomas' NHS Foundation Trust, London.)

Pathophysiology of ALI/ARDS

Pathology

In 1972 the National Institute of Health estimated the incidence of ARDS at 60 cases per 100 000 population per year (National Heart and Lung Institute, National Institute of Health (NHL, NIH) 1972). Several robust studies since then have demonstrated a wide range of incidence rates of ARDS from 1.5 to 8.3 cases per 100 000 per year (Villar and Slutsky 1989; Garber et al. 1996). Although it could therefore be considered a rare disease, the mortality of ARDS is high, estimated to be between 34% and 65% (Estenssoro et al. 2002; Herridge et al. 2003). The incidence of ALI, however, appears more common with many patients within high dependency settings having a PaO_2/FiO_2 of <40 kPa. It is therefore essential that critical care nurses have an understanding of the pathophysiology and management of ALI and ARDS. The major cause of death in patients with ALI/ARDS is multiple organ failure and irreversible respiratory failure, with 84% of deaths occurring more than three days after the onset of ALI/ARDS caused by multi-system organ failure (Ware and Matthay 2000).

   Acute lung injury is a term used to describe the response of the lungs to a broad range of insults with ARDS representing the most severe end of the spectrum. Its pathophysiology is driven by an aggressive inflammatory reaction which results in widespread changes throughout the lung. A broad variety of precipitating causes are recognised and these can be differentiated into those which cause injury to the lung directly and those which cause injury indirectly (see Table 1.3). A number of endogenous anti-inflammatory mechanisms are also initiated to counteract the effects of the aggressive pro-inflammatory response; however, these responses may be excessive and contribute to a state of immunoparesis (Doyle et al. 1995).

   Epidemiological literature indicates that the major risk factor for the development of ALI and ARDS is severe sepsis; 18–40% of patients with sepsis will develop ALI/ARDS, followed by pneumonia, aspiration of gastric contents, multiple blood transfusions, multiple trauma and pregnancy-related ALI/ARDS (Villar and Slutsky 1989; Ware and Matthay 2000).

   From Mr Kuan Yew's clinical history and initial presentation it appears that he may have developed an acute lung injury and subsequent ARDS from a direct cause such as lobar pneumonia. It is also important, however, to note that as Mr Kuan Yew is mechanically

Table 1.3   Risk factors for ARDS.

Direct causes	Indirect causes
• Aspiration of gastric contents	• Sepsis
• Pneumonia	• Massive blood transfusion
• Near drowning	• Disseminated intravascular coagulation
• Lung trauma, e.g. blast injury, lung contusions	• Pancreatitis
• Inhalation injury	• Cardiopulmonary bypass
• Fat emboli	• Pregnancy-related ARDS

ventilated and is critically ill, he is at a significant risk of developing a nosocomial infection and secondary sepsis (Vincent et al. 1995), a major risk factor for the development of ARDS, and at present he is indeed demonstrating signs of severe sepsis.

ALI and ARDS cause diffuse alveolar damage affecting all parts of the alveolus, including the epithelium, the endothelium and the interstitial space. It is a progressive condition with the pathological changes typically described as passing through three overlapping phases – an inflammatory or exudative phase, a proliferative phase and a fibrotic phase (Ware and Matthay 2000).

Exudative phase

Lasting for up to seven days following the onset of symptoms, the exudative or acute phase of ALI/ARDS is characterised by the influx of protein-rich oedema fluid into the alveolar air spaces, as a result of increased permeability of the alveolar–capillary membrane and the formation of hyaline membranes. The hyaline membranes contain necrotic epithelial cells, plasma proteins which have been deposited in the alveolar space as part of the inflammatory exudate that leaks across the alveolar–capillary membrane, immunoglobulin and complement. The alveolar–capillary barrier has focal areas of damage and the alveolar wall is oedematous. Neutrophils are increasingly found within the capillaries, interstitium and eventually airspaces. As the process of damage progresses, there is extensive necrosis of type 1 alveolar epithelial cells and further hyaline membrane formation (Figures 1.2a and 1.2b).

These pathological changes can be seen in Mr Kuan Yew's clinical picture by the presence of pulmonary oedema and his deterioration in lung function. Flooding of the alveoli with protein-rich fluid and debris has caused a decrease in lung compliance, reflected in the high airway pressures. It has also caused a significant reduction in the diffusion of oxygen, leading to a reduced arterial oxygen saturation and PaO_2. Fluid-filled

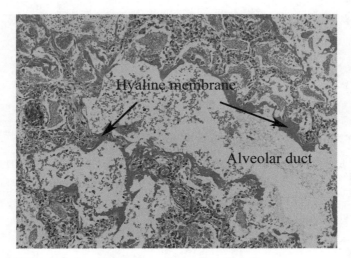

Figure 1.2 (a) Histopathology slide of lung tissue. (*Continued*)

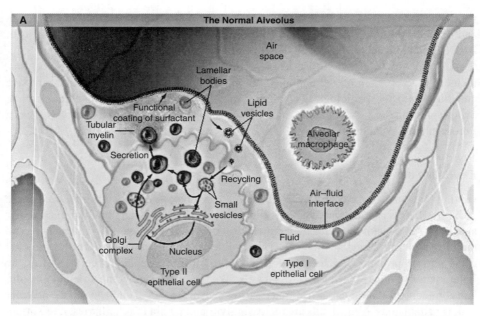

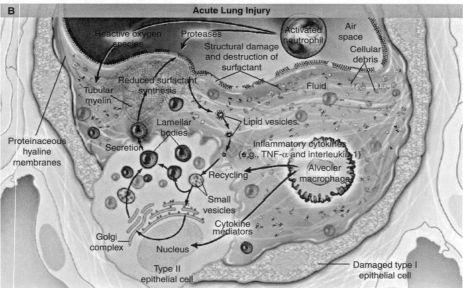

Figure 1.2   (*Continued*) (b) Diagrammatic illustration of cellular changes in ARDS. (Baudouin 2004). Used with permission of Massachusetts Medical Society.

and collapsed alveoli result in the development of a right to left intra-pulmonary shunt. The negative effects of this on Mr Kuan Yew's gas exchange are further compounded by loss of the normal compensatory hypoxic pulmonary constriction.

Proliferative phase

The proliferative phase is characterised by organisation of the hyaline membranes by proliferating fibroblasts, cell debris and inflammatory cells (Ware and Matthay 2000). Necrosis of type 1 alveolar cells exposes areas of the epithelial basement membrane and the lumens of the alveoli fill with leucocytes, red blood cells and fibrin. Type 2 alveolar cells, which are responsible for the production of surfactant, are also damaged but some proliferate along the alveolar wall in an attempt to cover damaged areas of the epithelium and differentiate into type 1 cells. Pulmonary oedema is less prominent at this stage; however, alveolar collapse becomes more marked and the alveolar ducts become narrowed and distorted. This then leads to a further increase in the degree of intrapulmonary shunt, leading to a further deterioration in gas exchange, and hypoxaemia resistant to oxygen therapy.

At this stage the process can be reversed and the lung parenchyma may return to normal. However, in some cases the damage is severe and the hyaline membranes become incorporated into the walls of the revised alveoli (Ware and Matthay 2000).

Fibrotic phase

The fibrotic phase can begin as early as ten days following the insult and is characterised by progressive thickening of the vasculature walls and an increase in the amount of lung collagen (Ware and Matthay 2000). Fibrosis results in a further reduction in lung compliance, increasing the work of breathing, decreasing the tidal volume and resulting in the retention of CO_2. As a result of the destruction of some alveoli and interstitial thickening, gas exchange is reduced and this contributes to further hypoxaemia and ventilator dependence.

Pathogenesis of ALI/ARDS

Inflammation

As a result of the initiation of an inflammatory response, there is increased leucocyte production and mobilisation to the inflamed site. Mediator cascades including the production of cytokines, chemokines, free radicals and complement and coagulation pathway components are also activated. There is also an anti-inflammatory response.

The neutrophil is the dominant leucocyte involved in the pro-inflammatory response. Neutrophils cause cell damage by the production of free radicals, pro-inflammatory mediators and proteases, and excessive quantities of these products, including cytokines, have been found in patients with ARDS (Chollet et al. 1996). The inflammatory response is in part driven by cytokines. Two of the major pro-inflammatory cytokines are tumour necrosis factor-α (TNF-α) and interleukin-1 (IL-1). The actions of these include (1) recruitment and localisation of macrophages to the lung parenchyma, (2) stimulation of other inflammatory cytokines such as IL-6 and IL-8 and (3) adherence of neutrophils to endothelium. Cytokines and other pro-inflammatory mediators such as endotoxin and thrombin have also been implicated in the increased vascular permeability that contributes to pulmonary oedema in ALI/ARDS (Ware and Matthay 2000).

This inflammatory response leads to surfactant dysfunction in ALI/ARDS (Baudouin 1997), with destruction and loss of type 2 cells resulting in decreased synthesis and recirculation of surfactants. Additionally, leakage of protein-rich fluid into the alveoli during the development of ALI/ARDS, as seen in Mr Kuan Yew's clinical picture, contaminates the surfactant, resulting in a further reduction in its ability to function. The degree to which lack of surfactant contributes to the pathogenesis of ALI/ARDS, however, remains unclear.

Fibroproliferative response and resolution of ARDS

The fibroproliferative response is part of a normal repair process; however, if not closely regulated, it can have serious consequences such as lung fibrosis. Mediators such as TNF-α and products of the coagulation cascade such as thrombin, fibrin and factor Xa fuel the fibrotic response and stimulate local fibroblasts to migrate, replicate and produce excessive amounts of connective tissue.

In some patients pulmonary fibrosis does not completely resolve and can lead to problems with weaning from mechanical ventilation. There does not appear to be a uniform response to injury in that some patients develop ALI, some develop ARDS and some do not develop pulmonary symptoms at all. The reason for this may lie in genetics and recent evidence suggests that there is a genetic susceptibility both to sepsis and ARDS (Wax and Angus 2000).

Holistic assessment and detailed management of all issues related to total patient care are fundamental in caring for patients such as Mr Kuan Yew who have ARDS. In early ARDS, however, difficulties with oxygenation can be the major physiological challenge requiring careful assessment, titration of therapy and meticulous monitoring.

Tests and investigations

Continuous pulse oximetry

Continuous pulse oximetry has become a vital part of monitoring the critically ill patient as it is readily available, is non-invasive and can be used in many different settings. Pulse oximeters shine red and infrared light through a finger or ear lobe using a probe. The proportion of light absorbed allows the amount of oxygenated and deoxygenated haemoglobin to be estimated. The pulsatile component of absorption corresponds to arterial blood, and therefore, arterial oxygen saturation can be deduced. When arterial oxygen saturations are greater than 80%, current pulse oximeters can detect arterial oxygen saturations to within a few percentage points and their use would, therefore, be beneficial in the assessment of Mr Kuan Yew's oxygenation. However, they are less accurate when arterial oxygen saturations are lower. It is also important to be aware that inaccurate values may be obtained in patients with shock, due to poor peripheral perfusion, by carboxyhaemoglobin, by low levels of haemoglobin and by the use of some dyes such as methylene blue which absorb wavelengths of light used by some pulse oximeters. After ruling out the possibility of any of these contraindications in Mr Kuan Yew's case, pulse oximetry will be a useful tool to rapidly detect periods of arterial hypoxaemia.

Arterial blood gas analysis

Arterial blood gas analysis is considered the gold standard in the assessment and management of ARDS patients such as Mr Kuan Yew. To ensure accuracy, however, it is important that the health professional obtaining the sample is aware of several key points. The sample must be taken and processed as quickly as possible to eliminate aerobic contamination; the current FiO_2 and temperature of the patient should be recorded at the time of sampling, the latter to allow temperature correction, and the sample rapidly analysed in a calibrated blood gas machine. If the arterial blood gas results are to reflect current ventilatory support, the sample should not be obtained until 15–20 minutes following any manipulation of ventilator settings. PaO_2, $PaCO_2$ and pH are measured during arterial blood gas analysis. Oxygen saturation may be measured by a co-oximeter built into a blood gas machine or estimated from the PaO_2 based on the oxygen-dissociation curve corrected for temperature, $PaCO_2$ and pH. This estimate is considered reasonably accurate for oxygen saturations greater than 80% but is significantly erroneous at lower saturations.

PaO₂/FiO₂ measurement

The sole use of PaO_2 in assessing Mr Kuan Yew has limitations. As a result calculation of the ratio of PaO_2 to FiO_2 is now commonly used as an additional measurement (see Chapter 2 on weaning for how to calculate the PaO_2/FiO_2 ratio). The usefulness of the PaO_2/FiO_2 ratio is clearly demonstrated in Mr Kuan Yew's arterial blood gas results. At first glance a PaO_2 of 10.8 kPa could appear to be an acceptable level; however, when the FiO_2 is taken into consideration, it is clear from the NAECC definition that he has ARDS as his PaO_2/FiO_2 ratio is 21.6 kPa.

Evidence-based management of a patient with ALI/ARDS

Airway and breathing

In patients like Mr Kuan Yew who have severe ARDS, the hallmark respiratory abnormality is hypoxaemia which gradually becomes more resistant to supplemental oxygen therapy as the condition progresses. Maintaining adequate arterial oxygenation is therefore a goal given a high priority and usually requires assisted/mechanical ventilation.

Assisted ventilation is generally carried out invasively via an endotracheal tube. However, a small subset of patients may be candidates for non-invasive ventilation (Hilbert et al. 2001). Non-invasive positive pressure ventilation (NIPPV) is finding increasing application in the management of acute respiratory failure in the high-dependency setting and it may be postulated that it would be successful in carefully chosen patients with ALI. It may aid in the recruitment of collapsed and fluid-filled alveoli, thereby reducing intrapulmonary shunt, and could also facilitate unloading of the respiratory muscles, reducing the work of breathing. It is important to highlight, however, that patients with ALI and ARDS are also frequently haemodynamically unstable, have severe hypoxaemia or have a rapidly progressive course of disease. Therefore, although NIPPV has been shown to be beneficial in some patients, there is little published experience or evidence of its benefits in patients with ARDS. It may therefore not be a good first choice for Mr Kuan Yew.

Approaches to mechanical ventilation

The pathophysiology of ARDS has been presented earlier in this chapter; however, it is important to highlight some important features which are relevant when discussing Mr Kuan Yew's ventilatory management. Computerised tomographic scanning (CT) has demonstrated that consolidation of lung tissue in ARDS is not uniform but rather is concentrated in dependent lung regions, leaving non-dependent areas relatively aerated. This distribution of aerated lung, described as 'baby lung' (Gattinoni et al. 1987), has important implications for mechanical ventilation strategies.

Traditional methods of mechanically ventilating patients with ALI and ARDS gave priority to the maintenance of oxygenation, while minimising the use of high concentrations of oxygen, and providing sufficient ventilation to maintain arterial pH and $PaCO_2$ within normal limits. These goals were achieved by the administration of increased levels of positive end expiratory pressure (PEEP) to enable a decrease in the FiO_2, and the use of relatively large tidal volumes of 10–15 mL/kg. This approach, however, results in high inspiratory pressures in patients who already have decreased lung compliance. The application of tidal volumes of 10–15 mL/kg can also lead to over-inflation of the normal 'baby lung' which has been shown to cause local damage and further inflammation (Dreyfuss and Sauman 1998). Present understanding of ventilator-induced lung injury suggests that a traditional mechanical ventilation strategy such as this, using high tidal volumes and is likely to enhance Mr Kuan Yew's lung injury. Lung injury is caused by excessive volumes rather than high airway pressure (Dreyfuss et al. 1988) and even healthy animals ventilated with high tidal volumes for several hours develop pulmonary oedema that is histologically identical to that seen in ARDS. Furthermore, in animal models with ALI, large lung volumes have been shown to cause increased oedema accumulation and cytokine production (Tremblay et al. 1997). Although evidence in humans is lacking, it is likely that ventilating with high tidal volumes results in similar effects.

Four randomised controlled trials of 'lung-protective' ventilation, directed at preventing over-distension of the lung in ARDS, have been published over the past ten years (Brochard et al. 1998; Stewart et al. 1998; Brower et al. 1999; Acute Respiratory Distress Syndrome Network (ARDSNet) 2000). Of these the ARDSNet (2000) study is the largest and the

Table 1.4   Summary of ARDSNet (2000) low tidal volume strategy.

Variable	Settings
Ventilator mode	Volume assist control
Set tidal volume (mL/kg)	Aim for 6 mL/kg (*if baseline tidal volume >8 mL/kg, then set initial tidal volume at 8 mL/kg and reduce by 1 mL/kg every 2 h until 6 mL/kg*)
Rate (breaths/min)	Set to approximate baseline rate of 6–35 breaths/min but not >35 breaths/min
Pressure (cmH$_2$O)	Aim for Pplat <30 cmH$_2$O or peak pressure <35 cmH2O
Inspiratory flow rate (L/min)	Above patient demand (>80 L/min)
Inspiratory:expiratory ratio	1:1–1.3
PaO$_2$ (kPa)	7.3–10.7
SpO$_2$ (%)	88–95
PEEP and FiO$_2$	Incremental FiO$_2$/PEEP combinations have been suggested with PEEP range from 5 to 24 cmH$_2$O (see Table 1.3)
pH	7.30–7.45

Source: Adapted from the NIH NHLBI ARDSNet low tidal volume ventilation strategy (ARDSNet 2000).

only one to date to demonstrate a mortality benefit of a lung-protective strategy in ARDS patients. Eight hundred and sixty one patients were randomised into two groups. One group received a tidal volume of 6 mL/kg if the plateau pressure (Pplat) did not exceed 30 cmH$_2$O and 4–5 mL/kg if the Pplat exceeded 30 cmH$_2$O and the other group received tidal volumes of 10–12 mL/kg if the Pplat did not exceed 50 cmH$_2$O and tidal volumes as low as 4 mL/kg if the Pplat exceeded 50 cmH$_2$O. A 9% mortality difference was observed in those patients who received the lower tidal volume ventilation strategy. Although the design of the ARDSNet trial has been heavily criticised, the ARDSNet lower tidal volume strategy has become accepted as the standard on which to base the ventilatory management of patients with acute lung injury (see Table 1.4 for protective lung ventilation protocol from the ARDSNet study) and this is how Mr Kuan Yew's ventilation should be managed.

Volume control versus pressure controlled ventilation

Traditionally, invasive mechanical ventilation has been provided by volume controlled modes, as in the case of Mr Kuan Yew, whereby a preset tidal volume is delivered at a preset rate and inspiratory flow. Volume control, has the benefit of maintaining a constant tidal volume and hence minute ventilation and PaCO$_2$ under changing respiratory system conditions and easy detection of changes in lung mechanics. Over the past decade, however, in light of research demonstrating the non-homogenous distribution of consolidation in ARDS and the focus on limiting alveolar distension, there has been a trend towards the use of pressure controlled modes of ventilation.

With pressure control, a decelerating inspiratory flow is applied to a preset pressure limit, allowing the critical care team to select both inspiratory and expiratory pressures with the advantage of limiting pressure to a set level. The critical care nurse has to be particularly vigilant when caring for a patient on pressure control ventilation as changes in lung compliance are not as easily detected. Close observation of the tidal volume and PaCO$_2$ is essential to detect changes in lung mechanics.

As a result of technological advances in mechanical ventilators, the distinction between volume- and pressure-controlled modes of ventilation has become slightly blurred. Parameters can now be adjusted within each of the different modes, such as pressure limitation within a volume-controlled mode of ventilation. The critical care teams are therefore faced with a number of different modes from which to choose. Several studies have attempted to compare the benefits of various modes; however, the majority of them have been too small to enable detection of an outcome benefit of either. In the ARDSNet (2000) study, a mortality benefit was detected between two groups of patients receiving volume-controlled ventilation which may suggest that it is more important to concentrate on the actual settings rather than the particular mode of ventilation.

Regardless of the mode of ventilation chosen, it is clear from the ARDSNet (2000) trial that we should aim for a tidal volume of 6 mL/kg, limiting the peak pressure to 35 cmH$_2$O or plateau pressure <30 cmH$_2$O if receiving volume-controlled ventilation (see Table 1.4).

Mr Kuan Yew is currently being ventilated on a volume-controlled mode which is acceptable when considering recent evidence. However, he is receiving greater than 6 mL/kg of tidal volume. In order to prevent further deterioration in Mr Kuan Yew's lung function and ventilator-induced lung injury, it would therefore be advisable to gradually decrease his preset tidal volume to closer to that suggested by the ARDSNet trial. When considering the most appropriate tidal volume, it is important to highlight that the ARDSNet (2000) study used predicted body weight which is based on the patient's sex and height rather than actual body weight.

Permissive hypercapnia

With traditional methods of mechanically ventilating patients with ALI/ARDS, attempts were made to maintain a normal PaCO$_2$ and acid–base balance. Reducing Mr Kuan Yew's tidal volume to 6 mL/kg, as advocated in the ARDSNet (2000) study, may result in an increase in his PaCO$_2$ and a corresponding decrease in pH, leading to a respiratory acidosis. Over the past ten years, increasing evidence suggests that allowing the arterial PaCO$_2$ to increase above 6 kPa, termed permissive hypercapnia, is safe when used in conjunction with a low-tidal volume, low-pressure ventilation strategy, as long as the pH remains >7.3. Although acidaemia has many physiological effects such as depression of myocardial contractility, systemic vasodilation, increased intracranial pressure and cellular metabolic dysfunction, these have not been demonstrated to be clinically significant. However, permissive hypercapnia is unlikely to be appropriate in patients who have a raised intracranial pressure. The question for the critical care nurse and critical team is therefore which puts the patient at more risk: a high PaCO$_2$ or alveolar distension? Current evidence would suggest that it is the latter. It is important, however, that the critical care nurse remains vigilant in monitoring the PaCO$_2$ and pH via arterial blood gas analysis, and responds to the results in a timely and appropriate manner.

Use of positive end expiratory pressure (PEEP)

PEEP has been shown to improve oxygenation in several ways, encouraging movement of fluid from the alveoli into the interstitial spaces, recruitment of small airways and collapsed alveoli and increasing functional residual capacity (FRC). Its application is now advocated during all modes of mechanical ventilation. Its use is particularly imperative for Mr Kuan Yew, not only as an adjunct to improve oxygenation, but also to prevent further ventilator-induced lung injury. It has been suggested that lung damage can be induced at low lung volumes as well as high lung volumes as a consequence of the production of shearing forces which can occur with the opening and closing of alveoli at low lung volumes during mechanical ventilation. The application of PEEP should reduce the volume of reopening–collapsing tissue and hence reduce the degree of damage (Gattinoni et al. 1995).

Mr Kuan Yew is currently receiving a PEEP of 5 cmH$_2$O. Controversy exists over what level to set the PEEP in patients with ALI/ARDS and indeed in respiratory failure in general. One method which has been used is to assess the pressure–volume relationship of the lungs (see Figure 1.3).

In theory, setting the PEEP above the lower inflection point (LIP) may prevent derecruitment and hence low-lung volume ventilator-associated injury; however, although the pressure–volume curve could give a physiological illustration of the mechanics of Mr Kuan Yew's lung, applying this technique in the clinical setting is difficult. Modern ventilators commonly display the pressure–volume relationship of the respiratory system but this is obtained under dynamic conditions where elasticity and resistance of the respiratory system as a whole are considered. In acute respiratory failure, the impairment of the respiratory mechanics involves mainly the elastic component of the respiratory system. As a consequence, the measurement of respiratory pressure–volume curves should be done under static or semi-static conditions in order to eliminate the resistive component.

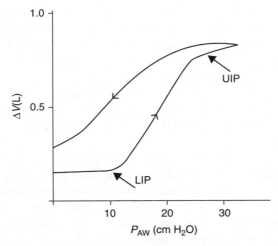

Figure 1.3 Pressure–volume relationship. (Adapted from Russell J and Walley K (eds) (1999) *Acute Respiratory Distress Syndrome: A Comprehensive Clinical Approach.* Cambridge University Press, Cambridge.)

Table 1.5   Titration of PEEP and FiO$_2$ in patients with ARDS.

FiO$_2$	0.3	0.4	0.4	0.5	0.5	0.6	0.7	0.7
PEEP	5	5	8	8	10	10	10	12
FiO$_2$	0.7	0.8	0.9	0.9	0.9	1.0	1.0	1.0
PEEP	14	14	14	16	18	20	22	24

Source: Adapted from the NIH NHLBI ARDSnet low tidal volume ventilation strategy (ARDSNet 2000)

Several research studies have attempted to quantify the appropriate level of PEEP for patients with ALI/ARDS. A small randomised controlled trial conducted by Amato and colleagues in 1998 suggested that high levels of PEEP should be adopted. Although this study demonstrated that the group of patients receiving higher than normal levels of PEEP had significantly lower mortality, it was difficult to conclude that the benefit was due to the high PEEP as there were many variables. The ALVEOLI study (ARDSNet 2004) conducted more recently found no difference in mortality between patients given higher levels of PEEP and those receiving traditional levels.

In light of the lack of conclusive evidence, a common approach is to choose the minimum level of PEEP likely to limit derecruitment, such as 10–15 cmH$_2$O. The ARDSNet trial protocol (ARDSNet 2000) also provides a useful guide to setting levels of PEEP in relation to FiO$_2$ (see Table 1.5) and this can be used by experienced critical care nurses when titrating FiO$_2$ and PEEP levels to oxygenation levels.

Prevention of ventilator associated pneumonia

It is important for the critical care nurse to appreciate that as an intubated patient, Mr Kuan Yew is at a high risk of developing nosocomial pneumonia. Preventing hospital-acquired infection is always important; however, the development of pneumonia associated with the use of mechanical ventilation is of particular concern. Ventilator-associated pneumonia (VAP) is an infection of the airways that develops more than 48 hours following intubation. It is the leading cause of death amongst hospital-acquired infections, exceeding the rate of death due to central line infections, severe sepsis and respiratory tract infections in the non-intubated patient. Hospital mortality of mechanically ventilated patients who do not develop VAP is 32% compared to 46% for ventilated patients who do develop VAP (Ibrahim et al. 2001). In addition, VAP increases the length of time patients spend on the ventilator, stay in the ICU and stay in hospital following discharge from the ICU (Rello et al. 2002), resulting in an estimated additional cost of approximately £20 000 to a hospital admission.

Prevention of VAP is therefore an essential component of caring for Mr Kuan Yew and he should be nursed according to the ventilator care bundle (Tablan et al. 2004). The ventilator care bundle is a series of evidence-based interventions which when implemented together aim to improve the outcome of ventilated patients. At the time of writing, a care bundle focusing specifically on preventing VAP was also undergoing consultation (DH 2010). The key components of both of these bundles are:

- Elevation of the head of the bed
- Daily 'sedation hold'
- Peptic ulcer prophylaxis

- Deep vein thrombosis prophylaxis
- oral hygiene with 2% chlorhexidine
- subglottic aspiration
- ventilator tube management
- tracheal tube cuff pressure monitoring.

A degree of debate exists between the literature and clinical practice in relation to the angle to which the head of the bed should be elevated. A meta-analysis by Hess (2005) concluded that the semi-recumbent position was the most effective position for preventing VAP, semi-recumbent being defined as elevation of the head of the bed to 45 degrees. A study by Grap et al. (2005) published at the same time as Hess (2005) suggested that elevation of the head of the bed at >30 degrees did not result in a statistically significant increase in the incidence of VAP. More recently, a prospective multicentre trial tested elevations of 45 and 10 degrees. The authors concluded that elevation to 45 degrees was not feasible, finding that in reality the mean elevation for ventilated patients was in fact closer to 30 degrees (Van Nieuwenhoven et al. 2006). On this basis elevation of the head of the bed to at least 30 degrees is the current recommendation (DH 2007).

Mr Kuan Yew's condition, as presented in the initial assessment, could be managed effectively by the aforementioned ventilatory strategies. If his condition were to deteriorate, however, with worsening oxygenation and ventilation, several adjuncts to conventional ventilation strategies have been described in the literature, which could be considered for him. These are discussed below.

Inverse ratio ventilation

Inverse ratio ventilation (IRV), which can be employed with either pressure- or volume-controlled modes of ventilation, involves prolongation of the inspiratory time, resulting in inspiratory/expiratory (IE) ratios of 1:1 or 2:1. Most studies using IRV demonstrate an improvement in the PaO_2 (Tharratt et al. 1988) with proposed mechanisms of improvement being related to increased alveolar recruitment, an increase in mean airway pressure and a more even distribution of mechanical ventilation. Unfortunately, not all patients respond positively and the use of IRV also has important implications physiologically. The critical care nurse is required to monitor the patient closely as lengthening the inspiratory time may result in a significant increase in the amount of gas that is trapped at the end of expiration, resulting in hyperinflation and an increase in the amount of intrinsic PEEP generated. These effects can then lead to a reduction in cardiac output in a patient who may already be compromised haemodynamically. With a lack of a clearly defined role IRV is usually adopted in those patients in whom hypoxaemia is refractory to more conventional approaches.

Recruitment manoeuvres

The use of recruitment manoeuvres evolved from traditional 'sighs' which are breaths two or three times greater than normal resting tidal volumes. Sighs occur approximately three to four times per hour in normal healthy subjects and increase the function of surfactants in stabilising the alveoli and preventing their collapse. The justification for use of recruitment manoeuvres in Mr Kuan Yew would be to recruit partially collapsed and

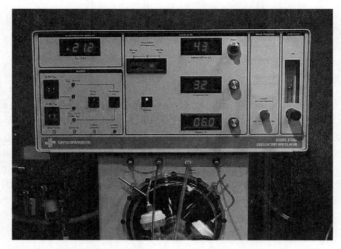

Figure 1.4   High-frequency oscillatory ventilator.

fluid-filled alveoli. These re-inflated alveoli could then be kept open by the application of PEEP, with the aim of improving oxygenation. Different methods of undertaking a recruitment manoeuvre have been described in the literature. Evidence that recruitment manoeuvres alone improve mortality, length of stay in ICU or ventilator-free days is, however, lacking. Complications of the manoeuvres have also been noted with transient hypotension and decreased SpO_2 being described. With this in mind the routine use of recruitment manoeuvres is not advocated within the literature and, if carried out, should be done so by an experienced member of the critical care team.

High-frequency oscillatory ventilation (HFOV)

Over the past few years there has been renewed interest in the use of HFOV (Figure 1.4) involving the administration of very small tidal volumes of approximately 80 mL at frequencies approaching 300 breaths per minute. The low tidal volume is generated by the movement of an oscillator within a ventilator circuit, similar to that used with continuous positive airway pressure (CPAP), and can be altered by adjusting the frequency of breaths, the IE ratio and the amplitude of the oscillator.

The repetitive movement of the oscillator results in an active expiratory phase which differs from conventional ventilators where expiration is passive and dependent on the elastic recoil properties of the lungs and chest wall. An active expiratory phase has been shown to aid in the clearance of CO_2, a common problem in patients such as Mr Kuan Yew who are ventilated using a low-tidal volume ventilation strategy. It is important that the critical care nurse is aware that altering the frequency of breaths in HFOV has the opposite effect on $PaCO_2$ when compared with conventional ventilation; that is, decreasing the frequency in HFOV can result in a decrease in $PaCO_2$ due to a slight increase in the tidal volume. Oxygenation is controlled simply by altering the mean airway pressure or the FiO_2.

On commencement of HFOV, the mean airway pressure is gradually increased to encourage lung recruitment. It is important during this stage that the critical care nurse closely monitors the SpO_2 as if the lung becomes over-distended, oxygen saturations can deteriorate. It is also imperative that the patient's haemodynamic status is closely monitored as increasing the mean airway pressure can result in an increase in intrathoracic pressure and decrease in venous return, with a subsequent decrease in cardiac output. Once it is felt that optimal recruitment has occurred, the mean airway pressure is then gradually decreased to an appropriate level.

HFOV has been used extensively and very successfully in neonates, but unfortunately, its application in the ventilation of adults with ALI/ARDS remains unclear. A study of the use of HFOV in adults, the MOAT trial, published in 2002 demonstrated a trend towards decreased mortality when compared to conventional ventilation (Derdak et al. 2002). The patients receiving conventional ventilation, however, were not ventilated using the ARDSNet (2000) guidelines and there were no significant differences in mortality at 30 days or 6 months. Furthermore, the mean airway pressure was significantly higher in the conventional ventilation group which raises the possibility of an increased risk of ventilator-induced lung injury in the control group. In order to obtain a definitive answer as to the application of HFOV in clinical practice, further research is clearly necessary to compare HFOV to the ARDSNet (2000) protocol and the recently commenced High Frequency Oscillation in ARDS (OSCAR) trial will hopefully provide the answer. Details of this trial, comparing conventional positive pressure ventilation with high HFOV for adults with ARDS can be found on the OSCAR website: http://duncanyoung.net/index.php.

Kinetic therapy

Kinetic therapy involves the use of specialised beds with low-air loss technology which can turn the critically ill patient in an arc of between 40 and 90 degrees (Figure 1.5). Rotation redistributes localised dependent oedema, helping to mobilise pulmonary secretions, therefore reducing atelectasis and respiratory tract infections associated with ALI/ARDS. Research studying the impact of kinetic therapy in patients with ALI/ARDS, however, is sparse.

A study by Pape et al. (1994) looked at the effects of kinetic therapy on lung function and pulmonary haemodynamics in patients with post-traumatic ARDS. Rotational therapy was commenced when the PaO_2/FiO_2 was 150 mmHg to angles of 30–62 degrees laterally with a two-minute pause in each position. Pape et al. (1994) demonstrated a significant improvement in oxygenation in the group receiving kinetic therapy with no notable adverse haemodynamic effects. Patients in this study were not commenced on kinetic therapy until they had severe hypoxaemia. The study was also conducted in a very specific group of patients. It is therefore difficult to apply these results to the general population of patients with ARDS. Further, the authors do not specify the exact angle patients were rotated to.

More recently McLean (2001) hypothesised that kinetic therapy could decrease the incidence of refractory hypoxaemia in a group of patients with risk factors for ALI/ARDS. Patients were rotated to 45 degrees laterally for a minimum of 18 hours per day. McLean

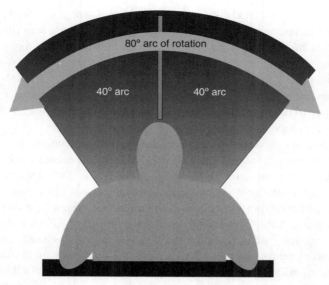

Figure 1.5   Diagrammatic representation of kinetic therapy.

(2001) concluded that kinetic therapy did have a positive effect on the lung function of severely injured trauma patients at risk of atelectasis, ALI and ARDS.

Kinetic therapy appears to have a role in the management of the critically ill patient with pulmonary complications resulting from prolonged immobilisation, who is at risk of VAP (NICE and NPSA 2008; MacIntyre et al. 1999). Further work is required, however, to establish the statistical significance of this therapy in influencing gas exchange in patients with ALI/ARDS.

Prone positioning

Mr Kuan Yew is currently being nursed in the supine position. However, multiple studies over the past 20 years have demonstrated an improvement in PaO_2/FiO_2 in two-thirds of patients with ARDS placed in the prone position (Langer et al. 1988; Pappert et al. 1994; Gattinoni et al. 2001) (Figure 1.6). Hypotheses offered to explain this improvement in oxygenation have included an increase in FRC, a change in the position of the heart and diaphragm allowing increased recruitment of lung units, increased clearance of secretions and redistribution of perfusion. Current thinking suggests that any improvement in oxygenation is mostly related to changes in the pleural pressure gradient from the dorsal to the ventral surface on turning to the prone position (Lamm et al. 1994). The gradient of pleural pressure from negative ventrally to positive dorsally is not completely reversed on turning prone which leads to a more even distribution of ventilation and improvement in ventilation/perfusion (V/Q) matching.

Unfortunately, although an improvement in oxygenation has been observed, a multi-centre randomised controlled trial published in 2001 failed to demonstrate any differences in clinical outcome between those nursed in the supine position and those nursed prone (Gattinoni et al. 2001). A recent systematic review by Alsaghir and Martin, which

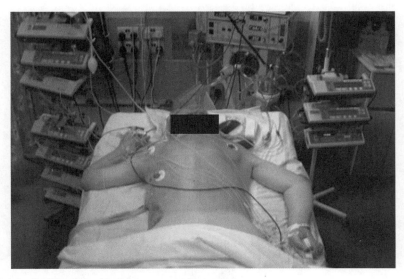

Figure 1.6 Patient placed in the prone position.

included five randomised controlled trials, further supports these findings (Alsaghir and Martin 2008). Turning a critically ill patient prone also has practical implications for the critical care nurse. A team of at least five members of the staff are required to safely turn the patient, and special attention and vigilance is required to prevent the development of pressure necrosis of the face, ears and genitals and to ensure maintenance and patency of the airway. With the lack of a randomised controlled trial supporting the routine use of the prone position, its use as an adjunct to mechanical ventilation strategies in patients with severe hypoxaemia has become a rescue therapy in many critical care units. However, the systematic review by Alsaghir and Martin (2008) did note a significant reduction in mortality in those with a higher illness severity, perhaps suggesting that it should be considered more frequently.

Inhaled nitric oxide/prostacyclin

Initially described almost 15 years ago, the use of inhaled nitric oxide (NO) as a potential therapy for ALI/ARDS has received a great deal of interest in the literature. Given continuously, via inhalation during mechanical ventilation, it selectively vasodilates pulmonary capillaries and arterioles which perfuse ventilated alveoli (Figure 1.7). This results in the diversion of blood from under-ventilated alveoli, subsequently improving V/Q matching and oxygenation. As a vasodilator, NO also has a function in decreasing pulmonary hypertension which can be present in patients with ARDS as a consequence of increased pulmonary vascular resistance caused by various pro-inflammatory mediators, hypoxia or thrombi. The systemic effects of inhaled NO are minimal due to its rapid inactivation on binding with haemoglobin, and there is little risk posed to the critical care team caring for patients receiving it as any NO present in exhaled gas is rapidly absorbed by scavenging systems. Unfortunately, as NO is rapidly deactivated by haemoglobin, any interruption in

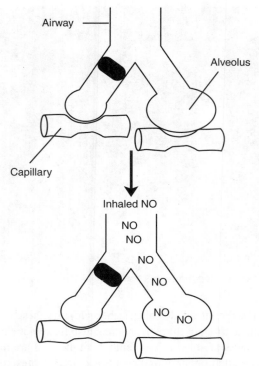

Figure 1.7   Schematic illustrating the vasodilatory effect of inhaled nitric oxide.

its supply, e.g. patient transport or supply exhaustion, can lead to a sudden decrease in
PaO_2 or rebound pulmonary hypertension which may precipitate right heart failure.

Randomised controlled trials of the use of NO in ARDS have shown that although NO
temporarily improves oxygenation and reduces pulmonary artery pressure in the majority
of patients, similarly to other therapies its use is not associated with an improved patient
outcome (Rossaint et al. 1995; Bigatello et al. 1994). Inhaled NO should not, therefore,
be considered as a standard treatment for Mr Kuan Yew.

Prostacyclin is an endothelium-derived prostaglandin vasodilator which inhibits platelet
aggregation and neutrophil adhesion when administered intravenously. Nebulised prostacyclin produces similar effects to inhaled NO with minimal side effects and without
measureable platelet dysfunction and appears to provide the same degree of improvement
in oxygenation as NO (Dahlem et al. 2004). Similarly to inhaled NO there are, however,
no large randomised controlled trials demonstrating an outcome benefit of its use in adults
with ARDS.

Extracorporeal membrane oxygenation (ECMO)/extracorporeal CO_2 removal (ECCO₂R)

During ECMO venous blood is removed via a cannula in the inferior vena cava or
right atrium, passed through a heart/lung machine and returned to either the right atrium

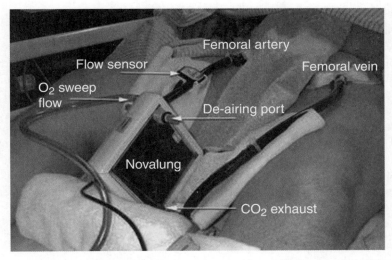

Figure 1.8 Novalung. (McKinlay, 2008). Reproduced with permission from John Wiley & Sons Ltd.

(veno-venous bypass) or aorta (veno-arterial bypass). The use of extracorporeal gas exchange techniques such as ECMO or $ECCO_2R$ in patients with ARDS is viewed as an attractive strategy since it allows the lung to remain at rest, hence preventing any further lung damage, whilst allowing adequate oxygenation and ventilation. ECMO has proven mortality benefit in neonatal ARDS; however, this benefit has not been demonstrated thus far in adult clinical studies. A randomised prospective controlled study of ECMO in 180 adult patients with ARDS (the CESAR trial) has recently been conducted in the UK and early results suggest that there is a survival benefit if it is used early. Further details of this trial can be found on the CESAR website: www.cesar-trial.org/.

$ECCO_2R$ involves the use of an extracorporeal veno-venous circuit with lower blood flows and with oxygenation still occurring via the patient's lungs. One such system is the Novalung (Bein et al. 2006) (Figure 1.8). However, randomised controlled trial of $ECCO_2R$ compared with conventional support in patients with severe ARDS reported no significant difference in survival (Morris et al. 1994).

Several centres have recently reported observational studies demonstrating high survival rates in adult patients managed with extracorporeal support. These encouraging results should, however, be interpreted in the context of a trend towards improved survival, generally in patients with ARDS.

Steroids

Corticosteroids reduce the production of a large number of inflammatory and profibrotic mediators and the importance of steroid therapy in the resolution of lung inflammation in animal models became apparent 20 years ago. Unfortunately, trials of high-dose steroid therapy have failed to show a survival benefit in patients with early ARDS and, in fact, some trials have shown an increase in infection rates and mortality.

The use of steroids in late ARDS (7–14 days from diagnosis) has been more closely studied in recent years. The rationale behind this interest is that much of the scarring that occurs during this phase of the illness is as a consequence of unattentuated inflammation that can cause severe damage to the affected alveoli. It has also been postulated that the use of steroids can have an effect on the fibrotic process seen in late ARDS. Unfortunately, however, a recent large multicentre prospective randomised controlled trial conducted by the ARDSNet failed to support the routine use of methylprednisolone for persistent ARDS (National Heart, Lung and Blood Institute (NHLBI) ARDSNet 2006a). In addition they demonstrated that commencement of methylprednisolone two weeks after the onset of ARDS may increase the risk of death. The routine use of corticosteroids in patients with ARDS is therefore not currently supported by the literature.

Circulation

Major emphasis is likely to be placed on ventilatory strategies for Mr Kuan Yew since hypoxaemia and hypoxia are of particular concern. ARDS, however, does affect the cardiovascular system, and cardiovascular management can have an effect on physiological status and outcome for several reasons. Firstly, oxygen delivery to the tissues is dependent not only upon arterial oxygen saturation but also upon the oxygen-carrying capacity of the blood and cardiac output. The management of cardiac output and haemoglobin is therefore as important as maintenance of arterial oxygen saturations via mechanical ventilation strategies. Mr Kuan Yew currently has a normal haemoglobin level, and infusion of packed red cells to increase his oxygen-carrying capacity would therefore not be indicated at this time. It is important, however, to ensure that he has an adequate cardiac output. Secondly, as previously discussed, ARDS is characterised by a degree of intra-pulmonary shunt, and in this situation, mixed venous oxygen saturations have an impact on arterial oxygen saturations. Cardiac output plays a key role in determining mixed venous oxygen saturations (SvO_2) and it is therefore imperative to ensure that an adequate cardiac output and SvO_2 is maintained. Thirdly, the initial stage of ARDS is characterised by pulmonary oedema which results in a decrease in oxygenation. A low PAOP may decrease the rate of oedema formation; therefore, finding the lowest possible PAOP which gives an adequate cardiac output may be a focus of cardiovascular management for Mr Kuan Yew. The measurement of PAOP would, however, require the insertion of a pulmonary artery catheter and the benefits of this are questionable when one considers the risks associated with its use.

The initiation of mechanical ventilation can also have an effect on the cardiovascular system. Pulmonary hypertension associated with ARDS may be exacerbated by the administration of positive pressure and this effect, combined with the direct application of positive pressure to the major vessels within the thoracic cavity, can significantly decrease venous return, leading to a reduction in cardiac output.

From the data presented in the initial assessment, Mr Kuan Yew is demonstrating signs of cardiovascular insufficiency. He has a mean arterial blood pressure (MABP) of <65 mmHg and a tachycardia of 115 beats per minute and is pyrexial. He is also warm to touch, suggesting that he is peripherally dilated with a low systemic vascular resistance. The management of Mr Kuan Yew's cardiovascular function presents a major challenge in that, as a consequence of ARDS, he also has non-cardiogenic pulmonary oedema, caused by increased pulmonary capillary permeability. On the one hand, intravenous fluid administration is critical to maintain an appropriate intravascular volume to ensure haemodynamic stability and organ perfusion. On the other hand, excessive fluid administration could worsen any pulmonary oedema and compromise gas exchange further. Fluid management practices within critical care units can vary greatly and are often guided by established practice ranging from the liberal 'wet' approach which prioritises perfusion to the very conservative or 'dry' approach which aims to prevent pulmonary oedema.

An associated challenge in managing Mr Kuan Yew's fluid status is the decision as to what is the most effective method of monitoring fluid status. Proponents of the pulmonary artery catheter argue that it is essential to measure the PAOP and cardiac output. However, others argue that the use of a pulmonary catheter carries a significant mortality risk and that fluids can be adequately managed using a central venous catheter in conjunction with clinical assessment. The FACTT study (Fluid and Catheter Therapy Trial), conducted by the NHLBI ARDS network (NIHB, ARDSNet 2006b) concluded that although there was no difference in mortality, patients receiving a conservative fluid strategy demonstrated improved lung function and had shorter duration of mechanical ventilation and intensive care stay. These results support the use of a conservative fluid management strategy for Mr Kuan Yew. With regards to the use of a pulmonary artery catheter versus a central venous catheter, although there were no differences in outcomes such as mortality, length of stay or number of ventilated days, patients with pulmonary artery catheters had twice as many catheter-related complications, and investigators concluded that the use of a pulmonary artery catheter is not indicated in the routine management of patients with ALI/ARDS. Alternative monitoring techniques such as use of a pulse-induced contour cardiac output (PiCCO; Cottis et al. 2003) (Figure 1.9) which measures both extravascular

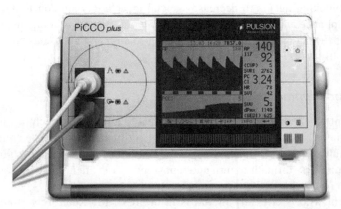

Figure 1.9   PiCCO plus monitor and example of information obtained. Reproduced with permission from Pulsion Medical UK Ltd.

and intravascular lung water (EVLW and IVLW) may also be used to enable more accurate measurement of the fluid status.

When deciding which fluid to administer, there is currently no conclusive evidence to suggest that choosing either a colloid or a crystalloid results in a significant improvement in outcome in patients with ARDS. The recent SAFE study, although not specifically related to patients with ARDS, suggested that either a colloid or a crystalloid may be used (Finfer et al. 2004). Regardless of the fluid chosen, it is essential that the critical care nurse pays strict attention to fluid balance whilst also closely monitoring gaseous exchange and the effects of the fluid infusion on Mr Kuan Yew's haemodynamic status.

Infused vasopressors and/or inotropic drugs are frequently used to increase a low MABP or cardiac output; however, the use of these should follow adequate and safe fluid resuscitation. Mr Kuan Yew is displaying signs of severe sepsis and the haemodynamic changes seen in ARDS patients are indistinguishable from those seen in sepsis and septic shock (please refer to Chapter 4 for further information on the cardiovascular management of sepsis).

Disability of the nervous system

In 2001, Van Den Berghe et al. demonstrated that strict attention to tight glycaemic control can reduce mortality in the critically ill patient. A continuous intravenous infusion of actrapid may therefore be considered in order to reduce Mr Kuan Yew's blood glucose to within the recommended level (see Chapter 7 for more information on blood glucose management).

Mr Kuan Yew will require sedation and analgesia in order to tolerate the ventilatory support he is receiving. It is important that the critical care nurse assesses pain and sedation requirements frequently in order to prevent over/under-sedation. As part of the ventilator care bundle discussed earlier in this chapter, it is also important that a daily sedation hold is implemented where possible. This will also facilitate a more accurate neurological assessment. A minority of patients with refractory hypoxaemia who are receiving more advanced forms of mechanical ventilation may also require the administration of neuromuscular blocking agents to decrease skeletal muscle oxygen consumption, improve thoracic compliance and favour redistribution of blood flow to vital organs (see Chapters 10 and 11 for further aspects of managing pain, sedation and neuromuscular blockade in the critically ill).

Exposure/environment

It is important when managing Mr Kuan Yew that a holistic approach to care is used as tissue hypoxia can lead to problems with skin integrity and this may be compounded by the use of multiple drug therapies. Respiratory and haemodynamic instability may also render Mr Kuan Yew difficult to turn and reposition. Strict attention to and assessment of the condition of his skin is therefore imperative.

As a patient who is critically ill and is in the ICU, Mr Kuan Yew is also at risk of developing further secondary infection and strict attention to infection control measures is therefore considered a high priority. These measures should include a high standard of hand hygiene, attention to line and wound care and effective eye and oral care (see Chapter 4 for further information on infection control).

Conclusion

This scenario has discussed the complex challenges associated with the care of a patient with ARDS. The condition does not just affect the respiratory system and a holistic approach to management, including titration of fluid support, titration of medication and a focus on general aspects of caring for a critically ill patient, is imperative.

Key learning points

- ARDS is the most severe form of a spectrum of respiratory disease and presents a great challenge to the multi-professional team within critical care.
- An evidence-based approach is essential, with strict attention being paid to appropriate ventilatory strategies as an initial priority and also the use of care bundles.

Critical appraisal of research paper

Drakulovic et al. (1999) Supine body position as a risk factor for nosocomial pneumonia in mechanically ventilated patients: a randomised trial. *The Lancet* **354**(9133), 1851–1858.

This prospective, randomised, controlled trial investigated whether use of the semi-recumbent position can reduce the incidence of nosocomial pneumonia in mechanically ventilated patients. Eighty-six intubated and mechanically ventilated patients in one medical and one respiratory ICU in a tertiary referral hospital in Spain were randomly assigned to supine ($n = 47$) or semi-recumbent ($n = 39$) position. The frequency of clinically suspected and microbiologically confirmed nosocomial pneumonia was assessed in both groups together with other known risk factors. These included the presence of enteral feeding, mechanical ventilation for seven days or more and a Glasgow Coma score of less than nine. Results of the study demonstrated that the frequency of clinically suspected nosocomial pneumonia was lower in the semi-recumbent group than in the supine group (8% vs. 34%, $p = 0.003$). This difference was also seen with microbiologically confirmed pneumonia (5% of those in semi-recumbent position vs. 23% of those in supine position, $p = 0.018$). The authors concluded that the semi-recumbent position reduces the risk and frequency of nosocomial pneumonia, especially in patients receiving enteral nutrition. They also concluded that the risk of nosocomial pneumonia is increased by decreased level of consciousness and long-duration mechanical ventilation.

Reader activities

1. Read the research article written by Drakulovic et al. (1999).
2. Using the critical appraisal framework in Appendix I, consider the methodological quality of the paper.

3. Reflect on this aspect of your own practice and the implications for future practice management that this paper arises.

A commentary on this paper has been provided by the chapter author in Appendix II.

References

Acute Respiratory Distress Syndrome Network (ARDSNet) (2000) Ventilation with lower tidal volumes as compared with traditional tidal volumes for acute lung injury and the acute respiratory distress syndrome. *The New England Journal of Medicine* **342**, 1301–1308.

Alsaghir A, Martin C (2008) Effect of prone positioning in patients with acute respiratory distress syndrome: a meta-analysis. *Critical Care Medicine* **36**(2), 603-609.

Amato M, Barbas C, Medeiros D (1998) Effect of a protective ventilation strategy on mortality in acute respiratory distress syndrome. *The New England Journal of Medicine* **338**, 347–354.

Ashbaugh D, Bigelow D, Petty T, Levine B (1967) Acute respiratory distress in adults. *Lancet* **2**, 319–323.

Baudouin S (1997) Surfactant medication for acute respiratory distress syndrome. *Thorax* **52**, S9–S15.

Bein T, Philipp A, Dorlac W, Taeger K, Nerlich M, Schlitt H (2006) A new pumpless extracorporeal interventional lung assist in critical hypoxaemia/hypercarbia. *Critical Care Medicine* **34**, 1372–1377.

Bernard G, Artigas A, Brigham K, Carlet J, Falke K, Hudson L, Lamy M, Legall J, Morris A, Spragg R (1994) The American-European Consensus Conference on ARDS. *American Journal of Respiratory and Critical Care Medicine* **149**, 818–824.

Bigatello LM, Hurford WE, Kacmarek RM, Roberts JD, Zappol WM (1994) Prolonged inhalation of low concentrations of nitric oxide in patients with severe adult respiratory distress syndrome. Effects on pulmonary haemodynamics and oxygenation. *Anaesthesiology* **80**(4), 761–770.

Brochard L, Roudot-Thoraval F, Roupie E, Delclaux C, Chastre Jean, Fernandez-Mondejar E, Clementi E, Mancebo J, Factor P, Matamis D, Ranieri M, Blanch L, Rodi G, Mentec H, Dreyfuss D, Ferrer M, Brun-Buisson C, Tobin M, Lemaire F (1998) Tidal volume reduction for prevention of ventilator induced lung injury in acute respiratory distress syndrome. *American Journal of Respiratory and Critical Care Medicine* **158**(6), 1831–1838.

Brower R, Shanholtz C, Fessler H, Shade, White P, Wiener C, Teeter J, Dodd J, Almog Y, Piantadosi S (1999) Prospective randomised controlled clinical trial comparing traditional versus reduced tidal volume ventilation in acute respiratory distress syndrome patients. *Critical Care Medicine* **27**(8), 1492–1498.

Chollet-Martin S, Jourdain B, Gibert C, Elbim C, Chastre J, Gougerot-Pocidalo MA (1996) Interactions between neutrophils and cytokines in blood and alveolar spaces during ARDS. *American Journal of Respiratory and Critical Care Medicine* **154**, 594–601.

Cottis R, Magee N, Higgins DJ (2003) Haemodynamic monitoring with pulse-induced contour cardiac output (PICCO) in critical care. *Intensive and Critical Care Nursing* **19**(5), 301–307.

Dahlem P, van Aalderen W, de Neef M, Dijkgraaf M, Bos A (2004) Randomised controlled trial of aerosolized prostacyclin therapy in children with acute lung injury. *Critical Care Medicine* **32**, 1055–1057.

Department of Health (DH) (2007) *Saving Lives: reducing infection, delivering clean and safe care*. Crown copyright, London. Available online at: www.dh.gov.uk/. Accessed 6 August 2009.

Department of Health (DH) (2010) High impact intervention no.5; care bundle to reduce VAP. Available online at: www.nric.org.uk. Accessed 26th November 2010.

Derdak S, Mehta S, Stewart E, Smith T, Rogers M, Buchman T, Carlin B, Lowson S, Granton J (2002) Multi-centre oscillatory ventilation for acute respiratory distress syndrome trial. High frequency oscillatory ventilation for acute respiratory distress syndrome in adults: a randomised controlled trial. *American Journal of Respiratory and Critical Care Medicine* **166**, 801–808.

Drakulovic MB, Torres A, Bauer TT, Nicolas JM, Nogue S, Ferrer M (1999) Supine body position as a risk factor for nosocomial pneumonia in mechanically ventilated patients: a randomised trial. *Lancet* **354**(9133), 1851–1858.

Doyle R, Szaflarski N, Modin G, Wiener-Kronish J, Matthay M (1995) Identification of patients with acute lung injury. Predictors of mortality. *American Journal of Respiratory and Critical Care Medicine* **152**, 1818–1824.

Dreyfuss D, Soler P, Basset G (1988) High inflation pressure pulmonary oedema: respective effects of high airway pressure, high tidal volume and positive end expiratory pressure. *American Review of Respiratory Disease* **137**, 1159–1164.

Dreyfuss D, Sauman G (1998) Ventilator induced lung injury: lessons from experimental studies. *American Journal of Respiratory and Critical Care Medicine* **157**, 294–323.

Estenssoro E, Dubin A, Laffaire E (2002) Incidence, clinical course, and outcome in 217 patients with acute respiratory distress syndrome. *Critical Care Medicine* **30**, 2450–2456.

Finfer S, Bellomo R, Boyce N, French J, Myburgh J, Norton R (2004) A comparison of albumin and saline for fluid resuscitation in the intensive care unit. *The New England Journal of Medicine* **350**, 2247–2256.

Garber B, Hebert P, Yelle J, Hodder R, McGowan J (1996) Adult respiratory distress syndrome: a systematic review of incidence and risk factors. *Critical Care Medicine* **24**(4), 687–695.

Gattinoni L, Pesenti A, Avalli L, Rossi F, Bombino M (1987) Pressure-volume curve of total respiratory system in acute respiratory failure. Computed tomographic scan study. *American Review of Respiratory Diseases* **136**, 730–736.

Gattinoni L, Pelosi P, Crotti S (1995) Effects of positive end expiratory pressure on regional distribution of tidal volume and recruitment in adult respiratory distress syndrome. *American Journal of Respiratory and Critical Care Medicine* **151**, 1807–1814.

Gattinoni L, Tognoni G, Pesenti A (2001) Effect of prone positioning on the survival of patients with acute respiratory failure. *The New England Journal of Medicine* **345**, 568–572.

Grap M, Munro C, Hummel R Elswick RK, McKinney J, Sessler C (2005) Effect of backrest elevation on the development of ventilator-associated pneumonia. *American Journal of Critical Care* **14**(4), 325–332.

Herridge M, Cheung A, Tansey C (2003) One-year outcomes in survivors of the acute respiratory distress syndrome. *The New England Journal of Medicine* **348**, 683–693.

Hess D (2005) Patient positioning and ventilator-associated pneumonia. *Respiratory Care* **50**(7), 892–897.

Hilbert G, Gruson D, Vargas F (2001) Non-invasive ventilation in immunosuppressed patients with pulmonary infiltrates, fever and acute respiratory failure. *The New England Journal of Medicine* **344**, 481–484.

Ibrahim E, Tracy L, Hill C, Fraser V, Kollef M (2001) The occurrence of ventilator-associated pneumonia in a community hospital: risk factors and clinical outcomes. *Chest* **120**(2), 555–561.

Lamm W, Graham M, Albert R (1994) Mechanism by which the prone position improves oxygenation in acute lung injury. *American Journal of Respiratory and Critical Care Medicine* **150**, 184–193.

Langer M, Mascheroni D, Marcolin R, Gattinoni L (1988) The prone position in ARDS patients: a clinical study. *Chest* **94**, 103–107.

MacIntyre N, Helms M, Wunderink R, Schmidt G, Sahn S (1999) Automated rotational therapy for the prevention of respiratory complications during mechanical ventilation. *Respiratory Care* **44**, 1447–1451.

McLean B (2001) Rotational kinetic therapy for ventilation/perfusion mismatch. *Critical Care Nursing in Europe* **1**, 113–118.

Morris A, Wallace C, Menlove R, Clemmer T, Orme J, Weaver L (1994) Randomised clinical trial of pressure controlled inverse ratio ventilation and extracorporeal CO_2 removal for adult respiratory distress syndrome. *American Journal of Respiratory and Critical Care Medicine* **149**, 295–305.

Murray J, Matthay M, Luce J (1988) An expanded definition of the adult respiratory distress syndrome. *American Review Respiratory Disease* **138**, 720–723.

National Heart and Lung Institute (NHLI), National Institute of Health (NIH) (1972) *Respiratory Distress Syndromes: task force report on problems, research approaches, needs*. US Government Printing Office, Washington, DC, **73-432**: 165–180.

National Heart, Lung and Blood Institute (NHBL) Acute Respiratory Distress Syndrome (ARDS) Clinical Trials Network (2004) Higher versus lower positive expiratory end pressures in patients with acute respiratory distress syndrome. *The New England Journal of Medicine* **351**, 327–336.

National Heart, Lung and Blood Institute (NHBL) Acute Respiratory Distress Syndrome (ARDS) Clinical Trials Network (2006a) Efficacy and safety of corticosteroids for persistent acute respiratory distress syndrome. *The New England Journal of Medicine* **354**(16), 1671–1684.

National Heart, Lung and Blood Institute (NHBL) Acute Respiratory Distress Syndrome (ARDS) Clinical Trials Network (2006b) Pulmonary artery versus central venous catheter to guide treatment of acute lung injury. *The New England Journal of Medicine* **354**, 2213–2224.

National Institute for Health and Clinical Excellence (NICE), National Patient Safety Agency (NPSA) (2008) Technical patient safety solutions for ventilator associated pneumonia in adults. Available online at: www.nice.org.uk. Accessed 26th November 2010.

Pape H, Regel G, Borgmann W, Sturm J, Tscherne H (1994) The effect of kinetic positioning on lung function and pulmonary haemodynamics in post traumatic ARDS: a clinical study. *Injury* **25**, 51–57.

Pappert D, Rossaint R, Slama K (1994) Influence of positioning on ventilation-perfusion relationships in severe adult respiratory distress syndrome. *Chest* **106**, 1511–1555.

Rello J, Ollendorf D, Oster G (2002) VAP Outcomes Scientific Advisory Group. Epidemiology and outcomes of ventilator-associated pneumonia in a large US database. *Chest* **122**(6), 2115–2121.

Rossaint R, Falke K, Lopez F, Slama K, Pison U, Zapol W (1993) Inhaled nitric oxide for the adult respiratory distress syndrome. *The New England Journal of Medicine* **328**, 399–403.

Rossaint R, Gerlach H, Schmidt-Ruhnke H, Pappert Dirk, Lewandowski K, Steudel W, Falke K (1995) Efficacy of inhaled nitric oxide in patients with severe ARDS. *Chest* **107**, 1107–1110.

Stewart T, Meade M, Cook D (1998) Evaluation of a ventilation strategy to prevent barotrauma in patients at high risk for acute respiratory distress syndrome. *The New England Journal of Medicine* **338**, 355–361.

Tablan O, Anderson L, Besser R, CDC Healthcare Infection Control Practices Advisory Committee (2004) Guidelines for preventing health care-associated pneumonia, 2003: Recommendations of CDC and the Healthcare Infection Control Practices Advisory Committee. *MMWR Recommendations and Reports* **53**(RR-3), 1–36.

Tharratt R, Allen R, Albertson T (1988) Pressure controlled inverse ratio ventilation in severe adult respiratory failure. *Chest* **94**, 755.

Tremblay L, Valenza F, Ribeiro S, Li J, Slutsky A (1997) Injurious ventilatory strategies increase cytokines and c-fos m-RNA expression in an isolated rat lung model. *Journal of Clinical Investigation* **99**, 944–952.

Van den Berghe G, Wouters P, Weekers F, Verwaest C, Bruyninckx F, Schetz M, Vlasselaers D, Ferdinande P, Lauwers P, Bouillon R (2001) Intensive insulin therapy in critically ill adults. *The New England Journal of Medicine* **345**, 1359–1367.

Van Nieuwenhoven C, Vandenbroucke-Grauls C, Van Tiel F, Joore H, Van Schijndel R, Van der Tweel I, Ramsay G, Bonten M (2006) Feasibility and effects of the semi-recumbent position to prevent ventilator associated pneumonia: a randomized study. *Critical Care Medicine* **34**, 396–402.

Villar J, Slutsky A (1989) The incidence of the adult respiratory distress syndrome. *American Review of Respiratory Disease* **140**, 814–816.

Vincent J, Bihari D, Suter P, Bruining H, White J, Nicolas-Chanoin M, Wolff M, Spencer R, Hemmer M (1995). The prevalence of nosocomial infection in intensive care units in Europe. Results of the European Prevalence of Infection in Intensive Care (EPIC) Study. *Journal of American Medical Association* **278**, 639–644.

Ware L, Matthay M (2000) The acute respiratory distress syndrome. *The New England Journal of Medicine* **342**(18), 1334–1350.

Wax R, Angus D (2000) The molecular genetics of sepsis. In: *Yearbook of Intensive Care and Emergency Medicine*, Vincent JL (ed). Springer, Berlin, pp. 3–17.

Chapter 2

The patient requiring complex weaning from mechanical ventilation

Dr. Cheryl Crocker

Introduction

With reference to two patient scenarios, this chapter discusses the knowledge and skills required by critical care nurses to mange the complex needs of the longer term patient requiring weaning from mechanical ventilatory support.

A number of studies have estimated the incidence of prolonged ventilation in an intensive care unit (ICU) to be between 5.5% and 15% (Brochard et al. 1994; Ely et al. 1996; Nevins and Epstein 2001). The hospital mortality of such patients is high, between 43% and 61% (Seneff et al. 1996; Kurek et al. 1997), and long-term patients are major resource users within critical care.

Weaning from mechanical ventilation is defined in the literature as the process of assisting the patient to breathe unaided (Knebel 1991) or the transition from ventilatory support to spontaneous breathing (Mancebo 1996). This process can take hours, days, weeks or months. Weaning from mechanical ventilation is not a new problem, but has now gained a higher priority in critical care largely as a result of the economic burden of long-term patients (Modernisation Agency 2002). This has provided the impetus for critical care units to review the weaning of patients from mechanical ventilation and presents an opportunity for nurses to further develop their role.

Scenario 1

John, a 30-year-old male with no co-morbidities, is admitted to the ICU with type 1 (hypoxic) respiratory failure, requiring ventilation. He is ventilated on 100% oxygen on synchronized intermittent mandatory ventilation (SIMV) with assisted spontaneous breathing (ASB) support, 5 cmH$_2$O PEEP, a mandatory respiratory rate of 12 breaths per minute and a preset tidal volume (Vt) of 700 mL (patient weighs 70 kg). He is receiving 8 mg/hour of morphine and 6 mg/hour of midazolam. He is unrousable. Arterial blood gases (ABGs) can be seen in Box 2.1.

Critical Care Nursing: Learning from Practice, 1st edition. Edited by Suzanne Bench and Kate Brown.
© 2011 Blackwell Publishing Ltd.

Box 2.1   John's arterial blood gas results.

pH	7.4
PaCO$_2$	4.5 kPa
PaO$_2$	13 kPa
HCO$_3$$^-$	25 mmol/L
Base excess (BE)	+1

By day three, John's sedation and ventilation remain unchanged, but his oxygen has been reduced to 60% (0.6 FiO$_2$). Organisms have been identified in his sputum and antimicrobial therapy has been commenced. Enteral feeding has also been started at 30 mL/hour. It is not until day eight that the sedation is discontinued and the inspired oxygen concentration is reduced further to 40% (0.4 FiO$_2$). John awakens quickly after sedation is discontinued. Active weaning is commenced on day nine. ABGs and laboratory results at this point can be seen in Table 2.1.

Table 2.1   John's assessment data.

Blood gases		Urea and electrolytes		Full blood count	
pH	7.48	Sodium	141 mmol/L	Haemoglobin	9.1 g/dL
PO$_2$	10.11 kPa	Potassium	3.9 mmol/L	White cell count	9.7
PCO$_2$	4.60 kPa	Magnesium	0.7 mmol/L	Haematocrit	0.28
HCO$_3$	24.0 mmol/L	Calcium	2.3 mmol/L	Platelets	66
BE	+1.0	Phosphate	1.06 mmol/L		
		Urea	4.7 mmol/L		
		Creatinine	49 mmol/L		
		Albumin	16 mmol/L		

Scenario 2

Peter, a 73-year-old gentleman is admitted with type II (hypercarbic) respiratory failure (non-pneumonic). He has chronic obstructive pulmonary disease (COPD) and smokes 30 cigarettes a day. He is normally quite well and has had no previous ICU admissions. His last hospital admission was one year ago for exacerbation of his COPD.

Following an unsuccessful trial of non-invasive ventilation (NIV) on a general ward, he was intubated and ventilated on biphasic positive airways pressure (BIPAP). An assessment of his status at this point can be seen in Box 2.2.

After 24 hours of ventilation on BIPAP, blood gases begin to normalise and weaning is commenced by reducing the mandatory respiratory rate to 8 breaths per minute. Peter is seen to be making an effort to breathe. Two hours later the ventilation mode is changed to continuous positive airways pressure (CPAP) of 5 cmH$_2$O with pressure support of 25 cmH$_2$O; however, Peter soon begins to tire. Tidal volumes drop from 500 to 300 mL

Box 2.2   Peter's initial assessment data.

pH	7.2
$PaCO_2$	11 kPa
PaO_2	7.5 kPa
HCO_3^-	30 mmol/L
Base excess (BE)	−6 mmol/L
FiO_2	0.4 (40%)
Inspiratory pressure	25 cmH_2O
PEEP	10 cmH_2O
Set respiratory rate	14 breaths per minute

---

and the total respiratory rate increases from 20 to 35. Peter's breathing appears laboured and he is using all his accessory muscles. He becomes tachycardic, hypertensive and restless.

Reader activities

Having read the two scenarios, consider the following questions:

- When should John's weaning have been commenced?
- What factors should you take into consideration when preparing to wean John?
- How would you wean John and Peter? Write a weaning plan for Peter.
- What parameters would you use to wean Peter and John?
- Do you think Peter would be difficult to wean?
- How would you know Peter had tired?
- Why are ABGs *not* the first sign of fatigue/respiratory distress?

Definition of weaning

Doctoral research has indicated that weaning is often defined, by nurses, according to the technology used and location of care (Crocker 2006). Moreover, the traditional view of weaning centres upon the eventual liberation of the patient from the ventilator (American College of Chest Physicians, the American Association for Respiratory Care and the American College of Critical Care Medicine (Collective Task Force) 2002). The method of respiratory support required and the geographical location are immaterial. Weaning may also be said to begin as soon as the decision to reduce the level of respiratory support is made.

There are two stages to weaning, pre-weaning or titrating ventilator support and active weaning (Crocker and Kinnear 2008). Pre-weaning involves preparation for weaning in order to optimise the weaning process and should begin as soon as the patient is ventilated. The weaning process should involve the patient. One single-weaning trajectory

Table 2.2   Classification of weaning.

Acute ventilatory dependence	6 hours a day, includes CPAP, NIV and IPPV
Weaning delay	Need for ventilation for >2 weeks in absence of non-respiratory factor
Chronic ventilatory dependence	CPAP by mask excluded, IPPV required regularly day or night irrespective of the number of hours
Weaning failure	Ventilation >3 weeks

Source: Modernisation Agency (2002).

is not possible; patients are individuals and, as such, weaning must be individualised. A description of patients' weaning trajectories as described by Egerod (2003) illustrates this. The Modernisation Agency (MA 2002) classifies weaning depending on the requirement for ventilatory assistance (Table 2.2).

For the purposes of this chapter weaning is defined as:

The gradual reduction of respiratory support (excluding oxygen) until the point has been reached when the patient either no longer requires assistance (for 24 hours a day) or has reached their maximum potential and has therefore come to a position when a further reduction of support cannot be achieved. In this case the patient may still require continuous or intermittent respiratory support.

In the past, patients with COPD have been associated with delayed weaning or failure to wean and, thus, clinicians have been reluctant to instigate invasive ventilation (Wildman et al. 2003). Recent research, however, has demonstrated that such patients can have a good outcome (Ai-Ping et al. 2005), and this has improved significantly with the introduction of NIV (Keenan et al. 2003) and the development of weaning centres (Quinnell et al. 2006).

Pathophysiology related to weaning

Initial weaning failure is usually due to incomplete resolution of the underlying illness which necessitated ventilation or the development of a new problem. Weaning depends on the strength of the respiratory muscles, the load applied to these muscles and central drive (see Table 2.3).

The adequacy of pulmonary gas exchange and the performance of the respiratory pump are important considerations during weaning assessment. The most common reason for failure to wean is an inadequate respiratory pump caused by either a decrease in the neuromuscular capacity of the respiratory muscles or an increased load (Krachman et al. 2001). For example, due to the COPD, Peter's lungs are hyperinflated, which results in a mechanically disadvantaged respiratory pump. Peter also has evidence of bronchospasm on auscultation. Any additional load such as this can lead to the development of respiratory muscle fatigue.

Table 2.3 The determinants of ventilation and common conditions associated with failure to wean.

Central drive	Respiratory muscle strength	Load
Sedation	Disuse atrophy	Left-ventricular failure
Metabolic alkalosis	Polyneuropathy	Pulmonary oedema
Delirium	Prolonged use of steroids, aminoglycosides and muscle relaxants	Hyperinflation
Raised intracranial pressure		
	Hypophosphatemia and hypomagnesia	Bronchospasm, upper airway obstruction
	Hyperinflation	Restrictive conditions, obesity, pleural effusions
	Ventilator-induced lung injury	Ventilator–patient dysynchrony
		Increased carbon dioxide production

Source: Adapted from Hemant et al. (2006).

Tests and investigations

Assessment of readiness to wean

There are no absolutes in weaning. Much of weaning is trial and error. There are two stages involved: pre-requisites or assessment of readiness for weaning and consideration of the method of weaning itself.

The first pre-requisite is that the reason for ventilation is resolving. A systematic assessment of the patient's readiness to wean should then follow. Many units have written guidelines to assist decision-making (for example, see Table 2.4). These will include parameters within which it is considered safe to wean. Many of these have been developed based on clinician experience rather than research evidence.

Using these pre-requisites, can you identify when John could have been assessed for weaning readiness? Can you see why it is important to have a two-stage approach to weaning? Preparing the patient for weaning is as important as weaning itself. The amount of oxygen and the level of sedation given to John could have been reduced much earlier and this would have allowed for weaning suitability to be assessed. There was a delay in preparing John to wean and this resulted in extending the number of ventilator days.

Inspiratory volumes

Normal Vt in an adult is 5–7 mL/kg. Therefore, a male of 70 kg would be expected to have a Vt of 350–490 mL. Compare this with John's set Vt of 700 mL a level at which acute lung injury could be triggered (see Chapter 1).

Table 2.4 Pre-requisites for weaning and readiness to wean.

Pre-requisites for weaning		
Physical	Respiratory	FiO_2 <0.5, FiO_2/PaO_2 150–300 mmHg, low levels of PEEP, acid–base balanced, ABGs acceptable and normal for patient, chest secretions acceptable. CXR acceptable.
	Cardio-vascular system	CVS stable (± inotropes), Hb >7, or 10 g/L for COPD, temp <38.5°C, >35°C
	Central nervous system	Respiratory drive in tact, pain controlled, sedation off or minimal amount, ICP within normal range
	GI tract	Feeding in progress or being considered, trace elements normalised, gut not distended
Psychological	Anxiety/mood/motivation	Patient prepared, involved, has rested, consider assessment of anxiety, mood, motivation, sleep, presence of delirium and treat appropriately
Readiness to wean		
Occlusion pressure (PO.1)	Normal value −3.4 to −4.5	Determines patient's level of support required and assessment of respiratory muscle function.
Rapid shallow breathing index (RSBI)	Below 105	*f* divided by TV
Spontaneous breathing trials (SBT)	30–120 minutes. T-piece or ventilator mode with or without PEEP and support/tube compliance	Once daily. If successful commence weaning, unsuccessful continue to ventilate.

Respiratory rate and Vt are sensitive indicators of respiratory fatigue. When Vt drops, respiratory rate increases in response, in order to maintain an adequate minute volume, as can be seen in Peter's data. Gas exchange may not be affected until the Vt drops to a level whereby effective ventilation is compromised, and at this stage ABGs change. It is therefore important to monitor the patient's respiratory observations closely and not rely solely on blood gases. In this way respiratory fatigue is picked up early and appropriate interventions can be applied.

A number of additional tools are available, which can be used to help predict the likelihood of successful weaning for John and Peter, and guide the speed at which weaning takes place.

Box 2.3 Calculation examples for PaO_2/FiO_2.

John's initial ABG showed a PaO_2 of 13kPa. Dividing this by his FiO_2, which was 0.1, gives a PaO_2/FiO_2 ratio of 130 kPa.

Peter's initial PaO_2 was 7.5 kPa. Dividing this by his FiO_2, which was 0.4, gives a PaO_2/FiO_2 ratio of 18.75 kPa.

A value less than 40 kPa would indicate inadequate gas exchange and thus would require an increase in support.

The ratio of PaO_2 to FiO_2 is commonly used as an additional measurement in assessing oxygenation in mechanically ventilated patients. The PaO_2/FiO_2 ratio is calculated by dividing the PaO_2 by the FiO_2 (see Box 2.3 for examples).

Rapid, shallow breathing is the frequency of breaths (f) divided by the tidal volume in litres (Vt) (Howie 1999). John's initial respiratory rate was 12 breaths per minute. Dividing this by his Vt, which was 700 mL, and multiplying it by 1000, to convert into litres, gives him an RSBI of 17. Further examples can be seen in Table 2.5. An RSBI of less than 105 has been widely accepted as an adequate value upon which to commence or progress weaning and extubation (Yang and Tobin 1991).

Airway occlusion pressure (P0.1) could also be used to assess John's and Peter's readiness to wean. Many acute diseases will increase the work of breathing (WoB) by altering compliance, airway resistance and carbon dioxide production. An increase in WoB also increases oxygen demand. The patient's ability to tolerate this is dependent on the power of their respiratory pump. This is dependent on the strength and endurance of the respiratory muscles. One way of measuring this is to use P0.1 (Whitelaw and Derenne 1993). This gives a measurement of the effect of all the respiratory muscles active at a given time and does not depend on resistance or compliance of the respiratory system. Many ventilators now have this measurement facility. It is operated by occluding the inspiratory limb for 0.1 second. This would not cause any adverse effect on Peter or John and they would be unaware that it was being measured. Normal values are between -3.5 to -4.5 cmH_2O (see Table 2.6). The interpretation of occlusion pressure must, however,

Table 2.5 Calculation examples for PaO_2/FiO_2.

(f divided by TV × 1000)		
	Respiratory rate	
Tidal volume	**20**	**30**	**40**
200 mL	100	150	200
300 mL	66.6	100	133.3
400 mL	50	75	100

Table 2.6   Interpretation of P0.1 and clinical applications.

P0.1 Value	Interpretation	Clinical application
−3.4 to −4.5	Normal range	Ventilation optimal
Below −3.5	Suggests patient is able to do more or ventilator providing too much support ventilator	Reduce support (e.g. reduce ASB) *Note*: A very low value (<1.0) may indicate the patient is unable to initiate a breath due to severe weakness or over sedation.
Above −4.5	Suggests patient requires more support	Increase support (e.g. increase ASB or add a rest period).
−6 or above	Suggests the patient is tired and may fail to wean	Rest and provide full ventilation for 24 hours.

be treated with caution. Although it is reliable in measuring output at the first part of inspiration, it should be used in conjunction with other measures and indices.

Spontaneous breathing trials (SBT)

Many units now include an assessment of the patient's readiness to wean using a daily spontaneous breathing trial (SBT). This can be achieved in two ways: either using a T-piece with 5 cmH$_2$O of PEEP or using a spontaneous mode on the ventilator with 5 cmH$_2$O PEEP and some level of support or tube compliance to counteract the extra WoB. The length of time the trial should last is a matter of debate. This ranges from 30 minutes to 2 hours. If there are no signs of fatigue, then weaning may begin. If the patient fails, then no further attempt at weaning should be made until the following day. Signs of fatigue have been defined by the Spanish Collaborative Group (Brochard et al. 1994; Esteban et al. 1995). These are:

- Respiratory rate (RR) > 35/minute or a change in RR > 50% above baseline
- SaO$_2$ < 90%
- Heart rate > 140 or sustained increase or decrease of 20% lower than baseline
- Systolic blood pressure > 180 mmHg or < 90 mmHg
- Increased agitation
- Signs of increased WoB.

Other available tools include the weaning continuum developed by Burns et al. (2000). The Burns Wean Assessment Programme (BWAP) is a computer application designed to help clinicians assess, evaluate and track factors important in weaning but has not been widely used in the UK (Burns et al. 1994).

Managing the patient during weaning

Following a decision to commence weaning, a number of issues need to be considered.

Methods of Weaning

A number of randomised controlled trials (RCTs) have been conducted in an effort to develop a body of evidence to support the systematic weaning of patients (for example, Esteban et al. 1995). The extensive research has not, to date, however, provided a clear answer as to the best method of weaning. This could be due to the inconsistencies in design. Firstly, patient groups were not homogenous and included short- and long-term patients, those following surgery and those with chronic disease. Secondly, the definition of successful weaning varied from 2 to 48 hours post-separation from the ventilator, with some studies including extubation as a criterion. Thirdly, weaning failure was inconsistently defined, and fourthly, outcome measures were not consistently applied. In a review by Meade et al. (2001), it was identified, however, that although all these factors may have obscured the impact of the ventilation mode, results do suggest that multiple daily T-piece weaning or pressure support may be superior to synchronized intermittent mandatory ventilation. Further, Meade et al. (2001) suggest that early extubation with the use of non-invasive positive-pressure ventilation as required may be a useful strategy in selected patients.

Peter is likely to be more difficult to wean due to his history of COPD. Butler et al. (1999) conducted a systematic review of the literature in difficult-to-wean patients in order to ascertain which of the three commonly used techniques of weaning (T-piece; SIMV or pressure support ventilation (PSV)) leads to the highest proportion of successfully weaned patients in the shortest time. Difficult-to-wean patients were determined by the length of time on the ventilator (over 72 hours) or a failed trial of spontaneous breathing after 24 hours of ventilation. Only 4 out of 667 identified studies met the criteria for the review.[1] Although individual trials reported outcomes in favour of a specific weaning mode, no mode was demonstrated to be consistently superior to the other two. Two of the four studies gave conflicting results, Brochard et al. (1994) supporting PSV and Esteban et al. (1995) supporting T-piece as the optimum method of weaning. Pooling of the results only highlighted the heterogeneity of the study designs.

Results of the reviews by Meade et al. (2001) and Butler et al. (1999) indicate that there is currently insufficient evidence to identify a clearly superior mode for weaning any group of patients. Furthermore, Butler et al. (1999) state that the manner in which the mode of weaning is applied may have a greater effect on the likelihood of weaning than the mode itself (Butler et al. 1999: 2332). Differences in clinicians' intuitive threshold for the reduction or discontinuation of ventilatory support appears to have a greater impact on the failure of SBTs, and on reintubation, than do modes of weaning (Meade et al. 2001). Clinical decisions regarding choice of mode may also be determined by the ventilators available within the department and the knowledge and competence of the healthcare staff utilising them.

---

[1]Criteria for review: (1) ventilation >72 hours or failed trial of spontaneous breathing >24 hours, (2) at least two of the three modes of weaning were compared, (3) outcomes based on one of the following were applied: weaning time (time from initiation of weaning to extubation), successful weaning rate (successfully off the ventilator for > 48 hours) and (4) controlled clinical trial.

Based on this evidence, the methods of ventilation used for John and Peter could both be considered suitable, although the parameters set need to be adjusted to ensure that that ventilation does not cause more harm than good (see Chapter 1 on ALI/ARDS for information on lung protective ventilation). Further, the decision to progress Peter from BIPAP to CPAP and PS appears justified.

The nursing role

Nursing research in this area has focused on patient communication whilst being ventilated (Bergbom-Engberg and Haljamae 1989; Hafsteindottir 1996), patients' recollections of stressful experiences whilst being ventilated (Gries and Fernsler 1988; Jablonski 1994; Rotondi et al. 2002) or patients' perceptions of fatigue (Higgens 1998). The patients' view of weaning has been under-investigated until recently (Cook et al. 2001). In a Canadian study of 20 patients undergoing ventilation and weaning, it was revealed that patients were actively engaged in a variety of physical, cognitive and emotional activities that contributed to successful weaning. These activities patients called work (Logan and Jenny 1997). The authors concluded that patients' work should be understood and supported by clinicians (nurses) in order to facilitate recovery from mechanical ventilation and weaning (Logan and Jenny 1997: 140). In a more recent study, Johnson (2004) interviewed nine Australian ICU patients undergoing weaning and identified four themes. Reclaiming the everyday world (the only theme discussed in the published literature) meant re-engaging with staff (and families) in the ICU, seeking control over treatments and attempting to communicate, question and interpret the environment (Johnson 2004). It is vital that these findings are taken into consideration if we are to understand and respond appropriately to the needs of patients like Peter.

The lack of consensus regarding the method of weaning has resulted in a change of focus in the literature to the use of protocols (for example, Blackwood et al. 2004; Tonnelier et al. 2005) and the role of the healthcare professional in weaning (for example, Blackwood 2003; Fulbrook et al. 2004; Gelsthorpe and Crocker 2004). Thorens et al. (1995) was the first paper (Swiss) to investigate the influence of the quality of nursing on the duration of weaning from mechanical ventilation in patients with chronic respiratory disease. Using an 'index of nursing', the effective workforce of nurses (indicated by the number of nurses and their qualifications) was compared with the ideal workforce required by the number of patients and their severity of disease. This index of nursing was then compared to the duration of weaning from mechanical ventilation. The study concluded that the quality of nursing appeared to be a measurable and critical factor in patients who were weaning with chronic respiratory disease. During the study, there were a number of changes, including an increase in medical staff and beds. These and other factors such as nurse education were not explored and these may have had bearings on the study. Despite this important research, there has not been any attempt to replicate or extend this work.

Despite many references to reducing weaning times using protocols (for example, Kollef et al. 1997), it is not clear whether nurse-led weaning strategies hasten weaning from mechanical ventilation compared to physician-led strategies. A systematic review of the literature by Price (2001) argues there is no evidence that nurses are leading weaning and therefore reducing weaning time, and suggests that it is the use of protocols rather than the person leading the weaning process that makes the difference (Price 2001). Recent research comparing protocol-led weaning by nurses to a historical matched cohort in a French ICU showed that nurse protocol-directed weaning does reduce the duration of mechanical ventilation and the length of stay in the ICU (Tonnelier et al. 2005). The incidence of ventilator-associated pneumonia (VAP), ventilator discontinuation failure rates and ICU mortality were similar in both groups.

Evidence of weaning effectiveness on its own does not guarantee that protocols will be used in practice (Blackwood 2003). Furthermore, there is a thought that protocols are too difficult to develop due to the unpredictability of patients' illnesses (Blackwood et al. 2004). The use of protocols or nurse-led weaning is not yet a common practice in ICUs in England (Blackwood 2003). A survey demonstrated that clinicians (doctors) were leading weaning in 152 units, with only 33 (17%) units using protocols (Modernisation Agency 2002: 16).

Fairman and Lynaugh (1998) found in their study of American intensive care nurses that the use of protocols strictly limited the scope of nurses' patient care decisions, but represented an enormous change in doctor–nurse relationships. Where protocols did not exist, nurses and doctors continued to make informal contracts defining boundaries of nurses' authority and responsibility. Protocols may be seen as a form of restraint applied by the intensivists. Nurses may appear happy to accept the use of protocols in order to extend their decision-making, which was previously limited (Crocker 2002). This was not found to be the case in a recent pilot study (Gelsthorpe and Crocker 2004). The authors demonstrated that nurses based the decision to wean on their professional judgement and disregarded the weaning protocols[2] (see Figure 2.1 for an example of a weaning protocol). The authors suggested that protocolised weaning may not be useful in the decision to commence weaning as individual judgement may override the protocol and cause variance in weaning (Gelsthorpe and Crocker 2004). The use of protocols in weaning may be a form of control; therefore, their use may be seen as not only limiting nurses' powers of decision-making but also reducing it to not much more than following a set of guidelines. Nurses, however, may not be in a position to accept this transfer of technology. Gelsthorpe and Crocker (2004) showed that nurses were delegating the responsibility for weaning to the medical staff. Experience was an influential factor in establishing the decision to wean, with less-experienced staff erring on the side of caution and delaying weaning. The study demonstrated that weaning followed a medical paradigm (systems approach) with a concentration on physiological factors which influenced the decision to wean. Blackwood et al. (2004) identified that physicians in the ICU had reservations regarding the use of protocols in weaning because of the variability of nursing experience and indicated that doctors should retain control over weaning. The transfer of technology from medicine to nursing, therefore, is not a simple one.

---

[2]In this study nurse-led weaning had been established for three years and this may have a bearing on the use of judgement rather than protocols.

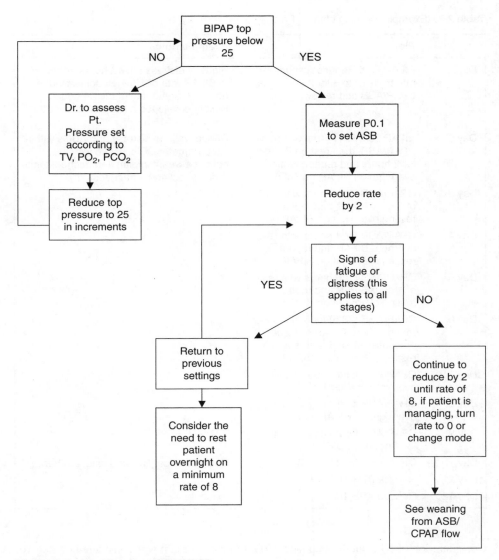

Figure 2.1   Weaning from BIPAP/ASB.

Rehabilitation during weaning

Assessment and planning for effective physical and psychological rehabilitation should be started as early as possible (NICE 2009) and should engage a holistic approach, which meets the needs of the individual.

Table 2.7 details a suggested weaning plan for Peter. The weaning plan should be written daily after a medical review and discussion with the multi-professional team. At any time, if Peter shows the ability to wean more quickly, this plan should be changed.

Table 2.7   Example weaning plan for Peter.

	Plan	Example notes
Day 1	BIPAP 25/5 Reduce respiratory rate from 12 to 8 for 2 hours trial CPAP/ASB and review	Signs of distress after 2 hours, returned to BIPAP rate of 12, then decreased to rate of 8 for the rest of the 24 hours. Patient developed a hospital-acquired pneumonia.
Day 2	BIPAP 25/5 RR 8, trial of 1 hour CPAP/ASB, then rest on BIPAP for 2 hours and repeat, resting overnight on BIPAP rate of 8	Coped well, no distress and ABGs within set parameters. Discussed with the patient a weaning plan and tracheostomy. Patient declined a tracheostomy.
Day 3	CPAP/ASB for 2 hours with rest of 1 hour BIPAP and repeat, resting overnight on BIPAP	
Day 4	CPAP/ASB for 4 hours with rest of 1 hour BIPAP and repeat, resting overnight on BIPAP	
Day 5	CPAP/ASB for 6 hours with rest of 1 hour BIPAP and repeat, resting overnight on BIPAP	
Day 6	CPAP/ASB (23/5) for 8 hours with rest of 1 hour BIPAP reduced pressures of 23/5 and repeat, resting overnight on BIPAP	
Day 7	CPAP/ASB for 10 hours resting overnight on BIPAP 21/5	
Day 8	CPAP/ASB for 12 hours resting overnight on BIPAP 19/5	
Day 9	CPAP/ASB for 20 hours resting for 4 hours on BIPAP 17/5	
Day 10	CPAP/ASB for 24 (17/5)	Could consider NIV and extubate here
Day 11	Reduce ASB 15/5	
Day 12	Reduce ASB 10/5	Extubate

Consideration of NIV should be made early. In Peter's case it was considered on day 10, but the decision was made to keep the conventional ventilator and extubate on day 12.

Documentation of Peter's progress in relation to the plan is important and should be recorded regularly. When possible, Peter should be encouraged to take an active part in decision-making and in evaluating his progress.

You may wish to discuss the issue of an early tracheostomy with colleagues. What would have been the benefits and disadvantages? The formation of a tracheostomy does not prevent NIV or long-term intermittent (at night) ventilation later if required. A recent study entitled 'TracMan' investigated the benefits of early (day 1–4) versus late (day 14) tracheostomy insertion, and found no benefit to early tracheostomy in relation to 30-day mortality. Further information about this multi-centre RCT can be found at www.tracman.org.uk. Specific information about the care and management of a patient

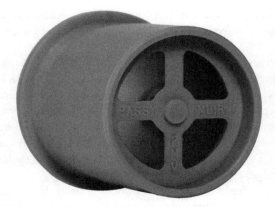

Figure 2.2 Passy–Muir valve. Photo courtesy of Passy-Muir Inc.

with a tracheostomy can be found in documents produced by St. George's Healthcare NHS Trust (2006) and NHS Quality Improvement Scotland (2007).

Should Peter have required a prolonged period of ventilation then use of a speaking valve such as the Passy–Muir valve (Figure 2.2) should be strongly considered (Dikeman and Kazandjian 1995). This valve allows phonation whilst being ventilated. Communication is essential to the motivation and psychological well-being of the patient, and all attempts should be made to facilitate this.

If Peter did have a tracheostomy inserted and continued to rely on ventilatory support, he is likely to have been kept nil by mouth until he could tolerate cuff deflation, and assessment of his ability to swallow. If he could demonstrate a competent swallow, then eating and drinking would be encouraged to avoid disuse atrophy. Long-term enteral feeding (PEG) might also need to be considered. Most published sources recommend oral intake only after cuff deflation and swallow assessment (St. George's Healthcare NHS Trust 2006). More recently, however, some units have, in close liaison with the speech and language therapists, considered allowing patients like Peter to have oral diet and fluid with the cuff inflated. To date, no published long-term studies have been undertaken investigating the potential effects of this strategy, although the key risks are cited to be aspiration and tracheal stenosis (St. George's Healthcare NHS Trust 2006). Implementing such a strategy needs careful vigilance by nursing staff and should be dependent on informed patient consent.

Loss of control is an identified problem affecting many longer term ICU patients (Maddox et al. 2001). Any intervention which increases sense of control has the potential to improve psychological well-being. Allowing patients to eat and drink normally may be one way of achieving this. Other ways include encouraging the patient to dress in their own clothes and allowing choices about care, for example, what time they want to wash.

Other problems which Peter could experience include feelings of hopelessness, sleep deprivation, cognitive dysfunction, pain, muscle weakness and night-time hypoventilation. Attention to all these factors is important in the development of a successful rehabilitation plan for Peter. Management will require effective communication and collaboration between the critical care nurse, the rest of the multi-professional healthcare team and the patient. For the longer term patient with complex needs, a case manager is imperative in order to co-ordinate an effective rehabilitation programme and to ensure regular reviews are in place.

Critical care nurses play a key role as they are at the bedside on a continual basis. Development of a relationship based on honesty and trust with both Peter and his family, and having a good understanding of his personality, and what motivates him will aid the rehabilitation process. The effective nurse will also recognise when Peter needs a rest. For example, if he has had bouts of diarrhoea or has not slept all night, sitting out in a chair may not be the most appropriate strategy, despite what it says on the weaning plan. Having the expertise and the confidence to instigate and defend such decisions requires a nurse with knowledge, expertise and experience.

Weaning is both a science and an art. One doctoral study demonstrated several nursing issues that affect weaning. These are continuity of care, knowing the patient, nursing expertise and patient-focused, individualised care (Crocker 2006). This ethnographic study observed nurses weaning patients from both NIV and invasive ventilation in one ICU and one high dependency unit. The study revealed that weaning patients were unpopular and nurses treated them not as partners in care but as recipients of care. As such there was little continuity of care as nurses requested to look after more 'critically ill' patients. Continuity of care was also affected by the nursing skill mix. More often than not, the most junior nurse would be allocated to look after the patient who was weaning whilst more experienced nurses cared for the sicker patients. This led to novice nurses, with little experience or understanding of weaning, caring for the most complex weaning patients. As such these nurses never got to know their patients; rather their knowing was framed by the technology but not the person (Crocker 2006) as described in the literature (May 1992; Radwin 1995, 1996; Henderson 1997) and, in particular, what this means in terms of weaning (Jenny and Logan 1992). These are important, but often overlooked, considerations which have the potential to greatly impact on weaning time and experience, and thus should be considered particularly during the management of longer term patients such as Peter.

Once Peter is ready to leave the ICU, nurses and other healthcare staff working outside of critical care must receive effective handovers and support to ensure Peter's individual needs continue to be addressed (NICE 2007, 2009).

Conclusion

Weaning from mechanical ventilation is complex and requires expert knowledge and skill. Research has tended to concentrate on trying to identify a superior method of weaning or a predictor of weaning success. There is little research exploring the patient's experience of weaning. What is known is that patients tend to be seen as passive recipients of care rather than active partners in care. Weaning protocols may have a place but, so far, we do not understand their exact role in weaning (Blackwood et al. 2010). The future may lie in the development of weaning centres as recommended by the Modernisation Agency (2002) which, so far, have failed to be implemented in the UK and the use of non-invasive ventilation. It is important to consider the long-term physical and psychological needs of patients who are difficult to wean at an early stage and to consider the possibility of domiciliary ventilation and how this may be achieved.

Key learning points

The two scenarios are different in terms of the age of the patient, the presence of co-morbidities, illness trajectories and ventilation/sedation strategies. These will all impact on weaning. It is important to understand that weaning can be complex as it is necessary to take account of both the physical and psychological factors.

- There are two phases of weaning: pre-weaning and active weaning.
- Weaning should be considered as soon as ventilation is commenced.
- Daily screening of the patient for readiness to wean is essential in order to optimise weaning and prevent a delay in commencing weaning.
- There is no best way to wean from mechanical ventilation. The approach is dependent on the context in which care is delivered and different approaches (nurse-led, protocolised, teams, etc.) may need to be tried and tested.
- The patient should be considered an active partner in care and included in the development of a weaning plan.
- Early extubation and the use of non-invasive ventilation, particularly in patients with moderate-to-severe COPD, should be considered.
- It is important to consider the nursing issues such as skill mix, continuity of care, nursing care activities and time of weaning. These may have a significant impact on weaning.
- If weaning is prolonged, then a psychological and physical rehabilitation programme must be in place.

Critical appraisal of research paper

Tonnelier et al. (2005) Impact of a nurse's protocol-directed weaning procedure on outcomes in patients undergoing mechanical ventilation for longer than 48 hours: a prospective cohort study with a matched historical control group. *Critical Care* **9**(2), 83–89.

Reader activities

1. Read the research article written by Tonnelier et al. (2005).
2. Using the critical appraisal framework in Appendix I, consider the methodological quality of the paper.
3. Reflect on this aspect of your own practice and the implications for weaning in your unit that this paper raises.

A commentary on this paper has been provided by the chapter author in Appendix III.

References

Ai-Ping C, Lee K, Lim T (2005) In-hospital and 5-year mortality of patients treated in the ICU for acute exacerbation of COPD: a retrospective study. *Chest* **128**(2), 518–524.

American College of Chest Physicians, the American Association for Respiratory Care and the American College of Critical Care Medicine (Collective Task Force) (2002) Evidence-based guidelines for weaning and discontinuing ventilatory support. *Respiratory Care* **47**(1), 69–90.

Bergbom-Engberg I, Haljamae H (1989) Assessment of patient's experience of discomforts during respirator therapy. *Critical Care Medicine* **17**, 1068–1072.

Blackwood B (2003) Can protocolised-weaning developed in the United States transfer to the United Kingdom context: a discussion. *Intensive and Critical Care Nursing* **19**, 215–225.

Blackwood B, Wilson-Barnett J, Trinder J (2004) Protocolised weaning from mechanical ventilation: ICU physicians' views. *Journal of Advanced Nursing* **48**(1), 26–34.

Blackwood B, Alderdice F, Burns KEA, Cardwell CR, Lavery G, O'Halloran P (2010) Protocolized versus non-protocolized weaning for reducing the duration of mechanical ventilation in critically ill adult patients. *Cochrane Database of Systematic Reviews* 2010, Issue 5. Art. No.: CD006904. DOI: 10.1002/14651858.CD006904.pub2.

Brochard L, Rauss A, Benito S, Conti G, Mancebo J, Rekik N, Gasparetto A, Lemaire F (1994) Comparison of three methods of gradual withdrawal from mechanically ventilatory support during weaning from mechanical ventilation. *American Journal of Respiratory Critical Care Medicine* **150**, 896–903.

Burns S, Burns J, Truit J (1994) Comparison of five clinical weaning indices. *American Journal of Critical Care* **3**, 342–352.

Burns S, Ryan B, Burns J (2000) The weaning continuum of APACHE II, Burns wean assessment programme, TISS and weaning index score to establish stages of weaning. *Critical Care Medicine* **28**(7), 2259–2267.

Butler R, Keenan S, Inman K, Sibbald W, Block G (1999) Is there a preferred technique for weaning the difficult-to-wean patient? A systematic review of the literature. *Critical Care Medicine* **27**(11), 2331–2336.

Cook D, Meade M, Perry A (2001) Qualitative studies on the patient's experiences of weaning from mechanical ventilation. *Chest* **120**(6), 469S–473S.

Crocker C (2002) Nurse-led weaning from ventilatory and respiratory support. *Intensive and Critical Care Nursing* **18**, 272–279.

Crocker C (2006) *The development of a nursing technology: making visible the nursing contribution to the development of critical care*. Unpublished Doctoral thesis, The University of Nottingham, Nottingham.

Crocker C, Kinnear W (2008) Weaning from ventilation: does a care bundle approach work? *Intensive and Critical Care Nursing* **24**(3), 180–187.

Dikeman KJ, Kazandjian MS (1995) *Communication and Swallowing Management of Tracheostomy and Ventilator-Dependent Adults*. Singular Publishing Group, Inc., San Diego.

Egerod I (2003) *Mechanical ventilator weaning in the context of critical care cursing: a descriptive, comparative study of nurses' decisions and interventions related to mechanical ventilation weaning*. PhD thesis, University of Copenhagen.

Ely EW, Baker AM, Dunagan DP, Burke HL, Smith AC, Kelly P (1996) Effect on the duration of mechanical ventilation of identifying patient capable of breathing spontaneously. *The New England Journal of Medicine* **335**, 1864–1869.

Esteban A, Frutos F, Tobin MJ, Alia I, Solsona JF, Valveruda I, Fernandez R, de la Cal MA, Benito S, Tomas R (1995) A comparison of four methods of patients who were weaning from mechanical ventilation. Spanish Lung Failure Collaborative Group. *The New England Journal of Medicine* **332**, 345–350.

Fairman J, Lynaugh J (1998) *Critical Care Nursing: A History*. University of Pennsylvania Press, Philadelphia.

Fulbrook P, Delaney N, Rigby J, Snowden A, Trevett M, Turner L, Whittam A (2004) Developing a network protocol: nurse-led weaning from ventilation. *The World of Critical Care Nursing* **3**(2), 28–37.

Gelsthorpe T, Crocker C (2004) A study exploring factors which influence the decision to commence nurse- led weaning. *Nursing in Critical Care* **9**(5), 213–221.

Gries M, Fernsler J (1988) Patient perceptions of the mechanical ventilator experience. *Focus on Critical Care* **15**(2), 52–59.

Hafsteindottir TB (1996) Patients' experiences of communication during the respirator period. *Intensive and Critical Care Nursing* **12**(5), 261–271.

Henderson S (1997) Knowing the patient and the impact on patient participation: a grounded theory study. *International Journal of Nursing Practice* **3**(2), 111–118.

Hemant H, Chacko J, Singh M (2006) Weaning from mechanical ventilation – current evidence. *Indian Journal of Anaesthesia* **50**(6), 435–438.

Higgens P (1998) Patient perception of fatigue while undergoing long term mechanical ventilation: Incidence and associated factors. *Heart & Lung* **27**(3), 177–183.

Howie A (1999) Rapid shallow breathing as a predictive indicator during weaning from ventilator support. *Nursing in Critical Care* **4**, 171–178.

Jablonski R (1994) The experience of being mechanically ventilated. *Qualitative Health Research* **4**(2), 186–207.

Jenny J, Logan J (1992) Knowing the patient: one aspect of clinical knowledge. *Image* **24**, 254–258.

Johnson P (2004) Reclaiming the everyday world: how long - term ventilated patients in critical care seek to gain aspects of power and control over their environment. *Intensive and Critical Care Nursing* **20**(4), 190–199.

Keenan S, Sinuff T, Cook D, Hill N (2003) Which patients with acute exacerbation of chronic obstructive pulmonary disease benefit from non-invasive positive pressure ventilation? *Annals of Internal Medicine* **138**(11), 861–870.

Knebel A (1991) Weaning from mechanical ventilation: current controversies. *Heart & Lung* **20**, 321–34.

Kollef HM, Shapiro SD, Silver P, St. John RE, Prentice D, Sauer S, Ahrens TS, Shannon W, Baker-Clinkscale D (1997) A randomised controlled trial of protocol-directed versus physician-directed weaning from mechanical ventilation. *Critical Care Medicine* **25**(4), 567–574.

Krachman S, Martin U, D'Alonzo G (2001) Weaning from mechanical ventilation: an update. *JAOA* **101**(7), 387–390.

Kurek CJ, Cohen IL, Lambrinos J, Minatoya K, Booth FV, Chalfin DB (1997) Clinical and economic outcome of patients undergoing tracheostomy for prolonged mechanical ventilation in New York state during 1993: analysis of 6353 cases under diagnosis-related group 485. *Critical Care Medicine* **25**, 983–988.

Logan J, Jenny J (1997) Qualitative analysis of patients' work during mechanical ventilation and weaning. *Heart & Lung* **26**, 140–147.

Maddox M, Dunn S, Pretty LE (2001) Psychological recovery following ICU: experiences and influences upon discharge to the community. *Intensive and Critical Care Nursing* **17**, 6–15.

Mancebo J (1996) Weaning from mechanical ventilation. *The European Respiratory Journal* **9**, 1923–1931.

May C (1992) Nursing work, nurses' knowledge, and the subjectification of the patient. *Sociology of Health and Illness* **14**(4), 472–487.

Modernisation Agency (2002) *Critical Care Programme: Weaning and Long Term Ventilation.* Department of Health, London.

Meade M, Guyatt G, Sinuff T, Griffith L, Hand L, Toprani G, Cook D (2001) Trials comparing alternative weaning modes and discontinuation assessments. *Chest* **120**(6), 425S–437S.

Nevins ML, Epstein SK (2001) Weaning from prolonged mechanical ventilation. *Clinical Chest Medicine* **22**, 13–33.

NHS Quality Improvement Scotland (2007) *Caring for the Patient with a Tracheostomy.* NHS Scotland, Edinburgh.

NICE (2007) *Acutely Ill Patients in Hospital: Recognition and Response to Acute Illness in Adults in Hospital.* National Institute for Health and Clinical Excellence. Available online at: http://www.nice.org.uk/. Accessed 20 March 2009.

NICE (2009) *Rehabilitation after Critical Illness.* National Institute for Health and Clinical Excellence. Available online at: http://www.nice.org.uk/. Accessed 09 September 2009.

Price A (2001) Nurse-led weaning from mechanical ventilation: where's the evidence? *Intensive and Critical Care Nursing* **17**, 167–176.

Quinnell T, Pilsworth S, Shneerson J, Smith I (2006) Prolonged invasive ventilation following acute ventilatory failure in COPD: weaning results, survival and the role of non-invasive ventilation. *Chest* **129**(1), 133–139.

Radwin L (1995) Knowing the patient: a process model for individualised interventions. *Nursing Research* **44**(6), 364–370.

Radwin L (1996) Knowing the patient: a review of research on an emerging concept. *Journal of Advanced Nursing* **23**(6), 1142–1146.

Rotondi A, C, Mendelsohn A, Schultz R, Belle S, Im K, Donahoe M, Pinski M (2002) Patient's recollections of stressful experiences while receiving prolonged mechanical ventilation in an intensive care unit. *Critical Care Medicine* **30**(4), 746–752.

Seneff MG, Zimmerman JE, Knauss WA, Wagner DP, Draper EA (1996) Predicting the duration of mechanical ventilation. The importance of disease and patient characteristics. *Chest* **110**, 469–479.

St. George's Healthcare NHS Trust (2006) *Guidelines for the Care of the Patients with Tracheostomy Tubes.* Smiths-Medical International, London.

Thorens JB, Rainer M, Jolliet P, Chevrolet JC (1995) Influence of the quality of nursing on the duration of weaning from mechanical ventilation in patients with chronic obstructive pulmonary disease. *Critical Care Medicine* **23**(11), 1807–1815.

Tonnelier J, Prat G, Le Gal G, Gut-Gobert C, Renault A, Boles J, L'Her E (2005) Impact of a nurse' protocol-directed weaning procedure on outcomes in patients undergoing mechanical ventilation for more than 48 hours: a prospective cohort study with a matched historical control group. *Critical Care* **9**(2), 83–89.

Wildman M, O'Dea J, Kostopoulou O, Tindall M, Walia S, Khan Z (2003) Variation in intubation decisions for patients with chronic obstructive pulmonary disease in one critical care network. *QJM* **96**(8), 583–591.

Whitelaw WA, Derenne JP (1993) Airway occlusion pressure. *Journal of Applied Physiology* **74**(4), 1475–1484.

Yang KL, Tobin MJ (1991) A prospective study of indices predicting the outcome of trials of weaning from mechanical ventilation. *The New England Journal of Medicine* **324**, 1445–1450.

Chapter 3

The patient with fever

Kate Brown

Introduction

Fever is present in between 30% and 50% of patients admitted to critical care units (Marik 2000; Ryan and Levy 2003). Fever is an elevation of core body temperature caused by infection or inflammatory processes and is a natural host defence mechanism. It is a symptom of underlying pathophysiology and not a disease process in itself. There is considerable debate concerning the most appropriate management of fever in the critically ill patient. This chapter examines the pathophysiology of fever and discusses aspects of the current controversies surrounding the assessment and management of a febrile patient.

Patient scenario

Mary O'Hara is a 64-year-old lady on a critical care unit, following admission with community-acquired pneumonia. Mary is self-ventilating on 40% oxygen, via facemask. During your shift Mary complains of feeling 'unwell'. She reports feeling cold and shivery. She is restless and tells you that she feels uncomfortable. A physical assessment of Mary is conducted, results of which can be seen in Table 3.1.

Reader activities

Having read this scenario, consider the following:

- How do Mary's symptoms support a diagnosis of fever?
- What stage of the fever cascade is Mary experiencing? Explain this using relevant pathophysiology.
- Mary has an altered respiratory pattern. Consider why this might be of concern at this time.
- Is tympanic thermometry a valid and reliable method of temperature assessment in the critically ill patient? Consider any other methods that might be used here and their possible advantages and limitations.

Critical Care Nursing: Learning from Practice, 1st edition. Edited by Suzanne Bench and Kate Brown.
© 2011 Blackwell Publishing Ltd.

• Fever is defined as a symptom of underlying pathology. What further assessment/investigations would be important?

Table 3.1 ABCDE assessment and findings.

Airway	Patent	Able to maintain own airway
Breathing	Respiratory rate	28 breaths per minute
	SpO$_2$	95% on 40% oxygen
	ABG	
	pH	7.32
	PaCO$_2$	3.4 kPa
	PaO$_2$	9.5 kPa
	HCO$_3$	22 mmol/L
	BE	−4
	SaO$_2$	95%
	Cough	Productive, yellow-green sputum
Circulation	Heart rate	105 beats per minute
	Blood pressure	165/85 mmHg
	Temperature via tympanic membrane thermometer	38.6°C
	Capillary refill time	> 2 seconds
	Peripheral circulation urine output 40 mls over previous 2 hours (weight 80 kg)	Pale and feels cool to touch
Disability	Level of consciousness	Alert and orientated: time place & person
Exposure/ environment	Skin	Generally intact. No wounds Arterial line in right radial artery Central line in right jugular neck vein Peripheral cannula left arm Indwelling urinary catheter
	Mobility	Able to transfer to chair, breathless on walking

Definition of fever

Mary's temperature has been recorded as 38.6°C via a tympanic thermometer. This is elevated above the normal core body temperature of 37°C in the human, thus supporting a diagnosis of fever (Ryan and Levy 2003). At present there is no clear agreement as to what temperature constitutes a fever however, temperatures of >38°C are generally regarded as clinically significant. The Society of Critical Care Medicine (ISCCM) and the Infectious Disease Society of America (IDSA) have recommended that temperatures of above 38.3°C should be regarded as representative of fever and should trigger a clinical review (O'Grady et al. 1998; Ryan and Levy 2003). Mary's temperature, at 38.6°C, fulfils the available diagnostic criteria of a clinically significant fever and should therefore prompt further investigation.

Fever is a normal host defence response arising from a number of stimuli, including infections (viral, bacterial or fungal), inflammation (trauma or autoimmune disease) or drug therapy, resulting in an elevation of the temperature set-point (T^{set}). Fever, as distinguished from hyperthermia, is classified as a controlled or regulated elevation of core body temperature above normal. In this state the hypothalamus is functioning normally and is responding to chemical mediators that stimulate an increase in the temperature set-point (Johnson Rowsey 1997a). It is crucial that fever is distinguished from hyperthermia, as in this state the elevation of body temperature is uncontrolled and arises from damage or failure of the temperature regulatory system, usually following head injury or spinal cord damage (Henker and Carlson 2007; Beard and Day 2008). In fever treatment is aimed at reducing body temperature through the use of antipyretic drugs whereas the management of hyperthermia is aimed at the physical cooling of the patient (Henker et al. 1997; Marik 2000; Beard and Day 2008).

The fever cascade

Mary has been admitted with a community-acquired pneumonia, suggesting that the likely cause of her fever is an infection. Infection involves the entry of microorganisms into the body from the external environment. Invading microorganisms will activate the fever cascade (Johnson Rowsey 1997a) comprising a complex physiological response involving cytokine-mediated temperature elevation (fever), acute phase and immunological stimulation and metabolic and endocrine responses (Plaisance and Mackowiak 2000). Microorganisms (exogenous pyrogens – heat-producing substances) induce monocytes to produce cytokines (endogenous pyrogens) (Ryan and Levy 2003), a group of heat-labile proteins that play a central role in the genesis of fever (Marik 2000). The cytokines known to be active in the development of fever include Interleukin (IL)-I, IL-6, tumour necrosis factor (TNF-α) and the interferons α, β and γ, with interferon being γ the most important of these (Johnson Rowsey 1997a; Marik 2000).

The interaction between cytokines and the exact mechanisms by which they affect neural tissue are complex and as yet are not entirely clear (Johnson Rowsey 1997a; Marik 2000; Ryan and Levy 2003). Cytokines bind to their own specific receptors in an area of the brain lacking the blood brain barrier, possibly the organum vasculosum laminae terminalis (OVLT) which lies in close proximity to the preoptic region of the anterior hypothalamus (Johnson Rowsey 1997a; Ryan and Levy 2003). A cytokine–receptor interaction occurs that activates the chemical phospholipase A_2. This liberates arachidonic acid, the substrate necessary for prostaglandin production. Prostaglandins directly modify the activity of thermosensitive neurons in the hypothalamus, raising the temperature set-point to a new setting (Marik 2000), resulting in a fever.

When hypothalamic set-point is raised and fever begins, core blood temperature lags behind and will only equal the new set-point when heat generating mechanisms have been activated. The person experiences the 'chill stage' of a fever, which lasts for about 10–40 minutes. During this stage all the physiological mechanisms for heat production and heat conservation are activated (Bruce and Grove 1992). Sympathetic activation, thyroid stimulation and shivering occur to increase basal metabolic rate and raise temperature. Heat loss from convection and radiation is reduced by diverting blood away from the skin surface (see Table 3.2 for definitions of heat loss processes).

Table 3.2   The four physical processes governing heat loss.

Physical process	Definition	Heat loss in human
Radiation	Process of heat loss into the atmosphere from emission of infrared radiation waves. All objects (unless at absolute zero) emit infrared radiation due to molecular collision.	Humans can lose large amounts of heat in this way, particularly when large areas of the body are exposed to the environment
Conduction	Process of kinetic heat exchange when one surface is in direct contact with another.	Humans do not lose a great deal of heat from conduction under normal conditions. Conductive heat loss increases significantly in immersion in water, or extended lying on cold surface following fall, unconsciousness etc.
Convection	The continuous process of heat loss through air currents. Air molecules are warmed as they come into contact with a warm body. Warm air rises towards the head and is replaced with cool air, which in turn is warmed.	Humans can lose significant amounts of heat via convection. Greatly enhanced by factors such as wind chill and fanning.
Evaporation	The process of heat loss from water evaporation. Kinetic heat is produced as a product of cellular metabolism this can be carried in water molecules to the skin surface and evaporated into the atmosphere.	When heat production is high (exercise, fever). Large quantities of heat can be dissipated by sweating in humans to restore heat balance

Related pathophysiology

Mary is demonstrating the cardinal signs of the chill stage of a fever. She is shivering as her body attempts to generate heat (thermogenesis) through shivering. Sweating ceases during this stage and 'goose bumps' (horripilation) appear on the skin, trapping warm air and reducing heat loss from convection and radiation (Bruce and Grove 1992; Johnson Rowsey 1997a). Shivering results in a substantial and costly increase in energy expenditure and may compromise cardiopulmonary function. Shivering should, therefore, be avoided in the critically ill and it is advisable to assist patients to warm themselves during this stage (Holtzclaw 2004).

Mary's sympathetic nervous system has been activated resulting in the release of the catecholamines, adrenaline and noradrenaline, increasing her heart rate and cardiac contractility and promoting vasoconstriction. An enlarged cardiac output is necessary to supply adequate oxygen to meet increased metabolic demand and there is a corresponding increase in the depth and rate of respirations to augment oxygen availability. A rising metabolic rate creates an initial cellular hypoxia as oxygen demand initially outstrips supply, lowering blood pH and PaO_2 levels and stimulating the respiratory centres in the medulla and pons to increase respirations. This would account for Mary's elevated respiratory rate of 28 breaths per minute and the metabolic acidosis evident in her blood gas analysis. Mary may find it difficult to cope with any increased demand on her respiratory system as she has an existing chest infection. A chest infection will decrease the efficiency of ventilation and decrease Mary's capacity to compensate for further demand. Mary is also receiving a high percentage of supplemental oxygen to meet present respiratory requirements.

Mary's skin is pale and feels cool to touch, indicating a noradrenaline-mediated vaso-constriction, and this also accounts for her increased capillary refill time of >2 seconds. Vasoconstriction effectively reduces the volume of blood present at the skin surface, thereby significantly reducing heat loss from convection and radiation and augmenting heat conservation.

During the chill stage of a fever, endocrine responses are also initiated. Sympathetic activation leads to stimulation of the thyroid gland to secrete thyroxines to raise the basal metabolic rate (BMR). An increased BMR promotes thermogenesis and also stimulates appetite, leading to sensations of hunger. Mary at this stage will be using large quantities of energy to maintain a high BMR and because of the substantial increase in energy used when shivering. This will, therefore, have implications for meeting her nutritional requirements.

As sentient beings, humans are also able to invoke behavioural responses to changes in body temperature. Feeling cold may provoke people to add extra clothing or blankets and to take hot food and drinks (see Table 3.3 for a summary of the responses evoked during the chill stage of a fever).

Table 3.3 Mechanisms activated by cold.

Heat gain	Physical responses: signs and symptoms
Shivering – promotes thermogenesis as a result of intense muscular contraction	Generalised, involuntary contraction of skeletal muscles Feels cold Increased energy expenditure
Activation of sympathetic activity – release of adrenaline and noradrenaline	Enhanced cardiovascular activity ↑HR,↑RR Vasoconstriction–↑BP
Activation of thyroid hormones to increase BMR- thermogenesis	Kinetic heat energy production from nutrient metabolism Hunger
Prevention of Heat loss Horripilation – reduction of heat loss from skin surface via convection, radiation	Goose bumps – cold sensors of skin stimulated, erectile tissue raises hairs on skin of arms, legs
Vasoconstriction – prevention of heat loss from convection, radiation at skin surface	Increased capillary refill time Pale skin Cool/cold peripheries Bluish tinge to fingers, nail beds
Sentient behaviour or voluntary activity	warmer clothing, blankets, curling up, desire for hot drinks, hot food

Skills-based knowledge

It is important to bear in mind that fever is a symptom of underlying disease, infection or inflammation and not a disease process in itself. Its presence should prompt investigations to determine its cause so that appropriate, targeted treatment can be commenced in a timely manner (O'Grady et al. 1998). Assessment of Mary at this stage would be focused on establishing the underlying cause of her fever by undertaking a septic screen: blood cultures, swabs and specimens for microbiological culture and sensitivity. Laboratory analysis might also include full blood count (FBC), white cell count (WCC), C-reactive protein (CRP) and procalcitonin (PCT). Ongoing assessment of her temperature should also be undertaken.

Temperature assessment

Temperature taking in clinical practice is often viewed as a relatively straightforward clinical assessment but recent studies reveal evidence of lack of consistency and accuracy in temperature taking (Holtzclaw 1998; Giuliano et al. 1999; Gilbert et al. 2002; Lefrant et al. 2003; Hooper and Andrews 2006; Kimberger et al. 2007; Moran et al. 2007). Errors arise from lack of reliability of temperature taking amongst nurses and health care assistants (Giuliano et al. 1999; Fisk and Arcona 2001; Evans and Kenkre 2006), and inadequate instrument reliability and validity in achieving accurate measurements across the range of temperatures assessed and at temperature-taking sites (Giuliano et al. 1999; Hooper and Andrews 2006; Moran et al. 2007).

Temperature assessment can be performed invasively or non-invasively. Invasive methods provide direct measurements of core temperature by placement of temperature probes in areas of core blood circulation. Invasive devices, if the equipment is functioning correctly, provide highly accurate and consistent measurements of core temperature. Non-invasive methods only give indications of core temperature by measuring the temperature of arterial blood peripherally. Invasive devices include pulmonary artery thermistor temperature measurement (often referred to as the gold standard as it provides direct measurement of blood temperature in the thoracic cavity), oesophageal or bladder devices. Rectal temperature equates well with core temperature but is considered unpopular for both aesthetic and infection control reasons. Non-invasive methods include oral (via chemical dot or electronic probe), tympanic membrane thermometry (via infrared spectrometry), axillary (via chemical dot or electronic probe) or temporal arterial devices (see Figures 3.1 and 3.2 for examples of non-invasive methods).

To achieve the most accurate temperature assessments, nurses should consider both the best method and the most appropriate site for an individual patient. It is not necessarily imperative that non-invasive temperatures replicate core temperatures exactly but they should reflect these and detect those outside of the normal ranges (hypothermia and fever/hyperthermia) (Erickson 1999).

Mary's temperature is currently being recorded non-invasively via a tympanic thermometer (Figure 3.1). Non-invasive measurements of shell temperature are more prone to variations due to user ability and may be affected by environmental factors (Gilbert

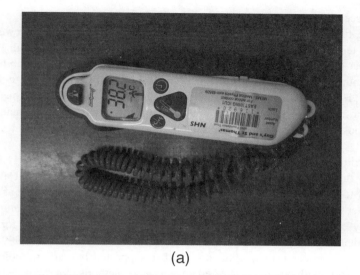

(a)

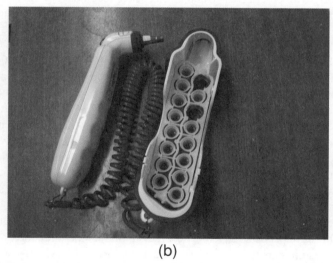

(b)

Figure 3.1   (a) Tympanic thermometer. (b) Tympanic thermometer open.

et al. 2002) but placement of an invasive device to record Mary's temperature at this stage would not be justified. Should very precise and more frequent temperature assessment become necessary, then placement of a urinary catheter with temperature probe or an oesophageal probe might become necessary. At present the use of the tympanic thermometer to measure Mary's temperature would be in keeping with accepted views of its accuracy and ease of use (Erickson and Kirklin 1993; Leon et al. 2005).

The tympanic membrane is an established site for non-invasive temperature assessment as it is well vascularised and is considered, therefore, to replicate the core temperature of blood in the intracranial cavity (Shinozaki et al. 1988, Erickson and Kirklin 1993). It is also an easily accessible site that can be used to obtain temperatures in a wide range of patients. In addition, tympanic temperatures record relatively quickly and may be viewed as being efficient in terms of nursing time (Erickson and Kirklin 1993; Giuliano et al. 1999).

A number of studies have demonstrated questionable accuracy and reliability of tympanic thermometry (Hooker and Houston 1996; Manian and Greisenauer 1998; Giuliano et al. 1999; Hooper and Andrews 2006; Moran et al. 2007). Hooker and Houston (1996) and Manian and Greisenauer (1998) both found that tympanic thermometers demonstrated a lack of sensitivity and were unable to detect fever in significant numbers of patients.

In the critically ill, Moran et al. (2007) suggest that it compares poorly to invasive pulmonary artery and bladder temperatures, possibly due to a significant alteration in blood flow to the tympanic membrane during critical illness, negating the ability of the thermometer to measure blood temperature accurately. Tympanic temperatures may be affected by cerebral blood flow and could be an inappropriate method for the head-injured patient or where cerebral ischaemia is suspected (Giuliano et al. 1999). The lack of accuracy of tympanic temperatures is further supported by earlier studies where it compared poorly with other invasive and non-invasive methods (Nierman 1991; Fisk and Arcona 2001), although these authors do not speculate as to the possible cause of its poor performance.

Giuliano et al. (1999), Fisk and Arcona (2001), Hooper and Andrews (2006) and Moran et al. (2007) have challenged whether tympanic thermometry is reliable or easy to use. Giuliano et al. (1999) and Fisk and Arcona (2001) highlighted the lack of adequate education and training in the use of tympanic thermometers, resulting in significant operator error even amongst experienced nurses. Giuliano et al. (1999) found that experienced nurses required more than ten minutes of intensive training to obtain an accurate reading. Fisk and Arcona (2001) recommended abandoning the expanded use of tympanic thermometry because it would be prohibitively expensive to provide hospital-wide training to maintain operator reliability. Evans and Kenkre (2006) further point out that the majority of temperature measurements in the acute setting are undertaken by healthcare assistants, who are often the least experienced and most poorly trained.

Oral temperature assessment (Figure 3.2) is a popular alternative to the tympanic method. Doubts have persisted as to the accuracy of oral temperature measurement in the critically ill as readings are thought to be subject to factors such as warmed and humidified oxygen, bradypnoea and oral intubation (Erikson and Kirklin 1993). Recent studies, however, have shown the acceptable performance of both chemical dot and electronic thermometers in intubated patients (Giuliano et al. 1999; Moran and Mendal, 2002; Potter et al. 2003; Hooper and Andrews 2006). Factors such as humidified oxygen and respiratory rates have also been discounted as statistically significant in oral temperature assessment (Hooper and Andrews 2007). Oral electronic thermometers with an appropriate probe cover have performed better than the chemical dot type in critically ill patients (Gilbert et al. 2002; Hooper and Andrews 2007).

Hooper and Andrews (2007) conclude that much of the available evidence on tympanic temperature taking is difficult to interpret because it is of generally poor methodological quality, concluding that its accuracy is yet to be established. They suggest that available studies investigating oral temperature were of greater methodological quality and support

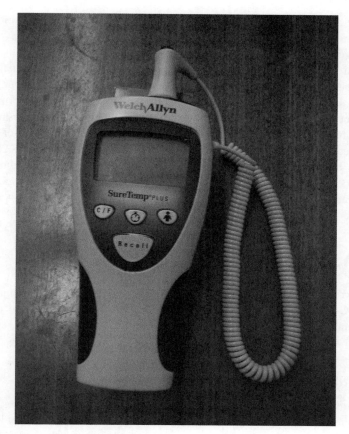

Figure 3.2 Electronic oral thermometer.

the use of this method as a more accurate and reliable method of non-invasive temperature assessment. Oral temperature taking was more quickly and easily taught to staff, thus potentially enhancing the cost-effectiveness of this method. Oral temperature measurement may not be suitable for all and should be avoided in patients with seizure activity or serious head and neck injuries.

Oral temperature measurement has generally performed better that other methods in most comparative studies and may reduce the incidence of operator error (Hooker and Houston 1996; Manian and Greisenauer 1998; Giuliano et al. 1999; Hooper and Andrews 2007). Axillary temperature measurement, via chemical dot or electronic probe, is not currently recommended for use in critically ill patients (Erikson and Kirklin 1993; Schmitz et al. 1995; Zengeya and Blumenthal 1996; O'Grady et al. 1998).

Axillary readings may be significantly affected by circulatory alterations in the critically ill and their validity and reliability has not been established for this patient population (Schmitz et al. 1995; Zengeya and Blumenthal 1996). Temporal artery thermometers have not been fully researched for use in adult critically ill patients and cannot currently be recommended for use in these patients (Kimberger et al. 2007).

Gilbert et al. (2002) found a lack of correlation between tympanic and oral measurements and advised against the mixing of methods and the importance of using the same site and device for all the readings taken on an individual patient.

At present the best site and device for taking non-invasive temperatures in the critically ill remains elusive. Regardless of measurement site, nurses should endeavour to maintain consistency in temperature taking as treatment decisions are based on abnormal readings and incorrect diagnosis of fever may lead to patients undergoing unnecessary tests and investigations. Accuracy can be improved by ensuring adequate training of the staff to eliminate frequent operator errors (Gilbert et al. 2002; Hooper and Andrews 2006; Moran et al. 2007). Temperature taking should also reflect individual patient's circumstances and requirements. Nurses should have a thorough knowledge of the advantages and limitations of the sites and devices for temperature taking to ensure the best method is selected for their patients.

Tests and investigations

New fevers require further investigation to establish whether an underlying infection is present (O'Grady et al. 1998). Nurses should follow local guidelines/protocols to determine temperatures which demand a septic screen but temperatures of $>38°C$ and certainly those $>38.3°C$ warrant consideration (O'Grady et al. 1998; Ryan and Levy 2003).

Blood cultures

Blood cultures are important in establishing a diagnosis of bacteraemia and identification of the specific pathogens present in the newly febrile patient (Department of Health (DH) 2007). The DH has produced guidelines on when and how to perform blood cultures as part of the Saving Lives care bundles (Saving Lives, DH 2007). The guidelines state that blood cultures should be taken from any patient suspected of having bacteraemia and have identified clinical symptoms that should alert clinicians to the need for blood cultures. These include:

- Core temperature out of normal range
- Focal signs of infection
- Abnormal heart rate (raised), blood pressure (low or raised) or respiratory rate (raised)
- Chills or rigors
- Raised or very low white blood cell count
- New or worsening confusion.

Mary should have blood cultures taken and these should be performed as soon as possible after confirmation of a temperature $>38°C$ (or $>38.3°C$) and preferably before commencing antibiotics (if the patient is already receiving antibiotics, cultures should be obtained before delivery of the next dose; DH 2007). Ideally two sets of cultures should be obtained from different sites at different times to maximise the possibility of obtaining positive cultures. If Mary's central venous catheter (CVC) is suspected as the source of infection, then cultures should be obtained from a peripheral site first and then from the CVC. Clinicians taking blood cultures should be properly trained and competent in performing this procedure and ensure that they follow the DH best practice guidelines for taking and adding samples to the culture medium (DH 2007).

Swabs and specimens

In addition to blood cultures, Mary should have a chest X-ray. Swabs from any wounds, her peripheral and CVC cannula sites, a catheter specimen of urine and a sputum specimen should also be obtained. These must be appropriately labelled and sent in a timely manner to the microbiology department for microscopy, culture and sensitivity (MCS). To reduce the risks of hospital-acquired infections, the Saving Lives guidelines recommend a strict daily review of all patients' invasive lines/devices and recommend removal of any that can no longer be clinically justified (DH 2007).

Biochemical markers of infection

The presence of fever can arise from infectious (viral, bacterial) or non-infectious causes (inflammatory conditions) and it is not currently possible to differentiate them in the first few hours following fever. This is problematic, as the prevention of sepsis by commencing early, targeted antibiotic therapy is of primary importance. The results of Mary's swabs, specimens and blood cultures will not be available for up to 72 hours delaying a definitive diagnosis of infection and the culture and sensitivity of the infective organism. If Mary's fever arose from a non-infectious cause, then antibiotics would be inappropriate and could contribute to the development of multi-resistant micro-organisms, so prevalent in critical care environments (O'Grady et al. 1998; Harbarth et al. 2001).

Blood testing for raised or low WCC and CRP should also be requested for Mary. Leukocytes (white cells) are produced in large quantities during the immune response and blood levels are normally elevated in patients with infections. The WCC is not a specific test for bacterial infection as leukocytes could also be increased in inflammatory conditions and viral and parasitic infections. Differentiation of the levels of leukocyte cell type may increase the specificity for bacterial infection; for instance, elevated neutrophil and monocyte levels are more indicative, but still cannot confirm the diagnosis (see Table 3.4 for normal values). In addition some patients with infection do not have elevated WCC and may even have an abnormally low WCC (Marik 2000).

CRP is an acute-phase protein that activates the classical complement pathway. It is normally present in the plasma at a concentration of less than 5 mg/L but increases quickly in response to tissue damage or inflammation and may double its concentration every 6 hours. High CRP levels are more indicative of bacterial than viral infections and Mary's raised CRP levels increase the evidence to confirm the presence of this. Measuring CRP levels is useful but lacks sufficient specificity and sensitivity to be a definitive diagnostic test.

Recent studies have identified Procalcitonin (PCT) PCT as a more accurate biochemical marker of infection. It has been shown to have greater sensitivity and specificity than CRP in differentiating between sepsis and inflammation. PCT is replacing CRP in many units as the preferred diagnostic marker of infection. It is more expensive than CRP but as it is likely to improve diagnosis and prevent inappropriate treatment of non-infectious fever,

Table 3.4 Biochemical markers of infection.

Biochemical marker	Normal range
Leukocyte (white cell count) Total WCC	$4.0–11.0 \times 10^9$/L
Neutrophils	$2.0–7.5 \times 10^9$/L
	40–75% WCC
Lymphocytes	$1.3–3.5 \times 10^9$/L
	20–45% WCC
Eosinophils	$0.04–0.44 \times 10^9$/L
	1–6% WCC
Basophils	$0.0–0.10 \times 10^9$/L
	0–1% WCC
Monocytes	$0.2–0.8 \times 10^9$/L
	2–10% WCC
Reticulocyte count	$25–100 \times 10^9$/L
Platelet count	$150–400 \times 10^9$/L
CRP	<5 mg/L
Individual laboratories vary in their ranges	

it may be more cost-effective in the long-term (Hatherhill et al. 1999; Muller et al. 2000; Vincent 2000; Harbarth et al. 2001).

Developing scenario

One hour later you observe that Mary is hot with a temperature 39.2°C; she is flushed and sweating. Her urine output has decreased and her blood pressure has fallen to 100/68 mmHg. Her respiratory status has also deteriorated.

Reader activities

- What stage of fever do Mary's symptoms indicate?
- Should Mary's temperature be treated? What would be the most appropriate method of achieving normothermia for Mary?
- What are the physiological advantages of fever for Mary?
- What are the detrimental effects of a high temperature for Mary?

Related pathophysiology

Mary is now in the hot, or plateau, stage of fever as her core temperature is now equivalent to the new set-point (Henker et al. 1997). This phase will continue until endogenous pyrogen activity ceases and the hypothalamus resets the temperature set-point. Heat is maintained at this time through the balance of heat gain and heat loss (Bruce and Grove 1992). Mary has hot, flushed skin and is sweating, as heat causes cutaneous vasodilatation, bringing blood to the skin surface, increasing heat loss from radiation and convection and sweating promotes heat loss through evaporation. BMR remains elevated during this phase and so Mary has remained tachypnoeic and tachycardic. Her blood pressure

Table 3.5 Mechanisms activated by heat.

Heat Loss	Clinical Signs and Symptoms
Cutaneous vasodilatation – increased heat loss via radiation, convection	Feels hot, dry skin initially Redness and flushing Warm peripheries Increased HR, RR Fall in BP
Sweating – increased heat loss through evaporation Exposure of more body surface to environment to promote heat loss from radiation, convection	Profuse sweating Increased respiration – water loss Fluid volume deficit, hypovolaemia, dehydration Decreased urine output Cool clothing, reduced bed coverings
Heat is energy and in the hot (febrile) patient heat is produced from elevated energy production – for every 1.0°C rise in body temperature BMR rises by 7–10%.	Increased HR Increased energy expenditure, sustained heat can result in significant reduction of energy stores, catabolism Weight loss
Decreased heat production Reduced thyroid stimulation of metabolic processes	Anorexia
Behavioural responses: Apathy/lassitude Activities to feel cooler	Lying still to minimise muscular activity and decrease heat generation Lying stretched out to increase heat loss surface Fluid intake – cold drinks, cool clothing

has dropped (100/68 mmHg) as generalised vasodilatation decreases vascular resistance. Cardiac output is increased and there is a 13% rise in oxygen consumption for every 1.0°C elevation in temperature. This places enormous demands on Mary's respiratory system to maintain adequate oxygen delivery and would account for her deteriorating respiratory function, as she is unable to meet increasing demand with suboptimal respiratory reserve as a consequence of her pneumonia. See Table 3.5 for a summary of the mechanisms activated by heat.

Patient-focused interventions

Airway/Breathing

Mary is able to maintain her own airway but observation should continue to detect any deterioration in her level of consciousness. Mary's respiratory function is now deteriorating and she is struggling to maintain an adequate oxygen delivery to keep pace with increased demand. Mary also has pneumonia and this will affect her ability to maintain adequate ventilation as areas of alveolar consolidation reduce gas diffusion. Improving Mary's oxygenation is, therefore, a priority of care.

Sitting Mary upright will improve inflation of lung bases augmenting alveolar ventilation and gas exchange. Care is needed, however, as Mary's blood pressure is falling and she may not tolerate a very upright position. Oxygen concentration and flow rate should be increased until a satisfactory SpO$_2$ of $\geq$94% has been restored. Oxygen should be given via a fixed delivery (Venturi) system to ensure delivery of an accurate oxygen percentage and this may need to be humidified to prevent drying of mucous membranes and pulmonary secretions. Physiotherapy referral should be considered if mobilisation of secretions is required or if areas of collapse or consolidation are present. A sputum specimen should be obtained for MCS and antibiotics commenced as per the unit protocol governing community-acquired infections. These are usually broad-spectrum antibiotics initially and these can be changed if positive culture and sensitivity becomes available from Mary's septic screen. As Mary has a significant fever and clinical signs of bacteraemia, antibiotics should be given intravenously.

Circulation

Interventions should be aimed at the restoration of an adequate circulating volume and maintenance of tissue oxygen delivery. Mary's blood pressure is falling due to vasodilatation and insensible fluid losses from sweating. Mary requires volume resuscitation with intravenous fluids to restore MAP $\geq$65 mmHg, CVP above 8 mmHg and urine output between 0.5–1.0 mL/kg/h. A crystalloid or colloid solution could satisfactorily be used. Controversy still exists over which type of fluid is preferable (see Chapter 4 for further discussion of fluid management). Hartmann's solution would expand Mary's extracellular fluid (ECF) compartment and closely resembles the components of the ECF, making it a good fluid choice. In addition, it does not lead to excessive sodium and chloride ion administration and resultant acidosis that can accompany the use of large volumes of normal saline (NaCl) (GIFTASUP 2009).

Monitoring of her fluid intake and output and hourly urine measurements are necessary to provide information to base ongoing fluid and electrolyte replacement. Accurate fluid balance assessment is difficult to achieve and even more so in patients where high volumes of insensible losses occur due to sweating. Crude estimates can seriously underestimate or overestimate fluid losses but there is no current evidence-based guidance on how to estimate insensible fluid loss (GIFTASUP 2009). A more accurate picture of Mary's fluid balance will be obtained if a combination of fluid intake, urine output, observation of skin, mucous membranes, extent of sweating, capillary refill, urine and serum biochemistry are performed (GIFTASUP 2009).

Mary may also require electrolyte replacement depending on levels obtained from blood samples. Water and sodium loss from sweating results in the triggering of the renin–angiotensin–aldosterone (RAAS) cascade. Aldosterone will cause reabsorption of sodium in exchange for potassium in the kidney, leading to hypokalaemia. If intracellular dehydration is suspected, additional 5% Dextrose or dextrose saline infusion would be appropriate to restore the intracellular fluid (ICF) volume.

Mary requires two- to four-hourly temperature assessment to monitor her febrile state, but as previously stated, interventions should be directed at discovering and treating the underlying cause of Mary's fever. The merits of treatments aimed at reducing Mary's temperature *per se* remain highly controversial (Henker et al. 1997; Henker and Carlson 2007) as some authors have suggested that aggressive fever management may worsen outcome in critically ill febrile patients (Greisman and Mackowiak 2002; Schulman et al.

2005; Ferguson 2007). There is, however, evidence that sustained fevers are detrimental to the patient (Ryan and Levy 2003; Ferguson 2007).

Fever is generally viewed as an evolutionary host defence mechanism important in enhancing an individual's resistance to infection. Left untreated, fever may lead to improved outcomes for patients suffering from infectious diseases (Marik 2000; Greisman and Mackowiak 2002). Humans also have self-regulatory responses that limit the height of fever and prevent an excess febrile response, possibly negating the need to treat most fevers (Henker and Carlson 2007). Clinicians have tended to view fever as a noxious process and have been generally more inclined to treat fever aggressively in the critically ill (Greisman and Mackowiak 2002; Schulman et al. 2005; Ferguson 2007).

Physiologically, fever has both beneficial and detrimental effects and treatment decisions regarding Mary's fever should be based on her clinical condition. The beneficial effects of fever include an enhanced host-defence response: improved macrophage function; increased lymphocyte and neutrophil proliferation; activation of acute phase proteins; sequestration of iron, zinc and copper (the substrates necessary to aid bacterial replication); and increased T-cell production, all of which aid in the control and elimination of invading micro-organisms. Increased heart rate, cardiac output and respiratory rate increase oxygen and nutrient delivery and circulate macrophages and antibodies (Johnson Rowsey 1997a; Marik 2000; Henker and Carlson 2007).

Fever also has detrimental effects. For instance, increased cardiac output and oxygen consumption may be poorly tolerated in critically ill patients, such as Mary, who has compromised respiratory function. Increased carbon dioxide production from cellular hypoxia and metabolic acidosis can arise and substantially elevated BMR results in vast increases in energy consumption. This has implications in achieving an adequate nutritional intake for Mary, which could result in catabolism (Johnson Rowsey 1997a; Marik 2000; Henker and Carlson 2007). Ongoing vasodilatation and sweating may worsen Mary's hypotension and hypovolaemia, decrease her urine output further and could lead to acute kidney injury (AKI).

Temperatures below 39.0°C may not always require intervention (Henker and Carlson 2007) but as Mary's temperature is now 39.2°C and she has cardiovascular and respiratory compromise, the administration of antipyretic medication to reduce her temperature should now be considered. (Henker and Carlson 2007). Drugs would be the most appropriate method to reduce Mary's temperature as she has a controlled rise in temperature with a normally functioning hypothalamus. Antipyretics inhibit prostaglandin synthesis, decreasing stimuli to the hypothalamus, resulting in reduction of the temperature set-point to normal (Plaisance and Mackowiak 2000; Ferguson 2007).

Paracetamol, aspirin and non-steroidal anti-inflammatory drugs (NSAIDs) are all antipyretic agents. Aspirin and NSAIDs inhibit prostaglandin synthesis directly and Paracetamol is believed to inhibit the formation of arachidonic acid, the substrate necessary for prostaglandin synthesis (Plaisance and Mackowiak 2000). Warwick (2008) suggests that Paracetamol is actually a very poor antipyretic agent with marginal effect when compared to placebo. It is, however, still the most favoured antipyretic agent in clinical practice as unlike aspirin and NSAIDs, it does not cause gastric irritation and can be used in patients on beta blocker drugs and in those with asthma. It can be administered orally, rectally or intravenously. Oral administration of 1 g of Paracetamol 4 hourly could be prescribed for Mary at this time, with ongoing assessment of her response.

External cooling by tepid sponging, fanning, cooling blankets or ice packs remains somewhat controversial in patients with fever (Keikkas et al. 2008). Aggressive physical cooling could generate intense shivering with subsequent increased heat generation and huge metabolic energy expenditure (Henker 1999; Holtzclaw 2004; Ferguson 2007; Keikkas et al. 2008). Cooling the skin can promote peripheral vasoconstriction and prevention of heat loss leading to rebound heat conservation and an increase in temperature. In addition, cooling Mary aggressively could result in a rapid defervescence (temperature drop) where heat loss mechanisms are accelerated and profound hypotension ensues (Bruce and Grove 1992; Johnson Rowsey 1997a).

Some studies have found a combination of antipyretic drugs and a degree of external cooling to be more effective in treating fever (Poblete et al. 1997). External cooling may be necessary in patients who are refractory to antipyretics and in those critically ill patients where more rapid cooling is necessary to prevent further cardiopulmonary compromise or where temperatures have exceeded 40°C (Schulman et al. 2005; Keikkas et al. 2008). Cooling should, however, be avoided during the chill stage of a fever and thermal wraps should be applied to the extremities during cooling activities to prevent shivering (Holtzclaw 2004; Ferguson 2007; Keikkas et al. 2008).

External physical cooling should be used in all patients with hyperthermia as antipyretics are ineffective in reducing temperature (Johnson Rowsey 1997b; Henker et al. 1997; Keikkas et al. 2008) and where recommended in patients with head injuries (see Chapter 12). The best method of performing external cooling has not yet been well established (Keikkas et al. 2008).

Nurses and clinicians could manage many uncomplicated fevers more conservatively as fever may have significant benefits in improving immune response and allowing the body to limit infectious disease naturally. Treatment should be reserved for patients who are unable to cope physically with the increased cardiovascular, respiratory and metabolic demands that arise in fever.

Disability of the central nervous system

Mary's level of consciousness should be assessed as she is mostly at risk of cerebral hypoxia due to cardiovascular and respiratory compromise, as fever rarely causes other neurological events such as seizures in adults (these can occur frequently in patients with hyperthermia) (Johnson Rowsey 1997b; Henker and Carlson 2007), but any neurological event must be managed as a matter of urgency. In Mary's situation, improving her oxygen delivery will improve her neurological function.

Patients may develop muscle and joint pain or headache with fever and this often necessitates pain relief. Mary should have a pain assessment performed and analgesia prescribed and administered as required. This, of course, often gives rise to an inadvertent antipyresis, as the drugs most commonly used for mild to moderate pain relief are also antipyretics (Paracetamol and NSAIDs).

Exposure

Mary's BMR is significantly elevated due to the effects of her fever and she is at risk of malnutrition. Mary may require referral to the dietician if she is not eating sufficient calories to meet her needs. Failure to meet nutritional energy requirements would ultimately result in catabolism and subsequent protein malnutrition with all the attendant problems of impaired immunity, wound healing and muscle weakness (leading to poor respiratory function) and decreased mobility.

Mary should have a nutritional assessment performed the Malnutrition Universal Screening Tool, (MUST) could be used (BAPEN 2003). Nutritional interventions for Mary would depend on her MUST score and her ability to take an adequate oral diet. Mary may have anorexia if she remains in the hot stage of fever and her nutritional requirements will remain high. If Mary is eating, she should be offered small meals regularly and may benefit from additional high-calorie supplements with a target calorie intake of 2000–2500, including 1.0–1.5 g protein daily (NICE 2006). A record of her nutritional intake should be recorded for three days and a review of her MUST score undertaken (BAPEN 2003). Should Mary stop eating or her oral intake is insufficient and her MUST score is ≥ 2, a dietician should review her nutritional requirements.

As discussed early in this chapter, it is important to reduce Mary's risk of further infection. Scrupulous attention to hand washing and aseptic management of her CVC are mandatory (Saving Lives, DH 2007), removal of unnecessary invasive lines and observation of wounds, catheters and line sites for clinical signs of infection (heat, redness, pain, swelling) and daily urinalysis will help to protect Mary from further hospital-acquired infection and assist in the early detection of infection (Saving Lives, DH 2007).

Mary is hot and sweating and will require assistance with hygiene to maintain her comfort and protect vulnerable pressure sites; urinary catheter care should also be done according to the local protocol. A pressure area assessment should be undertaken along with a physical examination of her skin for signs of damage or loss of skin integrity. Wounds and invasive line sites should be appropriately covered with sterile dressings.

Mary's risk of thromboembolism should be monitored and if she becomes relatively immobile, thromboprophylaxis measures should be considered, for example, measuring and applying thrombo-embolic stockings.

It is beyond the scope of this chapter to discuss detailed psychosocial interventions as these would be based on a more detailed assessment. It is, of course, important to consider Mary's emotional and psychological support at this time as she may be anxious and afraid as her condition has worsened.

Conclusion

Fever is a common symptom in the hospitalised patient and even more prevalent in the critically ill. Accurate assessment of temperature is vital as treatment decisions are based on findings. Non-invasive methods of temperature taking, however, often lack sufficient sensitivity or are prone to operator error undermining efforts to achieve accurate measurements. The treatment of fever remains controversial, not only in relation to its potential benefits versus detrimental effects but also in the best method of achieving antipyresis (drugs or external cooling). This chapter has focused on the care necessary for the patient with a fever and has highlighted the importance of discovering and treating the underlying cause of Mary's fever rather than aggressive management of the fever itself.

Key learning points from scenario

- Fever is common in critical illness arising from infection or inflammatory conditions. It is important to distinguish fever from hyperthermia as they are managed differently.
- Assessment of temperature is important but difficult to achieve reliably by non-invasive methods.
- Interventions should be aimed at eliminating the underlying cause of the fever.
- Fever has beneficial and detrimental effects and over-zealous treatment of fever should be avoided.

Critical appraisal of a research paper

Giuliano et al. (1999) Temperature measurement in critically ill orally intubated adults: a comparison of pulmonary artery core, tympanic and oral methods. *Critical Care Medicine* **27**(10), 2188–2193.

   This American-based study was performed by nurses in a 24-bed medical/surgical trauma intensive care unit. Its aim was to compare non-invasive oral and tympanic temperature measurements with those from a pulmonary artery (PA) catheter, largely accepted as the clinical 'gold standard' for temperature assessment. Instrument calibration for accuracy was performed and training of the operators undertaken to ensure reliability. Appropriate statistical analysis using the Bland and Altman repeated measurement technique was undertaken. Findings showed increased difficulty in training experienced nurses in the use of the tympanic thermometer compared to the electronic oral device. Results indicated a higher degree of agreement and less variability between oral temperatures and PA than between tympanic and PA. The authors conclude that oral temperatures are easier to perform and more accurate than tympanic in critically ill patients.

Reader activities

1. Read the research article written by Giuliano et al. (1999).
2. Using the critical appraisal framework in Appendix I, consider the methodological quality of the paper.
3. Reflect on this aspect of your own practice and the implications for future practice management that this paper raises.

   A commentary on this paper has been provided by the chapter author in Appendix IV.

References

BAPEN – Malnutrition Advisory Group (2003) *The Malnutrition Universal Screening Tool.* BAPEN. Available online at: www.bapen.org.uk. Accessed 19 January 2010.

Beard RM, Day MW (2008) Fever and hyperthermia: learn to beat the heat. *Nursing* **38**(6), 28–31.

Bruce JL, Grove SK (1992) Fever: pathology and treatment. *Critical Care Nurse* **12**(1), 40–49.

Department of Health (DH) (2007) *Saving Lives: Reducing Infection, Delivering Clean and Safe Care.* Available online at: www.clean-safe-care.nhs.uk. Accessed 28 January 2010.

Erickson RS, Kirklin SK (1993) Comparison of ear-based, bladder, oral and axillary methods for core temperature measurement. *Critical Care Medicine* **21**(10), 1528–1534.

Erickson RS (1999) The continuing question of how best to measure body temperature. *Critical Care Medicine* **27**, 2307–2310.

Evans J, Kenkre J (2006) Current practice and knowledge of nurses regarding patient temperature measurement. *Journal of Medical Engineering & Technology* **30**(4), 218–223.

Ferguson A (2007) Evaluation and treatment of fever in intensive care unit patients. *Critical Care Nursing Quarterly* **30**(4), 347–363.

Fisk J, Arcona S (2001) Comparing tympanic membrane and pulmonary artery temperatures. *Nursing Management* **32**(6), **42**, 45–48.

GIFTASUP: Powell-Tuck J, Gosling P, Lobo DN, Allison SP, Carlson GL, Gore M, Lewington AJ, Pearse RM, Mythen MG (2009) *British Consensus Guidelines on Intravenous Fluid Therapy for Adult Surgical Patients.* GIFTASUP. Available online at: www.bapen.org.uk. Accessed 25 January 2010.

Gilbert M, Barton AJ, Counsell CM (2002) Comparison of oral and tympanic temperatures in adult surgical patients. *Applied Nursing Research* **15**(1), 42.

Giuliano KK, Scott SS, Elliot S, Guiliano A (1999) Temperature measurement in critically ill orally intubated adults: a comparison of pulmonary artery core, tympanic and oral methods. *Critical Care Medicine* **27**(10), 2188–2193.

Greisman LA, Mackowiak PA (2002) Fever: beneficial and detrimental effects of antipyretics. *Current Opinion in Infectious Diseases* **15**, 241–245.

Harbarth S, Holeckova K, Froidevaux C, Pittet D, Ricou B, Grau GE, Vadas L, Pugin J and the Geneva Sepsis Network (2001) Diagnostic value of procalcitonin, interleukin-6 and interleukin-8 in critically ill patients admitted with suspected sepsis. *American Journal Respiratory Care Medicine* **164**, 396–402.

Hatherhill M, Tibby SM, Sykes K, Turner C, Murdoch IA (1999) Diagnostic markers of infection: comparison of procalcitonin with C reactive protein and leucocyte count. *Archives of Diseases in Childhood* **81**, 417–421.

Henker R (1999) Evidence-based practice: fever-related interventions. *American Journal of Critical Care* **8**(1), 481–487.

Henker R, Carlson K (2007) Fever: applying research to bedside practice. *AACN Advanced Critical Care* **18**(1), 76–87.

Henker R, Kramer D, Rogers S (1997) Fever. *AACN Clinical Issues* **8**(3), 351–367.

Hooper VD, Andrews JO (2006) Accuracy of noninvasive core temperature measurement in acutely ill adults: the state of the science. *Biological Research for Nursing* **8**(1), 24–34.

Holtzclaw B (1998) New trends in thermometry for the patient in the ICU. *Critical Care Nursing Quarterly* **21**(3), 12–25.

Holtzclaw B (2004) Shivering in acutely ill vulnerable populations. *AACN Clinical Issues* **15**(2), 267–279.

Hooker EA, Houston H (1996) Screening for fever in an adult emergency department: oral vs. tympanic thermometry. *Southern Medical Journal* **89**, 230–234.

Johnson Rowsey P (1997a) Pathophysiology of fever. Part 1: the role of cytokines. *Dimensions of Critical Care Nursing* **16**(4), 202–207.

Johnson Rowsey P (1997b) Pathophysiology of fever. Part 2: relooking at cooling interventions. *Dimensions of Critical Care Nursing* **16**(5), 251–256.

Kiekkas P, Brokalaki H, Theodorakopoulou G, Baltopoulos GI (2008) Physical antipyresis in critically ill adults. *American Journal of Nursing* **108**(7), 40–49.

Kimberger O, Cohen D, Illievich U, Lenhardt R (2007) Temporal artery versus bladder thermometry during perioperative and intensive care unit monitoring. *International Anaesthesia Research Society* **105**(4), 1042–1047.

Lefrant JY, Muller L, Emmanuuel Coussaye J, Benbabaali M, Lebris C, Zeitoun N, Mari C, Saissi G, Ripart J, Eledjam J-J (2003) Temperature measurement in intensive care patients: comparison of urinary bladder, oesophageal, rectal, axillary and inguinal methods versus pulmonary artery core method. *Intensive Care Medicine* **29**, 414–418.

Leon C, Rodriguez A, Fernandez A, Flores L (2005) Infrared ear thermometry in the critically ill patient. *Journal of Critical Care* **20**(1), 106–110.

Manian FA, Greisenauer S (1998) Lack of agreement between tympanic and oral temperature measurements in adult hospitalised patients. *American Journal of Infection Control* **26**(4), 428–430.

Marik PE (2000) Fever in the ICU. *Chest* **117**, 855–869.

Moran DS, Mendal L (2002) Core temperature measurement: methods and current insights. *Sports Medicine* **32**(14), 879–885.

Moran JL, Peter JV, Solomon PJ, Grealy B, Smith T, Ashforth W, Wake M, Peake SL, Peisach AR (2007) Tympanic temperature measurements: are they reliable in the critically ill? A study of measures of agreement. *Critical Care Medicine* **35**(1), 155–164.

Muller B, Becker KL, Schachinger H, Reckenbacher PR, Huber PR, Zimmerli W, Ritz R (2000) Calcitonin precursors are reliable markers of sepsis in a medical intensive care unit. *Critical Care Medicine* **28**, 977–983.

NICE and the National Collaborating Centre for Acute Care (2006) *Nutrition Support in Adults: Oral Nutrition Support, Enteral Tube Feeding and Parenteral Nutrition. Clinical Guideline 32.* London. Available online at: http://www.nice.org.uk/Guidance/CG32. Accessed 25 January 2010.

Nierman DM (1991) Core temperature measurement in the intensive care unit. *Critical Care Medicine* **19**, 818–823.

O'Grady NP, Philip SB, Bartlett JG (1998) Practice guidelines for evaluating new fever in critically ill adult patients. *Clinical Infectious Disease* **26**, 1042–1059.

Plaisance KI, Mackowiak PA (2000) Antipyretic therapy: physiologic rationale, diagnostic implication and clinical consequences. *Archives of Internal Medicine* **160**, 49–456.

Poblete B, Romand J-A, Pichard C, Konig P, Suter PM (1997) Metabolic effects of i.v. propacetamol, metamizol or external cooling in critically ill febrile sedated patients. *British Journal of Anaesthesia* **78**, 123–127.

Potter P, Schallom M, Davis S, Sona C, McSweeney M (2003) Evaluation of chemical dot thermometers for measuring body temperature of orally intubated patients. *American Journal of Critical Care* **12**(5), 403–407.

Ryan M, Levy M (2003) Clinical review: fever in intensive care unit patients. *Critical Care* **7**(3), 221–225.

Schmitz T, Bair N, Falk M (1995) A comparison of five methods of temperature measurement in febrile intensive care unit patients. *American Journal of Critical Care* **4**, 286–292.

Schulman CI, Namias N, Doherty J, Manning RJ, Li P, Alhaddad A, Lasko D, Amortegui J, Dy CJ, Dlugasch L, Baracco G, Cohn SM (2005) The effect of antipyretic therapy upon outcomes in critically ill patients: a randomized, prospective study. *Surgical Infections* **6**(4), 369–375.

Shinozaki T, Deane R, Perkins FM (1988) Infrared tympanic thermometer: evaluation of a new clinical thermometer. *Critical Care Medicine* **16**, 148–150.

Vincent JL (2000) Procalcitonin. The marker of sepsis? *Critical Care Medicine* **28**, 1226–1228.

Warwick C (2008) Paracetamol and fever management. *The Journal of the Royal Society for the Promotion of Health* **128**(6), 320.

Zengeya ST, Blumenthal I (1996) Modern electronic and chemical thermometers used in the axilla are inaccurate. *European Journal of Paediatrics* **155**(12), 1005–1008.

Chapter 4

The patient with severe sepsis

Suzanne Bench

Introduction

In Europe approximately 150 000 people die annually from severe sepsis and in the USA this rises to 200 000 (Angus et al. 2001). The Sepsis in European Intensive Care Units (SOAP) study reported mortality rates as >50% for patients in intensive care with septic shock (Vincent et al. 2006). This scenario will focus on the assessment and management of a patient who develops severe sepsis.

Patient scenario

Penelope Taylor, a 68-year-old lady, is admitted to the intensive care unit (ICU) following emergency laparotomy for a perforated caecum. She has been unwell for two weeks at home with nausea and vomiting. Peri-operatively she lost one litre of blood and had a temporary colostomy performed following a peritoneal washout. Four days post-operatively, Mrs Taylor remains sedated and intubated. Assessment data can be seen in Table 4.1.

Reader activities

Having read this scenario, consider the following:

- How do Penelope's symptoms support a diagnosis of sepsis?
- What stage of the sepsis continuum is Penelope experiencing? Explain this using relevant pathophysiology.
- Consider the possible causes of Penelope's sepsis. Outline the factors that make her high risk for the development of sepsis.
- Analyse the blood gas presented. Consider why Penelope might have altered gas exchange.
- Explain the possible reasons why Penelope has a raised lactate and hyperglycaemia. Why are these abnormalities of concern?
- What is $ScvO_2$? What is the normal value and why might it be altered in sepsis?

Critical Care Nursing: Learning from Practice, 1st edition. Edited by Suzanne Bench and Kate Brown.
© 2011 Blackwell Publishing Ltd.

Table 4.1   Clinical and laboratory data.

Cardiovascular	Heart rate (HR) 126 bpm (sinus rhythm) Mean arterial blood pressure (MABP) 55 mmHg Central venous pressure (CVP) 9 mmHg Tympanic temperature 38.5°C Peripherally feels hot to touch
Respiratory	Ventilated on synchronised intermittent mandatory ventilation–volume control (SIMV-VC) Set on 60% oxygen (FiO$_2$ 0.6) PEEP 5 cmH$_2$O Tidal volumes set at 450 mL (weighs 62 kg) Respiratory rate set at 18 bpm (no spontaneous effort) Bilateral air entry with coarse crackles throughout
Arterial blood gases	pH 7.31 PaCO$_2$ 6.2 kPa PaO$_2$ 10.3 kPa HCO$_3$$^-$ 18 mmol/L (standard) Base excess −4 SaO$_2$ 96% ScvO$_2$ 85%
Input/output	Hartmann's 1 L in progress over 4 hours 2 L of colloid administered over last 24 hours Nasogastric tube on free drainage Urine output 20–32 mL over previous 4 hours Rising urea and creatinine
Laboratory results	Sodium 142 mmol/L Potassium 4.1 mmol/L Lactate 3.8 mmol/L Glucose 11.4 mmol/L Haemoglobin (Hb) 8.2 g/L White cell count (WCC) 18 000 mm^2 C-reactive protein (CRP) 250 mg/dL suspected gram-negative rods in blood cultures

Definitions of sepsis

Sepsis has been defined as a 'systemic inflammatory response (SIRS) with a presumed or confirmed infectious process' (Bone et al. 1992). It is one step in a continuum originally described by the American College of Chest Physicians (ACCP) and the Society of Critical Care Medicine (SCCM) Consensus Conference in 1991 (see Table 4.2).

In 2001, an International Sepsis Definitions Conference added additional clinical signs and symptoms to reflect better the clinical response to infection (Levy et al. 2003). These include hyperglycaemia; altered mentation; the presence of considerable oedema; raised inflammatory markers, for example, white cell count (WCC) and C-reactive protein (CRP); altered haemodynamic parameters, for example, altered ScvO$_2$, oliguria and coagulation abnormalities; and finally altered tissue perfusion parameters such as a raised lactate and reduced capillary refill time.

Table 4.2 The sepsis continuum.

SIRS	Sepsis	Severe sepsis	Septic shock	Multiple organ dysfunction syndrome (MODS)
Patient displays at least 2 of the following: • Temp >38°C or <36°C • Respiratory rate >20/min or PaCO$_2$ <4.27 kPa • Heart rate >90/min • WCC >12 000/mm^3 or <4000/mm^3	SIRS with a presumed or confirmed infection	Sepsis with at least one acute organ dysfunction	Severe sepsis with hypotension refractory to adequate fluid resuscitation	At least two organ failures as a result of severe, persistent and generalised inflammation

Source: Adapted from Bone et al. (1992).

Based on these definitions, Penelope is presenting with severe sepsis, and possibly septic shock. She meets the criteria for SIRS. In addition, she has inadequate tissue perfusion evidenced by a metabolic acidaemia, raised lactate and an elevated SvO$_2$. She is also hypotensive with a mean arterial blood pressure (MABP) <65 mmHg, and her respiratory and renal function appear to be deteriorating (raised urea and creatinine). However, these abnormalities could be due to inadequate fluid resuscitation. This would need to be determined, ideally with the use of advanced haemodynamic monitoring, for example, pulmonary artery catheter, pulse-induced contour cardiac output (PiCCO) or oesophageal Doppler prior to assuming she is in septic shock.

The pathophysiology of sepsis

Sepsis can be caused by a multitude of invading organisms, and the clinical manifestation and outcome vary depending on the individual's immune response. This in turn will be modulated by factors such as their pre-morbid status, the severity of the infection and the ability to mount an appropriate host response. Although traditionally gram-negative bacteria such as *Escherichia coli* predominated as a cause of sepsis, gram-positive organisms such as the *Staphylococcus aureus* organism have now been shown to make up almost half of all cases of severe sepsis (Bochud and Calandra 2003; Vincent et al. 2006). The rates of fungal infections are also increasing in many countries (Bochud and Calandra 2003; Vincent et al. 2006). Additionally, the growing rates of multi-resistant organisms such as multi-resistant *Staphylococcus auerus* (MRSA) and vancomycin-resistant enterococci (VRE) further contribute to the high mortality seen in sepsis.

Nosocomial infections are a significant cause of sepsis in the critically ill population, with common primary sites being the lungs, abdomen and urinary tract (Vincent et al. 2006). Intubated patients, such as Penelope, have been shown to be at particularly high risk for the development of nosocomial pneumonia or ventilator-associated pneumonia (VAP) as it is commonly known (Pruitt and Jacobs 2006), with mortality rates of 46%

compared to 32% in those without VAP (Pruitt and Jacobs 2006). Critically ill patients are also at high risk of bacterial translocation within the gut, especially if they are unable to tolerate enteral nutrition. During gut hypoperfusion, intestinal bacteria multiply, and with protein malnutrition the integrity of the villi is disrupted and mucosal permeability increases. This subsequently allows passive movement of bacteria across the intestinal epithelium into the systemic circulation during periods of gut reperfusion (Pastores et al. 1996; Holland et al. 2005). Penelope is currently receiving no enteral nutrition. A further possible cause for sepsis in Penelope's case could be the presence of a central venous catheter, as catheter-related bloodstream infections are common in critically ill patients (Pronovost et al. 2006).

Regardless of the causative organism, the resulting process and mortality rates are similar. The pathophysiology associated with sepsis involves activation of inflammatory responses, endothelial dysfunction, disturbances of coagulation and fibrinolysis, and other factors such as the role of nitric oxide, neuro-endocrine activation and mitochondrial dysfunction.

Inflammation

A series of complex mechanisms are activated by the presence of the invading organism. These involve both the innate (non-specific) and specific immune mechanisms (see Thibodeau and Paton (2007) for an account of normal immune responses). Both pro-inflammatory and anti-inflammatory mediators are released, and the normal ability to activate and downregulate the inflammatory response to infection is impaired. The anti-inflammatory response renders the patient immuno-suppressed and thus prone to developing further infection (Hotchkiss and Karl 2003). The pro-inflammatory response leads to an increased metabolic rate and cardiac output, despite a reduction in contractility, increased capillary permeability resulting in loss of fluid from the intravascular space and an associated hypotension due to the effects of systemic vasodilation triggered via release of prostaglandins, bradykinin and nitric oxide. This leads to a reduced systemic vascular resistance (SVR). Initial clinical manifestations are therefore dependent on whether the patient presents with a predominant pro- or anti-inflammatory picture (Hotchkiss and Karl 2003).

These changes can be seen in Penelope's clinical presentation by the poor gas exchange and associated pulmonary oedema, the systemic hypotension, the warm peripheries and the increased heart rate. Pulses may also be bounding, indicating an increased cardiac output. In some patients, however, intravascular hypovolaemia due to fluid movement into the interstitial spaces and myocardial ischaemia leads to poor contractility and thus a drop in cardiac output. This will reduce oxygen delivery (DO_2) and lead to a lower-than-normal SvO_2, and an associated metabolic acidaemia.

Disturbance of coagulation and fibrinolysis

Endothelial damage caused by pro-inflammatory mediators such as IL-1, IL-6, IL-8 and tumour necrosis factor (TNF-α) causes the release of tissue factor which stimulates coagulation via both the intrinsic and extrinsic pathways. Thrombin and resultant fibrin clots within the vasculature are then formed. This contributes to poor blood flow, particularly within the micro-circulation and the typical perfusion deficits seen at the extremities. Anti-coagulation and fibrinolysis are also impaired exacerbating the problem. A key player in this pro-coagulant state is thrombin which is responsible for the ultimate conversion of fibrinogen to fibrin, and for the activation of further coagulation, and also for the suppression of anti-coagulant and fibrinolytic activities. Additionally, it has been shown that significant numbers of septic patients have decreased function or availability of protein C (Schulman and Hare 2003). Protein C has an important role in the body's response to inflammation and mediates many of the harmful responses seen in sepsis (Bernard et al. 2001). Protein C restricts the role of tissue factor on the clotting cascade and blocks thrombin formation by inhibition of factors Va and VIIIa. This prevents platelet and neutrophil activation and blocks the release of pro-inflammatory cytokines TNF-α, IL-1 and IL-6. In addition, it is pro-fibrinolytic through its role in the inactivation of plasminogen activation inhibitor type 1 (PAI-1) (Matthay 2001; Hotchkiss and Karl 2003).

The metabolic acidaemia seen in Penelope's case would in part be caused by inadequate tissue perfusion due to both the hypotension and reduced micro-circulatory blood flow because of the disruption of normal coagulation and fibrinolysis. Anaerobic metabolism would then ensue, causing the release of lactate, which contributes to hydrogen ion production, low bicarbonate and a drop in the blood pH. Organ perfusion deficits will be evident due to maldistribution of blood flow.

Other factors

In sepsis, inducible nitric oxide (NO) synthase production becomes abnormally elevated. This overproduction of NO causes mitochondrial inhibition, severe vasodilatation and decreased vasopressor responsiveness, which can lead to refractory hypotension. An acute-phase endocrine stress response is also triggered during sepsis involving the release of catecholamines, adrenocorticotrophin (ACTH), glucocorticoids and growth hormone (Trager et al. 2003; Gearhart and Parbhoo 2006). These factors promote hepatic glycogenolysis and gluconeogenesis (Brierre et al. 2004), causing elevated plasma glucose levels as seen in Penelope. Hyperglycaemia is also evident due to insulin resistance and thus the inability of some cells to utilise available glucose (Brierre et al. 2004; Gearhart and Parbhoo 2006), whilst other non-insulin-dependent cells become glucose toxic. This contributes to the mitochondrial damage and may explain why cells are unable to utilise oxygen made available to them (Singer 2005), resulting in a higher-than-expected SvO_2. Insulin resistance has also been linked with the development of critical illness neuropathy. Finally, some patients show evidence of adrenal insufficiency and thus reduced serum cortisol levels (Brierre et al. 2004).

Tests and investigations

Mixed venous and central venous oxygen saturations (SvO_2 and $ScvO_2$)

SvO_2 measurements are used to monitor the balance between oxygen delivery (DO_2) and oxygen consumption (VO_2). Normal values are approximately 75% as normal oxygen consumption is about 25% (Marx and Reinhart 2006). Blood from the pulmonary artery is required to obtain this measurement. However, with a reduction in the number of pulmonary artery catheters that are now used, this has become problematic. A central venous saturation ($ScvO_2$) obtained from the distal lumen of a central venous catheter has been suggested as an alternative. Although values are not transferable in patients with septic shock (Marx and Reinhart 2006), studies have demonstrated that $ScvO_2$ levels are a reliable alternative for monitoring trends with values of >70% associated with a reduction in mortality (Rivers et al. 2001). An $ScvO_2$ of <70% indicates an inadequate DO_2, allowing bedside clinicians to attempt to improve this by volume resuscitation, improvement in contractility and oxygen carriage. In sepsis, however, patients often present with higher-than-normal values as the cells become unable to utilise the oxygen made available to them due to the inflammatory process and associated mitochondrial dysfunction. The amount of oxygen which is returned to the right heart is therefore higher than that would be normally expected. This can be clearly seen in the results presented for Penelope.

Lactate

Lactate is produced as a by-product of anaerobic metabolism and is normally converted in the liver to bicarbonate. Thus, although elevated levels of lactate can indicate tissue hypoperfusion from any cause, or hepatic dysfunction, or a combination of factors, a raised lactate (normal lactate levels are considered to be <2 mmol/L) has been shown to be a useful early marker of critical illness. It is now recommended in the sepsis resuscitation guidelines that all patients presenting with suspected sepsis should have their lactate measured and acted upon within the first six hours of recognition and, regularly, thereafter to monitor their ongoing condition (Dellinger et al. 2008). Elevated levels of lactate will cause the patient to present with a metabolic acidosis due to lactic acid. Thus, as seen in Penelope's results, the pH will be low, and bicarbonate and base excess levels will be reduced as bicarbonate becomes utilised to buffer the acid produced.

Anion gap (AG)

Penelope will also have an increasing anion gap. Normal values for the AG are 8–16 mEq/L (Thelan et al. 1998). The AG represents the concentration of all the unmeasured anions in the plasma. The negatively charged proteins account for about 10% of plasma anions and make up the majority of the unmeasured anion represented by the anion gap under normal circumstances. The acid anions (e.g. lactate, acetoacetate and sulphate) produced during a metabolic acidosis are not measured as part of the usual laboratory biochemical profile. The H^+ produced reacts with bicarbonate anions (buffering) and the CO_2 produced is excreted via the lungs (respiratory compensation). The net effect is a decrease in the concentration of measured anions (i.e. HCO_3^-) and an increase in the concentration of unmeasured anions (the acid anions), so the AG increases.

AG can be calculated from the following formula:

Anion gap $= (Na - K) - (Cl - HCO_3^-)$

Short synacthen test

Adrenal sufficiency can be affected in septic patients, and is sometimes assessed by administering a small dose (usually 250 μg of adrenocorticotropic hormone (ACTH)) and monitoring to see if a normal serum cortisol concentration response is achieved (Brierre et al. 2004). However, following the CORTICUS study (Sprung et al. 2007), the use of this test prior to commencing steroid therapy is no longer recommended (Dellinger et al. 2008). Indeed, the use of any steroids in sepsis is now limited to those patients who do not respond to vasopressors (Dellinger et al. 2008).

See Chapter 3 for further discussion of investigations relevant to fever.

Developing scenario

Despite fluid resuscitation, guided by haemodynamic monitoring, Penelope's condition continues to deteriorate. She is now hypotensive with a MABP of 40 mmHg, is oliguric and has a worsening metabolic and respiratory acidaemia. Her cardiac output is 6.8 l/min (normal 4–6 l/min), and she has an SVR of 500 dynes/sec/cm^{-5} (normal 800–1200). She also has marked systemic oedema and evidence of clotting dysfunction (prolonged activated partial thromboplastin time (aPPT) and low platelets). Penelope is now in established septic shock and has evidence of MODS (see Table 4.2).

Managing septic shock

In 2003 international experts involved with the Surviving Sepsis Campaign developed evidenced-based guidelines for managing patients with sepsis, which were updated in 2007 (Dellinger et al. 2008). These were further developed into two care bundles (Table 4.3), one aimed at sepsis resuscitation during the first 6 hours, and one for ongoing

Table 4.3 Sepsis care bundles.

Sepsis resuscitation bundle (within 6 hours)	Sepsis management bundle (within 24 hours)
• Measure serum lactate • Blood cultures prior to antibiotic administration • Broad spectrum antibiotics within 3 hours • Treat hypotension and/or serum lactate >4 mmol with fluid • Apply vasopressors for ongoing hypotension • For septic shock, maintain CVP >8 mmHg and SvO$_2$ >70%	• Consider low-dose steroids • Consider activated protein C • Strict glycaemic control • Inspired plateau pressures <30 cmH$_2$O

Source: Surviving Sepsis Campaign (2009). Reproduced with permission. Copyright © 2009. European Society of Intensive Care Medicine, International Sepsis Forum and Society of Critical Care Medicines.

management of the patient with sepsis (Dellinger et al. 2008). These along with the Savings Lives Campaign document which discusses high-impact interventions produced by the Department of Health (DH 2007) provide a template for management of all patients at risk of or diagnosed with sepsis.

Airway and breathing

As Penelope is intubated, she is at high risk of developing a nosocomial pneumonia. Attention must be paid to the avoidance of this as a source of secondary sepsis. She should be nursed in accordance with the ventilator care bundle (Pruitt and Jacobs 2006). Furthermore, guidelines for managing patients with acute lung injury should be followed to reduce ventilator-induced lung injury and further exacerbation of the inflammatory response. A key aspect of this includes pressure-limited ventilation (ARDSnet 2000; Sevransky et al. 2004). Further details of these aspects of management can be found in Chapter 1.

Circulation

One of the key challenges in managing severely septic patients is the struggle to balance fluid requirements for a patient who has systemic hypotension alongside pulmonary fluid overload and deteriorating gas exchange. This problem is evident in the data presented for Penelope, showing respiratory dysfunction alongside hypotension, and associated oliguria, systemic oedema and a low SVR, and a metabolic acidaemia. The overall management aim must be to optimise tissue perfusion.

Initially, fluid resuscitation is paramount to ensure that the goals in Table 4.2 are reached, and during the first 24 hours, the patient will usually require large volumes of fluid (Dellinger et al. 2008). Which fluid should be utilised to do this remains controversial. Studies such as the SAFE study which showed no difference between the use of saline and albumin (Finfer et al. 2004) suggest that a colloid or a crystalloid may be utilised. However, many clinicians continue to prefer the choice of colloid for intravascular fluid repletion due to the reduced volume requirements. Colloid fluid challenges may therefore be used together with a restricted crystalloid maintenance fluid regime to avoid the associated pulmonary complications. The nursing role includes close monitoring of fluid balance and vigilance for signs of hypovolaemia and deteriorating gas exchange, as well as monitoring the effects of administered fluids. A central venous pressure (CVP) of 12 mmHg would be the target for optimal intravascular filling in Penelope as she is receiving positive pressure ventilation (Dellinger et al. 2008). However, the CVP may be unreliable in a patient with pulmonary oedema, and more advanced monitoring should therefore be instigated, for example, a PiCCO, Doppler or pulmonary artery catheter. Fluid loss into the interstitial space due to the increased vascular permeability will also be compounded by insensible losses associated with evaporation during sweating. Additionally, in spontaneously ventilating patients an increased respiratory rate and loss of water vapour in expired air will be evident. These factors, must be taken into consideration during fluid assessment.

The use of blood products is generally restricted with an aim to keep haemoglobin (Hb) 7–9 g/dL as this has been shown to reduce blood viscosity and improve micro-circulatory blood flow (Hebert et al. 1999). However, this has to be considered in relation to optimising DO_2, and in some patients, for example, those with acute cardiac insufficiency, a higher level may be more appropriate (Hebert et al. 2001). Examining haemoglobin (Hb) and haematocrit (HCT) levels alongside blood gases will help to ensure optimal DO_2 to the tissues is achieved. Additionally, the risk of the development of disseminated intravascular coagulation (DIC) must not be forgotten and the bedside nurse should be vigilant for signs of bleeding or tissue perfusion deficits, for example, poor distal limb perfusion and bruising, which may be associated with this condition. Laboratory data such as platelet count, aPTT and internationalised ratio (INR) should also be monitored closely for this reason.

Vasopressor and/or inotropic drugs will be required to maintain an adequate MABP (>65 mmHg) in a patient such as Penelope where fluid resuscitation alone has not been adequate. Agents of choice appear to be noradrenaline or dopamine for high-output states with a low SVR, with the possible addition of vasopressin, and dobutamine for inotropic support in patients presenting with a low cardiac output following fluid resuscitation (Dellinger et al. 2008). These patients must be nursed in a critical care facility where invasive blood pressure can be monitored and nurses are familiar with the actions and potential problems associated with the agents being used. Double pumping of such drugs is essential to avoid life-threatening periods of hypotension during syringe changes. The best methods of safely managing this have been studied by Morrice et al. (2004) and Trim and Roe (2004).

Both fluid therapy and vasoactive drug therapy should be guided by the use of an invasive haemodynamic device which calculates cardiac output, SVR, DO_2 and VO_2. Additionally, pulmonary data are available from some devices, for example, extravascular lung water (EVLW) from PiCCO (Cottis et al. 2003) which can be useful in decision making regarding fluid and drug therapy.

Penelope could meet the criteria for the administration of recombinant activated protein C (rhAPC), a drug aimed at restoring normal coagulation and limiting thrombin production. Following a study by Bernard et al. (2001), which showed that rhAPC significantly reduced mortality, it is now recommended for use in patients presenting with severe sepsis and septic shock, who have a high risk of death unless contraindications associated with bleeding are identified (Dellinger et al. 2008). The bedside nurse must ensure a high degree of vigilance during administration of this agent for signs of bleeding. This should include neurological assessment for signs of cerebral haemorrhage. Further, the drug must be administered through a dedicated line, preferably central, and should be withheld for at least two hours prior to and after any invasive procedure being carried out. Laboratory data need to be examined, but it should be noted that although the aPPT is likely to increase, this may not affect the risk of bleeding, so clinical assessment should take priority in deciding whether to stop the infusion before the 96 hours it is usually administered for has elapsed (Schulman and Hare 2003).

The management of fever would also be an important issue to consider as part of the care of Penelope. The data presented suggest that she is currently compromised from both a respiratory and a metabolic perspective. This in itself should justify the use of antipyretics and/or physical cooling interventions in this case (see Chapter 3 for further details of fever management).

Disability of the nervous system

Regular assessment of Penelope's neurological status and sedation level should be undertaken. Penelope is at high risk of the development of critical illness neuropathy due to insulin resistance and hyperglycaemia. Paralysing agents should be avoided for these reasons, and regular assessment using a peripheral nerve stimulator (with an aim of maintaining one to two twitches) should be undertaken if continuous administration is necessary (Murray et al. 2002).

Strict attention to tight glycaemic control is also vital (Van den Berghe et al. 2001). This may be further complicated as an infusion of steroids to counter any suspected adrenal insufficiency may be in progress (Annane et al. 2002), although use of steroids is controversial with a recent research multi-centre trial (the CORTICUS trial) failing to demonstrate any mortality benefit (Sprung et al. 2007). Problems controlling plasma glucose levels may also arise during attempts to administer enteral nutrition. This is a high priority in the prevention of bacterial translocation and secondary sepsis but the presenting condition, and the use of opiates for sedation and analgesia may impair gut motility leading to enteral feed and absorption rates varying over time, and substitution glucose infusions being utilised. Frequent assessment of plasma glucose levels and appropriate titration of infusions using a validated protocol is vital to prevent undesired hypoglycaemia from occurring. Numerous studies have examined the use of a variety of protocols to try and increase both the effectiveness and safety of such a regime (Wilson et al. 2007). Dellinger et al. (2008) recommend maintaining blood glucose levels <8.3 mmol rather than the 4.4–6.1 mmol suggested by Van den Berghe et al. (2001) to reduce the risks of such problems occurring (see Chapter 7 for more information on altered blood sugar management).

Exposure/environment

A holistic approach to the management of Penelope is vital as many of the above factors will lead to problems associated with poor perfusion such as impaired skin integrity. Eye, oral care and effective positioning are paramount to prevent secondary infection, as is the importance of appropriate psychological care to reduce anxiety and stress, which in turn will reduce the metabolic demands on the body (Frazier et al. 2003; Adam and Osborne 2005). Additionally, continued attempts to establish enteral feeding should be made (Heyland et al. 2003), alongside the use of stress ulcer prophylactic agents to prevent upper gastrointestinal bleeding (Dellinger et al. 2008). The nurse should prioritise strict infection control measures and should be continuously vigilant for potential causes of sepsis, performing septic screens as indicated, and minimising risks wherever possible. This should include appropriate wound management and effective care of invasive lines and tubes. The central venous catheter care bundle (DH 2007) should be applied to Penelope's management to help prevent catheter-related bloodstream infection. The two elements of this bundle focus on catheter insertion actions and ongoing care. The latter element makes reference to effective hand hygiene, regular catheter site inspection, maintaining intact dry dressings on insertion sites, aseptic technique and chlorhexidine 2% for cleaning ports and guidelines for administration set replacement. It also recommends against routine catheter replacement (DH 2007). The National Patient Safety Agency (NPSA) offers further guidelines for central venous catheter care to prevent bloodstream infection as part of the recent Matching Michigan project initiative (NPSA 2009).

The other relevant high-impact interventions included in the DH (2007) Saving Lives document should also be applied to Penelope's care. These include guidelines on the management of peripheral lines, urinary catheters and best practice with regards to prevention and management of clostridium difficile, antibiotic use and obtaining blood cultures. As sepsis is a thrombotic disorder, attention should also be paid to effective anti-thrombotic measures such as the use of thrombo-embolic stockings and systemic anticoagulation (Dellinger et al. 2008).

Conclusion

This scenario has discussed the complex challenges associated with caring for a patient with severe sepsis.

Key learning points

- Severe sepsis is part of a continuum of illness which starts with a patient's normal inflammatory response being triggered, which can then become out of control, with the end result being multiple organ dysfunction syndrome and death.
- Management of patients with severe sepsis can be optimised using an evidence-based approach, implementing care bundles such as those related to sepsis, ventilator care and central venous catheter care (DH 2007; Dellinger et al. 2008; NPSA 2009).
- Early recognition of infection and its consequences and prevention is vital.
- Appropriate use and titration of ventilatory support, fluid and drugs within a holistic framework of care which encompasses the DH (2007) high-impact interventions offers the patient the best chance of recovery.

Critical appraisal of research paper

Pronovost et al. (2006) An intervention to decrease catheter related bloodstream infections in the ICU. *The New England Journal of Medicine* **355**(26), 2725–2732.

This American prospective cohort study studied the impact of a number of interventions, one being related to central-line management, in 103 ICUs across 67 hospitals in Michigan. Interventions specific to the reduction of catheter-related bloodstream infection included hand washing, full barrier precautions during central-line insertion, chlorhexidine use to clean line sites, avoidance of the use of the femoral access and removal of unnecessary catheters. Results indicated that following the implementation of the interventions, the median rate of catheter-related bloodstream infection per 1000 catheter days had decreased significantly at both 3 months and 18 months ($p < 0.002$). Their conclusions suggest that the use of these evidence-based interventions result in a large and sustained reduction of central venous catheter-related infection in both adult and paediatric intensive care.

Reader activities

1. Read the research article written by Pronovost et al. (2006).
2. Using the critical appraisal framework in Appendix I, consider the methodological quality of the paper.
3. Reflect on this aspect of your own practice and the implications for future practice management that this paper raises.

A commentary on this paper has been provided by the chapter author in Appendix V.

References

Adam S, Osborne S (2005) *Critical Care Nursing; Science and Practice*, 2nd edn. Oxford Medical Publications, Oxford.

Annane D, Sébille V, Charpentier C, Bollaert PE, François B, Korach JM, Capellier G, Cohen Y, Azoulay E, Troché G, Chaumet-Riffaut P, Bellissant E (2002) Effect of treatment with low doses of hydroscortisone and fludrocortisone on mortality in patients with septic shock. *Journal of the American Medical Association (JAMA)* **288**, 862–872.

Angus D, Linda-Zwirble W, Lidicker J, Clermont G, Carcillo J, Pinsky MR (2001) Epidemiology of severe sepsis in the United States: analysis of incidence, outcome and associated costs of care. *Critical Care Medicine* **29**(7), 1303–1310.

ARDSnet (2000) The Acute Respiratory Distress Syndrome Network: ventilation with lower tidal volumes as compared with traditional tidal volumes for acute lung injury and the acute respiratory distress syndrome. *The New England Journal of Medicine* **342**, 1301–1308.

Bernard GR, Vincent JL, Laterre PF, LaRosa SP, Dhainaut JF, Lopez-Rodriguez A, Steingrub JS, Garber GE, Helterbrand JD, Ely EW, Fisher CJ Jr (2001) Efficacy and safety of recombinent human activated protein C for severe sepsis. *The New England Journal of Medicine* **344**(10), 699–709.

Bone RC, Balk RA, Cerra FB, Dellinger RP, Fein AM, Knaus WA, Schein RM, Sibbald WJ (1992) ACCP/SCCM Consensus Conference: definitions for sepsis and organ failure and guidelines for the use of innovative therapies in sepsis. *Chest* **101**(6), 1644–1655.

Bochud P, Calandra T (2003) Pathogenesis of sepsis: new concepts and implications for future treatment. *British medical Journal* **326**, 262–266.

Brierre S, Kumari R, Deboisblanc B (2004) The endocrine system during sepsis. *The American Journal of Medical Sciences* **328**(4), 238–247.

Cottis R, Magee N, Higgins DJ (2003) Haemodynamic monitoring with pulse-induced contour cardiac output (PiCCO) in critical care. *Intensive and Critical Care Nursing* **19**(5), 301–307.

Dellinger RP, Levy MM, Carlet JM, Bion J, Parker MM, Jaeschke R, Reinhart K, Angus DC, Brun-Buisson C, Beale R, Calandra T, Dhainaut J-F, Gerlach H, Harvey M, Marini JJ, Marshall J, Ranieri M, Ramsay G, Sevransky J, Thompson B, Townsend S, Vender JS, Zimmerman JL, Vincent J-L (2008) Surviving Sepsis Campaign: international guidelines for management of severe sepsis and septic shock: 2008. *Critical Care Medicine* **36**(1), 296–327.

DH (2007) *Saving Lives: Reducing Infection, Delivering Clean and Safe Care*. Department of Health. Available online at: http://www.clean-safe-care.nhs.uk/public/default.aspx?level= 2&load=Tools&NodeID=181. Accessed 12 December 2009.

Finfer S, Bellomo R, Boyce N, French J, Myburgh J, Norton R (The SAFE study investigators) (2004) A comparison of albumin and saline for fluid resuscitation in the intensive care unit. *The New England Journal of Medicine* **350**(22), 2247–2256.

Frazier SK, Moser DK, Daley LK, McKinley S, Riegel B, Garvin BJ, Kyungeh A (2003) Critical care nurses' beliefs about and reported management of anxiety. *American Journal of Critical Care* **12**, 19–27.

Gearhart M, Parbhoo S (2006) Hyperglycaemia in the critically ill patient. *AACN Clinical Issues* **17**(1), 50–55.

Hebert PC, Wells G, Blajchman MA, Marshall J, Martin C, Pigliarello G, Tweeddale M, Schwitzer I, Yetisir E (1999) A multicenter, randomised, controlled clinical trial of transfusion requirements in critical care. *The New England Journal of Medicine* **340**, 409–417.

Hébert PC, Yetisir E, Martin C, Blajchman MA, Wells G, Marshall J, Tweeddale M, Pagliarello G, Schweitzer I (The Transfusion Requirements in Critical Care Investigators for the Canadian Critical Care Trials Group) (2001) Is a low transfusion threshold safe in critically ill patients with cardiovascular diseases? *Critical Care Medicine* **29**(9), S181–S188.

Heyland DK, Dhaliwal R, Drover JW, Gramlich L, Dodek P (2003) Canadian clinical practice guidelines for nutrition support in mechanically ventilated, critically ill adult patients. *Journal of Parenteral and Enteral Nutrition* **27**(5), 355–373, 383.

Holland J, Carey M, Hughes N, Sweeney K, Byrne PJ, Healy M, Ravi N, Reynolds JV. (2005) Intraoperative splanchnic hypoperfusion, increased intestinal permeability, down-regulation of monocyte class II major histocompatibility complex expression, exaggerated acute phase response and sepsis. *American Journal of Surgery* **190**, 393–400.

Hotchkiss R, Karl I (2003) The pathophysiology and treatment of sepsis. *The New England Journal of Medicine* **348**, 138–150.

Levy M, Fink M, Marshall JC, Abraham E, Angus D, Cook D, Cohen J, Opal SM, Vincent JF, Ramsay G (2003) 2001 SCCM/ESICM/ACCP/ATS/SIS International Sepsis Definitions Conference. *Intensive Care Medicine* **29**(4), 530–538.

Marx G, Reinhart K (2006) Venous oximetry. *Current Opinion in Critical Care* **12**, 263–268.

Matthay MA (2001) Severe sepsis: a new treatment with both anticoagulation and anti-inflammatory properties. *The New England Journal of Medicine* **344**, 759–62.

Morrice A, Jackson E, Farnell S (2004) Practical considerations in the administration of intravenous vasoactive drugs in the critical care setting: part II – how safe is our practice? *Intensive and Critical Care Nursing* **20**(4), 183–189.

Murray MJ, Cowen J, DeBlock H, Erstad B, Gray AW Jr, Tescher AN, McGee WT, Prielipp RC, Susla G, Jacobi J, Nasraway SA Jr, Lumb PD (2002) Clinical practice guidelines for sustained neuromuscular blockade in the critically ill adult. *Critical Care Medicine* **30**(1), 142–156.

National Patient Safety Agency (NPSA) (2009) *Matching Michigan Project*. Available online at: http://www.nrls.npsa.nhs.uk/matchingmichigan/. Accessed 26 January 2010.

Pastores SM, Katz DP, Kvetan V (1996) Splanchnic ischemia and gut mucosal injury in sepsis and the multiple organ dysfunction syndrome. *American Journal of Gastroenterology* **91**, 1697–1710.

Pronovost P, Needham D, Berenholtz S, Sinopoli D, Chu H, Cosgrove S, Sexton B, Hyzy R, Welsh R, Roth G, Bander J, Kepros J, Goeschel C (2006) An intervention to decrease catheter related bloodstream infections in the ICU. *The New England Journal of Medicine* **355**(26), 2725–2732.

Pruitt B, Jacobs M (2006) Best practice interventions: how can you prevent ventilator associated pneumonia? *Nursing* **36**(2), 36–41.

Rivers E, Nguyen B, Havsted S, Ressler J, Muzzin A, Knoblich B, Peterson E, Tomlanovich M (2001) Early goal directed therapy in the treatment of severe sepsis and septic shock. *The New England Journal of Medicine* **345**(19), 1368–1377.

Schulman C, Hare K (2003) New thoughts on sepsis; the unifier of critical care. *Dimensions of Critical Care Nursing* **22**(1), 20–30.

Sevransky JE, Levy MM, Marini JJ (2004) Mechanical ventilation in sepsis-induced acute lung injury/acute respiratory distress syndrome: an evidence-based review. *Critical Care Medicine* **32**, S548–S553.

Singer M (2005) Metabolic failure. *Critical Care Medicine* **33**(12), S539–S542.

Sprung C, Annane D, Briegel J *et al.* (2007) Corticosteriod therapy of septic shock (CORTICUS). *American Review of Respiratory Critical Care Medicine* **175**, A436.

Surviving Sepsis Campaign (2009) Available online at: http://www.survivingsepsis.org. Accessed 2 December 2009.

Thelan L, Urden L, Lough M (1998) *Critical Care Nursing; Diagnosis and Management*, 3rd edn. Mosby, London.

Thibodeau G, Paton K (2007) *Anatomy and Physiology*, 6th edition. Mosby, Elselvier Ltd.

Trager K, DeBacker D, Radermacher P (2003) Metabolic alterations in sepsis and vasoactive drug-related metabolic effects. *Current Opinion in Critical Care* **9**(4), 271–278.

Trim J, Roe J (2004) Practical considerations in the administration of intravenous vasoactive drugs in the critical care setting: the double pumping or piggy back technique – Part one. *Intensive and Critical Care Nursing* **20**(3), 153–160.

Van den Berghe G, Wouters P, Weekers F, Verwaest C, Bruyninckx F, Schetz M, Vlasselaers D, Ferdinande P, Lauwers P, Bouillon R (2001) Intensive insulin therapy in critically ill patients. *The New England Journal of Medicine* **345**(19), 1359–1365.

Vincent J-L, Sakr Y, Sprung CL, Ranieri VM, Reinhart K, Gerlach H, Moreno R, Carlet J, Le Gall J-R, Payen D (2006) Sepsis in European intensive care units: results of the SOAP study. *Critical Care Medicine* **34**(2), 344–353.

Wilson M, Weinreb J, Soo Hoo G (2007) Intensive insulin therapy in critical care: a review of a dozen protocols. *Diabetes Care* **30**, 1005–1011.

Other useful resources

www.survivesepsis.org

This website, and the accompanying training programme, highlights the importance of sepsis recognition and provides useful resources to support education and practice outside of the intensive care unit.

Chapter 5

The patient following cardiac surgery

Dr. Maureen Coombs

Introduction

This chapter is predicated on two statements. Firstly, an effective cardiovascular system is vital to the performance of many other body systems. Secondly, that cardiovascular disease remains the main cause of death in the United Kingdom (216 000 per annum) with an estimated 345 000 angina and 66 000 heart failure cases newly diagnosed each year (Allender et al. 2006). Many of the general population, therefore, will have cardiac disease. In hospital, there will be patients whose primary admission diagnosis is cardiac (e.g. post-myocardial infarction) and those whose admission diagnosis is non-cardiac (e.g. post-trauma, diabetes) but who have underlying cardiac problems. For all these patients, wherever they are cared for, the impact of their cardiac disease will require consideration.

This chapter will follow the format of previous sections and use a patient case study to explore cardiac critical care issues. The case study will evolve to allow specific cardiac management issues to be identified and the underpinning pathophysiology, assessment, diagnostics and interventions to be discussed. This is not intended to be a comprehensive review of all cardiac disease states and management challenges; instead, key principles will be introduced and applied to critical care settings.

The case study will begin with cardiac surgical principles and then evolve to explore aspects of non-surgical patient management. In this way, content can be utilised by those working in general intensive care, cardiac intensive care, coronary care and high-dependency clinical areas. The chapter closes with a critique of primary research in cardiac care and signposts further sources of information on the critically ill cardiac patient.

Patient scenario

Mrs Raipul is a 68-year-old lady who has had elective coronary artery bypass grafts ×3. She arrives on the critical care unit with an anaesthetist and technician. She came off bypass on dopamine at 4 mcg/kg/min. Instructions are to 'wake, wean and extubate' (see Figure 5.1 for example of post-cardiac surgery patient).

Critical Care Nursing: Learning from Practice, 1st edition. Edited by Suzanne Bench and Kate Brown.
© 2011 Blackwell Publishing Ltd.

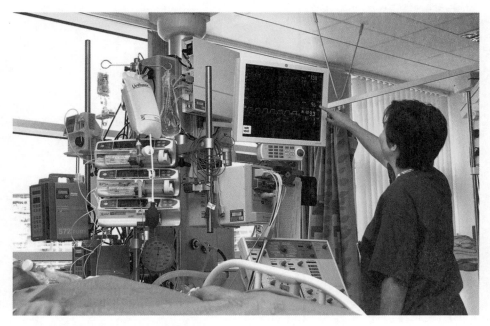

Figure 5.1   Post-operative cardiac surgery patient.

Reader activities

Having read this scenario, consider the following:

- What are the key anatomical and physiological concepts for the cardiovascular system?
- In relation to cardiac anatomy, physiology and disease, what other clinical information needs to be ascertained from handover with the theatre team?

Applied anatomy and pathophysiology

In order to competently care for Mrs Raipul, there must be sound understanding of the underlying anatomy, physiology and disease aetiology. This subject area is well explored in a range of texts (Levick 2003; Noble et al. 2005), so a concise introduction to key issues pertinent to the case study follows.

The cardiovascular system has a vital role in delivering oxygen (metabolic substrate) to cells and removing carbon dioxide (metabolic waste). Functioning organs are maintained by pulsatile blood flow from the heart and the linking of pulmonary and systemic circulatory systems. The heart is situated in the mediastinum with the base of the heart (point of origin of great arteries) located behind the sternum at the level of the second intercostal space. The apex of the heart (left ventricle) is approximately located at fifth intercostal space left mid-clavicular line. Considering its vital function, the heart is only the size of a clenched hand and often weighs <0.5 kg/lb (Filer and Hatchett 2007).

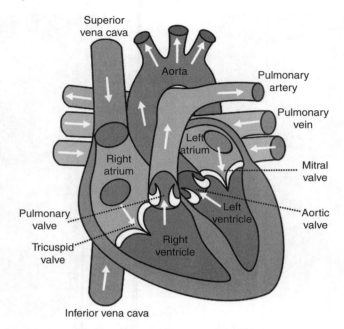

Figure 5.2   Cardiac anatomy. (Courtesy of Wikimedia Commons.)

Simplistically, the heart can be visualized as a hollow, fibromuscular organ. The right side of the heart pumps blood to the pulmonary circulation via the main pulmonary artery, and the left side pumps to the systemic circulation via the aorta. The heart comprises four chambers: two thin-walled atria chambers that act to collect blood returning to the heart, and two thicker walled ventricles that act to contract and eject blood out into the systemic and pulmonary circulations via the great arteries. The chambers are separated by a dividing structure, the septum. This ensures that deoxygenated blood in the right side of the heart, and oxygenated blood in the left side, remains isolated. The cardiac valves ensure blood only travels forward through the heart (see Figure 5.2).

The wall of the heart comprises three layers: pericardium, myocardium and endocardium. The outer layer (pericardium) is a two-layered fibrous sac which, attached to the base of the heart, stabilises the heart position whilst allowing free movement of the apex. The myocardium is mainly muscle (myocytes) together with specialised autorhythmic conduction cells. The endocardium is the inner lining of squamous epithelial cells.

Whilst the endocardium can obtain metabolic nutrients from direct blood contact, other layers of the heart require supply via the coronary circulation. There are two main coronary arteries (left coronary and right coronary artery) that arise from anterior and posterior sinuses of the ascending aorta, and from these a diffuse capillary system ensures optimal oxygen supply to the myocardium. The majority of coronary blood drains back to the heart via the cardiac veins into the coronary sinus, located between the right atrium and ventricle.

In considering cardiac physiology, there are three main physiological principles that need attention for any patient with cardiac disease: preload, afterload and contractility.

Preload is the volume of blood in the ventricles at the end of diastole (i.e. emptied from the atria). It is therefore affected by circulating volume, atrial contraction, left ventricular compliance and length of time of diastole (relaxation phase of cardiac cycle). Afterload is defined as resistance to ventricular ejection and is affected by the resistance in and around the outflow tract area, and in the peripheries. Contractility is the strength of myocardial contraction. In optimising preload and afterload through manipulation of the autonomic nervous system and inotropic therapy, contractility (and cardiac output) is increased. It is manipulation of the relationship between preload and contractility that is explored in Starling curves.

Assessment

Practitioners first meet critically ill patients through clinical handover. It is such communication between healthcare professionals that has been the focus of recent healthcare policy initiatives (National Institute for Health and Clinical Excellence (NICE) 2007). Information gained in patient transfer is important to understand retrospective events, to promote continuity of care and to inform prospective care planning through anticipation of future patient problems.

The arrival of any patient into a critical care area usually heralds great activity. However, once the patient is monitored and is safe, active listening to patient handover is paramount. In the handover of Mrs Raipul, key essentials (name, age, sex, reason for admission and plan) are outlined, but there is additional useful information to be gained, for example, the site from which the coronary artery grafts were taken and subsequently placed; length of time on cardiopulmonary bypass (CPB) and aortic cross-clamp time. Knowledge of graft donor site will direct post-operative observations and management. Knowledge of coronary arteries grafted will give some indication as to the severity of existing cardiac disease. Furthermore, longer CPB times are associated with increased systemic inflammatory and hematological problems, whilst longer aortic cross-clamp times are associated with increased organ ischaemia (Carter 2003). Additional useful information includes Mrs Raipul's pre-operative left ventricular function (an indirect measure of contractility) and filling pressures required to come off CPB. Mrs Raipul's central venous or capillary wedge pressures can be used as indicators of preload (Starling curve) and used post-operatively to optimise cardiac output. Excessive volume loading beyond these preload values could result in reduced cardiac output and pulmonary oedema.

Further useful patient information can be deduced from Mrs Raipul's past medical history, pre-operative medications and social history. Such detail can be integrated into patient assessment through the use of a history-taking model (Bickley and Szilagyi 2005). Additional past medical history (previous myocardial infarctions, asthma, hypertension, diabetes, renal failure, epilepsy, stroke) is important and may inform Mrs Raipul's post-operative care. For example, in patients with asthma, the choice of ventilation mode, respiratory observations and bronchodilator medications need consideration. Pre-existing disease will also be reflected in pre-operative medications taken. If Mrs Raipul is prescribed beta-blockers, aspirin/clopidogrel or angiotensin-converting enzyme (ACE) inhibitor drugs, these may influence her post-operative pathway. Pre-existing disease and the use of medications could give rise to an increased risk of bleeding, need for pacing or more complex fluid management. Similarly, if Mrs Raipul has any drug allergies, these must be noted, together with the nature of the reaction.

An understanding of any significant issues in Mrs Raipul's family or social history can also be useful in planning her care, and this can usually be gained from admission and nursing notes. Details regarding Mrs Raipul's next of kin/dependents, history of smoking, use of recreational drugs or excessive alcohol and her occupation can be helpful in building a holistic assessment and package of care. This information, integrated with initial patient assessment and routine cardiovascular observations (heart rate, rhythm, systolic/mean/diastolic pressures, central venous pressures, peripheral inspection) can ensure that the three cardiac principles of preload, afterload and contractility can be individually optimised for Mrs Raipul.

Developing scenario – bleeding and hypovolaemia

On undertaking routine observations on Mrs Raipul, you note:

- Heart rate 98 beats per minute. Sinus rhythm.
- Blood pressure 95/55 mmHg.
- Central venous pressure (CVP) 3 mmHg.
- Core temperature has not markedly risen over the past hour (35.8–36.0°C) and Mrs Raipul, who was warm to mid thigh, is now only warm to knee.
- Chest drain losses have risen from 50 mL over the first 2 hours to 100 mL over the past 30 minutes.

Reader activities

Consider the following:

- What physiologic terms describe Mrs Raipul's clinical signs?
- Why is Mrs Raipul especially at risk of bleeding?
- How can a clotting screen help determine the cause of bleeding?
- What drugs can be administered to reverse clotting abnormalities?
- What other treatment options can be used to minimise blood loss?

Applied pathophysiology

Mrs Raipul's clinical signs indicate hypotension due to hypovolaemia. Her blood pressure is low, and certainly lower than when it was measured pre-operatively at 145/95 mmHg. Her right-sided filling pressure (CVP) reading is also low, indicating reduced venous return. Hypovolaemia occurs when circulating blood volume is insufficient to fill intravascular spaces. The resultant reduction in venous return to the right heart leads to a decreased cardiac output, and reduced systolic and mean arterial pressure. A 10%

reduction in circulating volume will initiate compensatory mechanisms including tachycardia and peripheral vasoconstriction with higher diastolic blood pressure values (Ganong 2005), as evidenced in Mrs Raipul's observations. Losses resulting in a 20% or more reduction of circulating volume will lead to clinical signs and symptoms of hypovolaemic shock including reduced renal, cerebral and splanchnic perfusion with impaired function.

Any patient who sustains injury or trauma (post surgery, burns, road traffic accident), is dehydrated or has gastrointestinal obstruction is at risk of hypovolaemic shock unless the underlying cause is well managed. Mrs Raipul has undergone cardiac surgery and has a number of risk factors for hypovolaemia. Pre-operatively, Mrs Raipul will have been nil by mouth prior to surgery and will have a degree of dehydration, especially if receiving high dose diuretics. She will have sustained some blood loss peri-operatively and this may not have been fully replaced. Fluid volume deficit could have been further aggravated by the interstitial fluid shifts that occur post-CPB. During cardiac surgery, patients are centrally cooled to 32°C for cerebral and myocardial protection, and when re-warming begins, judicious volume replacement is required to ensure further hypovolaemia does not result.

Hypovolaemia due to blood loss is clearly a key consideration in Mrs Raipul's case. Factors that increase risk of post-operative bleeding include the pathophysiology of CPB and cardiac surgical techniques. CPB activates whole body inflammatory responses resulting from blood contact with non-endothelial CPB circuitry. Such contact activates plasma protein systems and intrinsic and extrinsic coagulation pathways, with the risk of clotting. To counteract this, intra-operative heparin is administered and this requires reversal post-surgery. CPB also activates platelet activity, decreasing overall platelet numbers and function. Cardiac surgery also requires suturing of key blood vessels and placement of cannulae into major cardiac structures. A sub-optimal surgical technique or excessive force (high systemic pressures) on these sites increases risk of post-operative bleeding. These are all major contributors to risk of post-operative bleeding.

There are many other specific factors that may pre-dispose Mrs Raipul to bleed post-operatively. In line with current secondary prophylactic practice, Mrs Raipul will have received pre-operative aspirin and anti-platelet therapy (clopidogrel) to reduce the risk of myocardial infarction (Antiplatelet Trialists' Collaboration 1994). Even with discontinuation of these prior to surgery, some residual anti-coagulation effect remains, increasing potential for blood loss. Furthermore, as the patient re-warms post-operatively, residual heparin given during CPB and trapped in vasoconstricted peripheries will be washed back into the systemic circulation and have an anti-coagulation effect (heparin rebound). If autotransfusion is used in theatre, or if blood drained from CPB is transfused (pump blood), these will contain heparin and/or citrate phosphate; whilst volume replacement will restore normovolaemia, further coagulation problems can result.

Critical care assessment and diagnostics

Whilst there are key diagnostics to assist in the treatment of blood loss, patient assessment can also offer pointers for management. Chest drains are routinely placed at the end of surgery to aid the flow of serous and blood losses away from the heart, thereby preventing clot formation. It would be standard for Mrs Raipul to have a minimum of one Portex

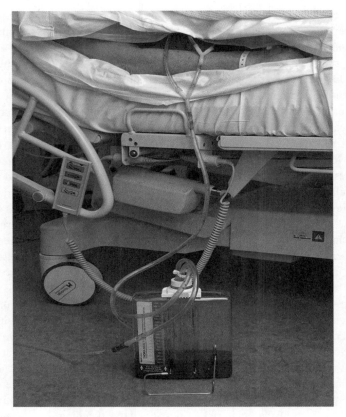

Figure 5.3   Post-operative chest drains.

mediastinal drain but Redivac drains may also be present. Chest drains are initially placed on low suction (2–4 kPa) and frequent observations undertaken on losses from, and patency of, the drains post-theatre (see Figure 5.3). Whilst there is little robust evidence base for the care of such drains, some practice guidelines are available. Clamping of chest drains (especially if air leaks are present) should be avoided, and routine milking or stripping of chest tubing should not occur due to the high negative pressures generated, and the stress placed on surgical anastomoses and healthy clot formation (Thorn 2006).

Blood loss is usually greatest immediately post-surgery and should reduce to near zero 6–12 hours post-surgery. With some local unit variation, acceptable blood loss values are 2 mL/kg/hour for the first 2–3 hours, up to 1 mL/kg/hour for the next 3 hours, and then under 0.5 mL/kg/hour by 12 hours post-surgery. There would be concern if blood loss substantially increased beyond these levels, or if blood loss appeared arterial, or if blood was observed advancing up the drain tubing against gravity. Surgical teams should attend haemodynamically unstable patients, especially those with increasing CVP readings as this may herald the surgical emergency of cardiac tamponade.

In contrast, a generalised coagulopathy is evidenced by increasing blood loss from any incision and/or line insertion sites. In this instance, and in all but the most urgent surgical

Table 5.1 Tests of haemostasis.

Name of test	Normal value	Clinical significance
Haemoglobin (Hb)	Males 13.5–17.5 g/dL Females 11.5–15.5 g/dL	Increased value associated with dehydration Decreased with anaemia, blood loss, vitamin deficiency, etc.
Red blood cell (RBC)	Males 4.5–6.5 $\times$ 10^{12}/L Females 3.9–5.6 $\times$ 10^{12}/L	As above
Packed cell volume (PCV)	Males 40–52% Females 36–48%	As above Test also known as haemotocrit
Activated partial thromboplastin time (APTT)	30–40 seconds	Increased in liver disease, vitamin K deficiency Test used to direct heparin therapy – APTT goal set per patient
Prothrombin time (PT)	10–14 seconds	Increased in liver disease
Thrombin time (TT)	14–16 seconds	Increased in liver disease
International normalised ratio (INR)		Test used to direct warfarin therapy Normal value aim with 2.0–3.0 on warfarin
Platelet count	150–400 $\times$ 10^9/L	Increased in malignant bone marrow disorders Decreased post-bypass, if receiving intra-aortic balloon therapy, in acute leukaemia, cytotoxic drugs Platelets may be dysfunctional if patient on aspirin pre-operatively

emergency, clotting studies are an important diagnostic tool. In theatre, activated clotting time (ACT) is routinely measured to determine the impact of heparin whilst on CPB and the effectiveness of protamine to reverse heparin once off CPB. In critical care areas, clotting tests include full blood count (FBC) and full clotting screen (see Table 5.1 for tests of haemostasis). Furthermore, some centres are increasingly using thromboelastograms (TEGs) to give rapid assessment of clotting (Wenker et al. 2000).

A final diagnostic test to check for bleeding post-cardiac surgery is the chest X-ray. The most common view for chest X-rays is the posteroanterior (PA) film undertaken in the radiology department. In this view the scapulas are rotated away from the lung fields and mediastinal shadowing of the lung fields is reduced. The PA film offers the highest quality chest view; however, it is not always practical to transport critically ill patients to radiology departments and so portable X-rays (anteroposterior (AP) films) are often used. Supine AP films are always used post-operatively. These still yield valuable information, although some caution must be exercised when interpreting mediastinal widening. Either all sequential AP or PA views should be used for comparison purposes (see Fig 5.4 for and example of a chest x-ray).

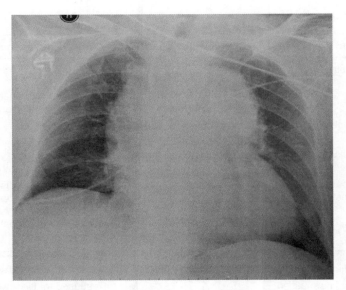

Figure 5.4   Widened mediastinum on CXR. (Courtesy of Wikimedia Commons.)

Excessive blood loss post-cardiac surgery will accumulate in the mediastinal space, producing a widening of the mediastinum (Figure 5.4). A haemothorax (blood in the pleural space) may also be present if one or both pleura were opened peri-operatively. Such collections move freely in the pleural space and shift with the patient's position. In the supine position, blood will layer out over the posterior surface of the chest, producing a diffuse shadow that makes, by comparison, the unaffected lung look denser in appearance. Echocardiography may also be useful to assess cardiac function/structure in these situations. The transthoracic (TTE) or transoesophageal echocardiography (TOE) approach can be used to give information about cardiac structures and any obstruction to ventricular filling or pericardial collection.

Critical care interventions

The management of bleeding can be addressed surgically, haematologically and through general measures. If blood loss is excessive (500 mL in 30 minutes) or there is evidence of cardiac tamponade, then surgical intervention is required. In cardiac tamponade, blood collects around the heart, usually in the pericardial sac, constricting the heart. This leads to increased left- and right-sided filling pressures, reduced flow of blood through the heart and reduced cardiac output, and hypotension with a resultant tachycardia. Chest drain patency should be maintained to enable free drainage of blood until surgical intervention occurs.

The most frequent sites of venous bleeding include atrial cannulation site, mammary bed, bone marrow along the sternum and the innominate vein. Key arterial bleeding sites usually include aortic cannulation site, aortotomy, left atriotomy, coronary artery

Table 5.2 Blood replacement products.

Product	Key practice points
Blood	Normally supplied as red blood cells, can be supplied in 20 minutes 1 unit of blood will increase Hb by 1 g/dL (70-kg adult) In emergencies, O-negative blood used without risk of incompatibility
Platelets	Do not require cross matching Must be ABO compatible and Rhesus matched in females of child-bearing age 1 unit/bag increases platelet count by 10^9/L (70-kg adult)
Fresh-frozen plasma (FFP) 1 unit = 150–250 mL	Contains all coagulation factors except platelets Will raise most clotting factors by 1% in 70-kg adult. Normally 5–10 mL/kg required Must be ABO compatible and Rhesus matched in females of child-bearing age Thawed over 20 minutes and must be discarded if not used within 2 hours

anastomosis and cardiac vent sites. Re-sternotomy rates for bleeding or tamponade are required in approximately 5% of patients (Chikwe et al. 2006), and emergency chest opening is a cause of stress and anxiety for patients, relatives and staff and requires careful and well organized management. If time permits, patients will be returned to theatre, but some circumstances require re-opening of the chest on the unit. In any event key practice pointers would include:

- Ensure blood is available for patient.
- Notify theatre staff and perfusionist.
- Ensure good lighting available.
- Prepare to attach theatre suction tubing to wall suction.
- Ensure defibrillator is available, including facilities for internal defibrillation.
- Notify consultant surgeon of events – if not already present.
- Ensure resuscitation, anaesthetic and inotropic drugs are available.
- Consider when to notify patient family members.
- Ensure other patients and staff are supported.

If diagnostics reveal a coagulopathy, surgical intervention is not indicated and blood products or pharmaceutical agents will be used. If the volume lost is blood, then it is obviously best to replace like with like (see Table 5.2). However, any colloid fluid (e.g. Vulpix) can be used to maintain systolic blood pressure in an emergency. Dependent on laboratory results, cryoprecipitate containing fibrinogen and factors VII and VIII, or prothrombin complex concentrates (PCCs), may be required in cases of severe bleeding (e.g. Beriplex, Nova 7). These contain concentrated amounts of a number of clotting factors and substances (FII, FVII, FIX, FX and protein S and C) and achieve more effective, rapid clotting (Preston 2002). They are, however, extremely expensive and are used only following consultation with a senior haematologist (Preston et al. 2002). All practitioners must understand current best practice guidelines to ensure patient safety in this area (National Health Service Executive 2002) and large infusions of volume should always be warmed as hypothermia further diminishes platelet function.

Some units empirically administer 2 units of platelets and 4 units of fresh-frozen plasma or administer an aprotinin infusion (0.5 million units per hour intravenously) to reduce post-operative bleeding. Aprotinin inhibits mediators of the systemic inflammatory response and decreases fibrinolysis, thereby reducing bleeding and blood transfusion requirements. It is particularly useful for those receiving pre-operative anti-platelet agents (Mannucci 1998). Additional protamine (50–100 mg) may also be given post-theatre to correct prolonged ACT and reverse any remaining systemic heparin. Protamine must be slowly administered intravenously as transient systemic hypotension can result, as can specific protamine-type reactions. Some centres will administer desamino-D-arginine-vasopressin (DDAVP) 16–20 mg intravenously slowly over 30 minutes, or vitamin K 10 mg, similarly administered, for post-operative bleeding.

There are also some general measures that can be used to control or minimise bleeding including maintaining systolic blood pressure <100 mmHg with sedative or antihypertensive agents and increasing positive end expiratory pressure on the ventilator (7.5–10 cmH$_2$O) to tamponade bleeding points. The best treatment option, however, is effective and efficient pre/peri/post-operative management by surgical, anaesthetic and nursing teams.

Developing scenario – cardiac dysrhythmias

Mrs Raipul's bleeding has reduced to 50 mL/hour following administration of blood products. She is now normothermic and cardiovascularly stable. She is on reducing amounts of anaesthesia (Propofol) with a view to assessing her neurological status and her readiness for ventilator weaning. She has received a total of 4 mg of intravenous morphine sulphate for post-operative pain management.

As you are talking with Mrs Raipul, orientating her to time and place, you notice some dysrhythmias on the cardiac monitor. They appear irregular and of varying morphology (shape). During these beats, there is reduction in her blood pressure.

Reader activities

Consider the following:

• What may have predisposed Mrs Raipul to cardiac rhythm problems?
• Which are the common dysrhythmias for patients with cardiac disease?
• Why are certain electrolytes important for cardiac stability?
• How does an electrocardiogram (ECG) help diagnosis?
• How do cardiac drugs work on cardiac cells?

Applied anatomy and pathophysiology

Cardiac conduction occurs through specialised excitatory conducting cardiac tissue. This is different in structure to the contractile muscle tissue in the atria and ventricles. The

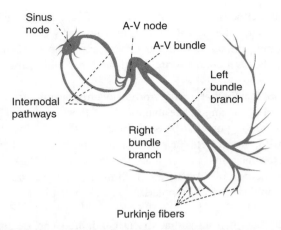

Figure 5.5 Cardiac conduction system. (Courtesy of Wikimedia Commons.)

conducting tissue acts to generate and conduct cardiac electrical activity, and is found in specific areas within the heart (Figure 5.5). These cardiac cells have inherent properties of automaticity and rhythmicity. The heart will continue to beat even when denervated because these cells have an intrinsic ability to depolarise. This occurs due to changes in cell membrane permeability allowing ionic flows. These alter the electrical charge across the membrane and lead to an impulse, the action potential. An action potential at one end of a conducting tissue propagates (continues) the action potential along the fibre in the same direction, and this leads to depolarisation of the fibre membrane, leading to large amounts of calcium release within the muscle cells (myofibrils in the heart), resulting in cardiac contraction.

Each cardiac cell (sinoatrial node, ventricles) has a specific action potential but all cardiac action potentials share some key principles. The action potential comprises five key stages (Figure 5.6) and starts with a negative membrane potential. This value represents the voltage difference across the cell membrane. It is mostly due to the difference in potassium and sodium ion concentrations inside and outside the cell. Phase 0 is a period of rapid depolarisation due to sudden influx of sodium into the cell. This diminishes the transmembrane potential, causing it to become positive in value. With closure of the sodium channels, the membrane potential begins to fall (Phase 1). Rapid repolarisation is prevented by calcium entering the cell (plateau or Phase 2). This stage

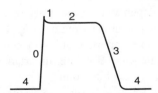

Figure 5.6 Cardiac cell action potential.

is also known as the effective refractory period. In Phase 3, repolarisation returns the cell to its resting membrane potential. This is caused by an increased permeability of the cell membrane to potassium, leading to its exit from the cell. Once repolarisation is complete, potassium channels are inactivated and the resting phase (Phase 4) is achieved.

It is clear there are factors that modify normal electrophysiological functioning. These affect the rate of voltage changes, the magnitude of these changes or the timing intervals of the cardiac action potential phases; for example, catecholamines (intrinsically released through pain, anxiety etc. or extrinsically administered as inotropes) increase both the rate and the magnitude of cardiac depolarisation of Purkinje and sinus node cells, and increase the rate of repolarisation. Similarly, acidosis and electrolyte imbalances impact on depolarisation and repolarisation with potential to cause cardiac rhythm problems.

Dysrhythmias are common in cardiac disease and, after cardiac surgery, where over a third of patients develop rhythm problems (Cheng and David 2006). Pre-operative dysrhythmias may exist, particularly in the older patient, and these may be exacerbated post-operatively. Patients with chronic dysrhythmias may succeed in coming off CBP in sinus rhythm but will usually revert back to established pre-operative cardiac conduction pathways (e.g. atrial fibrillation). The site of cardiac disease can also influence the nature of rhythm disorders. Patients with established mitral valve disease are likely to present in atrial fibrillation, whereas those with large left ventricles (aortic stenosis) are more likely to present with ventricular ectopics. Ineffective cooling/cardioplegia or incomplete myocardial revascularisation can further aggravate rhythm problems. Post-operatively, hypovolaemia, hypoxia, acidosis, anxiety/pain and intravenous cannula within the cardiac chambers can all predispose to cardiac ectopy and irregularities. Whilst some such problems may be tolerated for a short time, tachyarrhythmias (little time for diastolic filling) are poorly tolerated by those with stiff, non-compliant ventricles. In addition, loss of atrial kick in atrial dysrhythmias may further reduce stroke volume by up to 30%. Prompt diagnosis and management of cardiac rhythm disorders is important.

Critical care diagnostics

There are two diagnostic tests clinically available to assist in the management of cardiac rhythm problems: serum electrolyte levels to optimise a healthy cardiac cell environment and the ECG to diagnose dysrhythmias.

Plasma electrolyte levels have a fundamental impact on the working of the heart. Effective cardiac function is dependent on the movement of ionic currents across cell membranes to generate action potentials, conduct impulses and enable contraction of the myocardium. Two of the most important electrolytes routinely monitored in cardiac disease are potassium and magnesium. Both are important in contributing to ionic fluxes that affect cardiac and smooth muscle functioning.

The concentration of extracellular (i.e. serum) potassium is 3.5–4.5 mmol/L, whilst the intracellular concentration is higher at 140 mmol/L. The resting membrane potential of the heart is relative to the ratio of potassium concentrations in the intracellular and extracellular fluids. A decrease in serum potassium decreases the extracellular-to-intracellular potassium concentration ratio, causing the resting membrane to become more negative. Cells are then less responsive to stimuli than normal and more prone to abnormal escape beats. Hypokalaemia also increases the rate of depolarisation of cardiac cells, effectively destabilizing the membrane potential, leading to further increased risk of atrial and ventricular ectopy.

Magnesium is also primarily an intracellular ion, and similarly for potassium, only the serum levels of magnesium are monitored. Normal levels of serum magnesium are 0.8–1.2 mmol/L. Intracellular magnesium is important for many enzymes (including ATPases) that regulate intracellular potassium myocardial levels. The effects of hypomagnesaemia are similar to those of hypokalaemia, for instance, shortening of the absolute refractory period and lengthening of the relative refractory period. Hypomagnesaemia can cause coronary artery spasm and potentiate digoxin toxicity. For cardiac patients, it is therefore important frequently to monitor serum potassium and magnesium.

If an action potential is a representation of the electrical activity of one cardiac cell, the ECG depicts total cardiac cell electrical activity. Electrodes (leads) placed on the body detect the depolarisation and repolarisation of all myocardial cells. ECGs can be continuously monitored through 3 leads (standard limb), 5 leads (standard limb leads plus neutral, plus chest lead for left ventricular diagnosis if in V5 position) and 12 leads for full diagnosis of the location of the ischemic and injury pattern. The 12-lead ECG is not used for continual monitoring of the patient.

In the following section on critical care diagnostics, the three key common cardiac rhythms of atrial ectopics, atrial fibrillation and ventricular ectopics are discussed. Atrial ectopics may be isolated in nature or may precede the onset of atrial tachycardias including atrial fibrillation. The stimulus for an atrial ectopic is initiated by an irritable atrial cell. The resultant conduction pathway is aberrant and the shape of the P wave abnormal and premature. Once the conduction stimulus reaches fully repolarised ventricles, a normal QRS will follow (Figure 5.7a).

Atrial fibrillation (AF) is a common cardiac dysrhythmia found in 10% of the population over the age of 80 (Freestone and Lip 2003). In AF, multiple foci in the atria fire at a highly chaotic and disorganised rate (over 350/min). As the impulses bombard atrioventricular and ventricular cells, some stimuli are conducted by fully repolarised cells, whilst others are not conducted onwards to the ventricles. This leads to the characteristic ECG finding of irregularly irregular QRS complexes and no well-defined P waves (Figure 5.7b).

Ventricular ectopics (also known as premature ventricular contractions) are due to early depolarisation of the ventricles from an irritable ventricular cell. This sets up a depolarisation wave away from the normal fast depolarisation channels with a resultant abnormal, broad QRS complex (Figure 5.7c). Ventricular ectopics can occur in isolation, alternating with every other sinus beat (bigeminy), or in groups of three or more (salvos). Myocardial ischemia, hypoxia, cardiac failure, increased catecholamine and hypokalaemia/hypomagnesaemia can all initiate ventricular ectopics. If the ectopic beat depolarises just after the relative refractory phase (T wave) of the preceding sinus beat, the cells are at their most vulnerable and are potentially irritable. There is evidence that this phenomenon, known as 'R on T', can potentiate ventricular fibrillation.

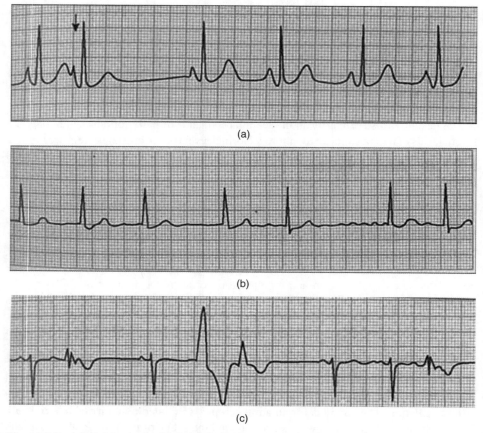

(a)

(b)

(c)

Figure 5.7   (a) Atrial ectopic. (b) Atrial fibrillation. (c) Ventricular ectopic.

Critical care interventions

In order to treat non-threatening cardiac rhythm disturbances, the simplest intervention is electrolyte supplementation and correction of any obvious precipitating causes. Hypokalaemia can result from a decreased potassium intake resulting from poor dietary intake or excessive diarrhoea. Non-potassium-sparing diuretic use (especially loop and thiazide diuretics) without potassium cover can lead to profound hypokalaemia, as can aggressive haemofiltration without sufficient potassium replacement. This has led to nurse-led protocols to optimise patient management (Brooks 2006). Other situations that induce low serum potassium include alkalotic states, large transfusion of red blood cells, and rapid correction of acidotic states, sliding scale insulin therapy, and hypomagnesaemia. Catecholamines also cause potassium ions to shift into cells and any of these causes should be identified and managed appropriately. On-going monitoring of the serum potassium level must be maintained, especially in patients with renal failure, as potassium levels can rise dramatically requiring equally prompt treatment.

As Mrs Raipul is a cardiac patient, serum potassium would normally be kept slightly higher ($\geq$4.5 mmol/L), as severe hypokalaemia (potassium <3.0 mmol/L) can result in life-threatening dysrhythmias. For patients taking oral diet, potassium management can occur through intake of food rich in potassium (bananas, prunes, apricots, orange juice) or adjustment of diuretics, for example, furosemide (frusemide) to furosemide (frusemide) and amiloride combination). Oral supplementation is also useful, although slow K^+ (1 tablet = 12.5 mmol potassium chloride) is usually better tolerated than the effervescent Sando K^+ (1 tablet = 20 mmol potassium). If intravenous supplementation is required with peripheral access, a maximum of 40 mmol of potassium in 1 litre of fluid over 8 hours can be administered. As Mrs Raipul has central-line access, 20 mmol of potassium chloride can be safely administered in 50 mL of fluid over 30 minutes, although local practices will vary. Storage and supply of potassium has received great scrutiny over recent years, and the staff should be familiar with best practice guidelines (National Patient Safety Agency 2003).

Hypomagnesaemia is commonly seen in patients with a high alcohol intake, following CPB, those receiving non-sparing potassium diuretics or with congestive cardiac failure and congested splanchnic beds (impaired uptake of magnesium). Most units will aim to maintain serum magnesium above 1 mmol/L. Normal corrective administration is with 2–4 g of magnesium sulphate in 50 mL 5% dextrose as per unit policy.

The goals of treatment for cardiac dysrhythmias are directed at rate control, restoration of sinus rhythm and prevention of thrombo-embolic complications. This is particularly applicable if the patient is in AF and compromised (i.e. low blood pressure/cardiac output). Interventions can be pharmacological or electrical. Initial treatments include supplementation of potassium and magnesium, and correction of any hypoxia, hypovolaemia or acidosis. If Mrs Raipul is receiving any medications/infusions that are dysrhythmogenic, then these should be reduced or reconsidered. Amiodarone 300 mg over 1 hour via a central line is usually the subsequent choice of therapy for patients with good to moderate cardiac function. This is followed by a maintenance dose of 900 mg over 23 hours, diluted as per local unit policy. Amiodarone prolongs the action potential duration and repolarisation time by inhibiting potassium fluxes. This gives it both Class I and Class III (Vaughn Williams's classification) anti-arrhythmic properties. Digoxin is usually the second-line choice of drug, particularly for patients with poor left ventricular function. It acts to decrease conduction through the atrioventricular node, thereby slowing the ventricular response rate. Regular heparin should be considered if atrial fibrillation continues, as the risk of cerebrovascular accident is 5–6 times higher in these patients (Choudhury and Yip 2005), with the risk of embolism highest in the first year after onset of AF (PRODIGY 2003).

If Mrs Raipul was acutely compromised, synchronised DC cardioversion (BiPhasic DC shock) may be considered following administration of sedation. Initially 100 J of energy is delivered, increased by 50–100 J (maximum 360 J). There are clear clinical guidelines available to direct this intervention (Resuscitation Council UK 2010).

This section has detailed diagnosis and interventions associated with the common, often non-life-threatening, dysrhythmias experienced by cardiac patients. Whatever the rhythm problem, the most important patient assessment is whether the dysrhythmia interferes with cardiac output. This means, is Mrs Raipul responsive? Does she have a palpable major pulse? If the answer is no, then immediate interventions should begin using current Advanced Cardiac Life Support guidelines (Resuscitation Council UK 2010). All clinicians should ensure they are familiar with and have received recent updates on these guidelines, and are familiar with the local emergency equipment. Finally, it is important to remember that it is not just physiological support that is required. During clinical emergencies, psychological support will be required by Mrs Raipul, her family and, at times, the clinical staff.

Conclusion

This chapter has introduced key principles in caring for those patients with cardiac problems. Although a surgical case study has been presented, aspects of cardiac care that transcend care settings have been discussed. In addition, many of the other chapters within this book are important and useful resources in caring for patients with cardiac problems. Finally, whatever the physiological concern for the cardiac patient, attendance to mental well-being is equally important. Readers should consider the chapters on the management of pain (Chapter 10) and care of the patient with long-term needs in critical care (Chapter 16) as important additions to the nursing armoury when caring for the critically ill cardiac patient.

Key learning points

- No patient is ever 'just a cardiac patient'. This is not the nature of critical care nursing, and this is not the nature of cardiac disease.
- Patient care following surgery can be optimised by an effective clinical handover.
- Critical care nurses need to be aware of the common complications post-cardiac surgery, how to recognize these and how best to manage them. These complications include hypovolaemia secondary to bleeding and dysrythmias.
- Where available, local departmental and national evidence-based guidelines should be utilised to guide care for patients post-cardiac surgery.

Critique of research paper

De Laat E, Schoonhoven L, Grypdonck M, Verbeek A, de Graaf R, Pickkers P, van Achterberg T (2007) Early postoperative 30° lateral positioning after coronary artery surgery: influence on cardiac output. *Journal of Clinical Nursing* **16**, 654–661.

In the high-technology world in which we work, it is easy to forget how the most fundamental of interventions impact on patient outcome. Even the most well-informed, expert nurse can cause harm to the critically ill if intelligent thinking is not applied to every aspect of patient care, including patient positioning. It is for this reason that the primary research chosen for critique is a clinical trial on the effects on cardiac output of early post-operative 30° lateral positioning after coronary artery surgery.

Reader activities

1. Read the research article authored by De Laat et al. (2007).
2. Using the critical appraisal framework in Appendix I, consider the methodological quality of the paper.
3. Reflect on whether the issues and findings of this paper have implications for your own practice.

A commentary on this paper has been provided by the chapter author in Appendix VI.

Recommended further reading

The following resources may be of interest to readers:

Cohn LH, Edmunds LH (2004) *Cardiac Surgery in the Adult*, 2nd edn. Full text free online at http://cardiacsurgery.casebooks.org/.

Higgins C (2007) *Understanding Laboratory Investigations for Nurses and Health Professionals*, 2nd edn. Blackwell Publishing, Oxford.

SCTS (2005)*The Evidence Base for Cardiothoracic Surgery*, Treasure T, Hunt I, Keogh B, Pagano D, (eds). tfm Publishing Limited, Shrewsbury, UK.

Tang A, Ohri SK, Stephenson LW (2005) *Key Topics in Cardiac Surgery*. Taylor & Francis, Abingdon.

Woods SL, Sivarajun Froelicher ES, Underhill Motzer S (2000) *Cardiac Nursing*, 4th edn. Lippincott Williams and Wilkins, Philadelphia.

www.bhf.org.uk

www.cardiologysite.com.

www.ctsnet.org

References

Allender S, Peto V, Scarborough P, Boxer A, Raynor M (2006) *Coronary Heart Disease Statistics*. British Heart Foundation, London.

Antiplatelet Trialists' Collaboration (1994) Collaborative overview of randomised trials of anti platelet therapy. Prevention of death, myocardial infarction, and stroke by prolonged antiplatelet therapy in various categories of patients. *British Medical Journal* **308**, 81–106.

Bickley LS, Szilagyi PG (2005) *Bates' Guide to Physical Examination and History Taking*, 9th edn. Lippincott Williams and Wilkins, Philadelphia.

Brooks G (2006) Potassium additive algorithm for use in continuous renal replacement therapy. *Nursing in Critical Care* **11** (6), 273–280.

Carter R (2003) Current trends and techniques in OPCAB surgery. *Journal of Cardiac Surgery* **18**, 32–46.

Cheng DCH, David TE (2006) *Perioperative Care in Cardiac Anaesthesia and Surgery*. Lippincott Williams and Wilkins, Philadelphia.

Chikwe J, Beddow E, Glenville B (2006) *Cardiothoracic Surgery. Oxford Specialist Handbooks in Surgery*. Oxford University Press, Oxford.

Choudhury A, Yip GYH (2005) How good is anticoagulant control in non-valvar atrial fibrillation? Observations on the elderly, ethnicity, patient perceptions and understanding of AF thromboprophylaxis. *Heart* **91**, 425–426.

De Laat E, Schoonhoven L, Grypdonck M, Verbeek A, de Graaf R, Pickkers P, van Achterberg T (2007) Early postoperative 30° lateral positioning after coronary artery surgery: influence on cardiac output. *Journal of Clinical Nursing* **16**, 654–661.

Filer L, Hatchett R (2007) Cardiac nursing. A comprehensive guide. Chapter 4. In: *The Applied Anatomy and Physiology of the Cardiovascular System*, Hatchett R, Thompson DR (eds). Churchill Livingstone, Edinburgh, pp. 55–77.

Freestone B, Lip G (2003) Epidemiology and costs of cardiac arrhythmias. In: *Cardiac Arrhythmias: A Clinical Approach*, Lip Y, Godtfredsen J (eds). Mosby, Edinburgh, pp. 3–24.

Ganong WF (2005) *Review of Medical Physiology*, 22nd edn. Lange Medical Publishers, Los Altos, CA.

Levick JR (2003) *An Introduction to Cardiovascular Physiology*, 4th edn. Oxford University Press, Oxford.

Mannucci PM (1998) Hemostatic drugs. *The New England Journal of Medicine* **339**, 245–465.

National Health Service Executive (2002) *Better Blood Transfusion*. Health Services Circular 2002/9. HMSO, London.

National Institute for Health and Clinical Excellence (2007) Acutely ill patient in hospital: recognition of and response to acute illness in hospitals. Guide No. 50. London. National Institute for Health and Clinical Excellence.

National Patient Safety Agency (2003) *Update on the Implications of Recommended Safety Controls for Potassium Chloride in the NHS*. Available online at: http://www.npsa.nhs.uk/patientsafety/alerts-and-directives/alerts/potassium-chloride/. Accessed 1 March 2008.

Noble A, Johnson R, Thomas A, Bass P (2005) *The Cardiovascular System. Systems of the Body Series*. Elsevier Churchill Livingstone, Edinburgh.

Preston FE, Laidlaw S, Sampson TB and Kitchen S (2002) Rapid reversal of oral anticoagulation with warfarin by a prothrombin complex concentrate (Beriplex): efficacy and safety in 42 patients. *British Journal of Haematology* **116** (3), 619–624.

PRODIGY (2003) www.prodigy.nhs.uk/guidance.asp?gt=Atrial%20fibrillation. Accessed 18 April 2008.

Resuscitation Council UK (2010) *Resuscitation Guidelines*. Resuscitation Council UK, London.

Thorn M (2006) Chest drains: a practical guide. *British Journal of Cardiac Nursing* **1**, 180–185.

Wenker OC, Wojciechowski Z, Sheinbaum R, Zisman E (2000) *Thrombelastography*. Available online at: http://www.ispub.com/ostia/index.php?xmlFilePath=journals/ijpf/vol1n1/teg.xml. Accessed 13 October 2010.

Chapter 6

The patient with severe upper gastrointestinal bleeding due to oesophageal varices

Suzanne Sargent

Introduction

This chapter provides an overview of the emergency care of a patient with an acute oesophageal variceal bleed, secondary to liver cirrhosis, and the development of portal hypertension. Variceal bleeding is one of the most frequent causes of mortality in patients with cirrhosis and portal hypertension, whereby approximately 30–50% of patients die within six weeks of the first variceal bleed (McCormick and O'Keefe 2001). This scenario focuses on a patient presenting with an acute variceal bleed who goes on to develop hypovolaemic shock. It will review and examine the current evidence base for both medical and nursing management.

Patient scenario

A 56-year-old Caucasian male, Mr Smith was admitted initially to the emergency department following a large haematemesis. He vomited fresh blood twice prior to seeking medical treatment and has had a further haematemesis (700 ml frank blood) since his admission. He has a known history of liver cirrhosis and portal hypertension due to a past history of alcohol-related liver injury. On physical examination he is noted to have mild jaundice to his sclera, a tense abdomen, shifting ascites on percussion and spider nevi to his upper torso.

He has no significant previous hospital admissions/past medical history and has abstained from alcohol for the last five months. He has no history of recreational drug abuse. He is currently only on oral spironolactone 200 mg daily for the management of his ascites, which he admits to taking intermittently. Other significant features of his clinical presentation can be seen in Table 6.1.

In view of his profuse bleeding, tachypnoea and decreased oxygen saturations, Mr Smith is electively intubated with a size 8.0 endotracheal tube prior to the insertion of a balloon tamponade tube, pending the arrival of the on-call endoscopy team. To manage his hypovolaemia, two 16-gauge cannulae are inserted in the emergency department and he is given intravenous colloids, whilst awaiting the arrival of

Critical Care Nursing: Learning from Practice, 1st edition. Edited by Suzanne Bench and Kate Brown.
© 2011 Blackwell Publishing Ltd.

Table 6.1   Clinical and laboratory assessment data.

Cardiovascular	BP: 87/40 mmHg (MABP 55 mmHg)
	Pulse: 123 bpm
	Sinus tachycardia
	Temperature: 36.1°C
Respiratory	Self-ventilating on 0.60 (60%)
	FiO$_2$ via a facemask
	Respiratory rate: 23 bpm
	SpO$_2$: 94%
Laboratory results	Hb 6.5 g/dl
	INR 1.3 seconds
	Prothrombin (PT) 18 seconds
	Platelets 47,000 ($\times 10^9$/l)
	Bilirubin 52 μmol/l
	Albumin 28 g/l
	AST 80 IU/l
	ALT 63 IU/l

cross-matched blood. After stabilisation Mr Smith is transferred to intensive care where a central venous catheter and an arterial line are inserted. Mr Smith receives in total 1 litre of colloid, 3 units of packed red blood cells, 1 unit of fresh frozen plasma (FFP) and one pool of platelets. He is commenced on intravenous terlipressin, omeprazole and antibiotic therapy (Ciprofloxacillin).

Reader activities

Having read this scenario, consider the following:

- What do you consider to be the priorities for the management of Mr Smith on arrival to intensive care?
- What is the optimal level of haemoglobin for this patient?
- What additional complications might be associated with his hypovolaemia?

Pathophysiology of cirrhosis, portal hypertension and oesophageal varices

Liver cirrhosis can occur as a consequence of any chronic liver disease whereby repeated hepatocyte damage results in the formation of fibrous tissue and the development of nodules (cirrhosis) (Sargent 2007).

The natural history of cirrhosis is characterised by an asymptomatic phase (compensated cirrhosis). Over time, as the disease progresses this eventually leads to the 'decompensated stage' whereby the development of portal hypertension leads to major complications; hepatic ascites, hepatorenal syndrome, infections, coagulopathy, hepatic encephalopathy

Table 6.2   The Child–Pugh score.

Clinical and biochemical measurements	Points scored for increasing abnormalities		
	1	2	3
Encephalopathy (grade)	None	1 and 2	3 and 4
Ascites	Absent	Slight	Moderate
Albumin (g/l)	>35	28–35	<28
INR	<1.7	1.7–2.2	>2.2
Bilirubin (μmol/l)	<34	34–50	>50
Bilirubin (for primary biliary cirrhosis) (μmol/l)	<69	69–170	>170
Top score	Child–Pugh class	Survival in chronic liver disease at 12 months	
5–6	A	84%	
7–9	B	62%	
10–15	C	42%	

Source: Adapted from Bacon et al. (2006).

and variceal bleeding (Mihas and Sanyal 2006). The Child–Pugh score (Table 6.2) is used to assess the prognosis and appropriate treatment in cirrhosis. Patients with a class C Child–Pugh score are more likely to die from the effects of a variceal bleed compared to Child–Pugh class A (Jalan and Hayes 2000). Based on the data available in Table 6.1, Mr Smith would be categorised as class A.

The normal anatomical relations of the liver and hepatic vein and branches are shown in Figure 6.1. The portal vein carries approximately 1.5 litres of blood from the small intestine, spleen and liver at a pressure of 5–10 mmHg (Wong 2009). As the liver becomes cirrhotic, there is an increase in intra-hepatic resistance, thus leading to portal hypertension with portal pressures exceeding 12 mmHg (Krige and Beckingham 2001). This increased pressure opens up a 'collateral circulation' whereby for blood flow to return to systemic circulation, portal blood flow needs to divert around the liver, especially the instrinsic veins around the gastro-oesophageal junction. These veins then dilate and become varicosed (varices) (Mihas and Sanyal 2006). These collateral vessels are inelastic and become thinner and more fragile as they enlarge and are at high risk of rupturing (Figure 6.2) (McArdle 1999).

Further information

In intensive care, Mr Smith is closely monitored with no further clinical signs of bleeding. As he continues to remain haemodynamically stable, the balloon tamponade tube is removed and he undergoes an upper gastrointestinal endoscopy, where two grade lll varices are found. These are treated with endoscopic variceal band ligation (EVL). Twenty-four hours later with no further bleeding, Mr Smith is extubated and later transferred to a ward setting.

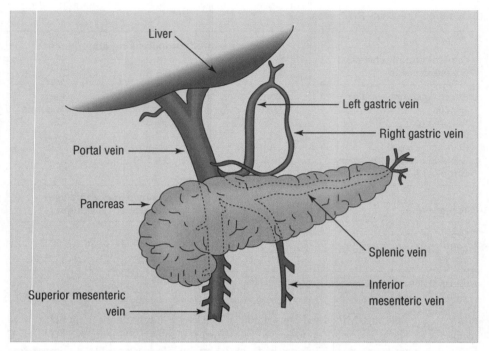

Figure 6.1   Anatomical relations of portal vein and branches. (Krige 2001). Used with kind permission of the BMJ)

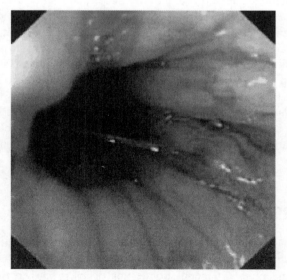

Figure 6.2   Endoscopic view of bleeding varix. (Krige 2001). Used with kind permission of the BMJ)

Laboratory tests and investigations

Liver function tests (LFTs) are the first line in diagnosing liver disease. They provide valuable information regarding the liver synthetic function and cellular damage and enable any biliary tree involvement to be identified (Stonesifer 2004). Other immediate investigations that are necessary for patients presenting with an acute variceal haemorrhage are full blood count, clotting screen, blood group and cross match, urea and electrolytes, and blood glucose (Wong 2009). Mr Smith already has an established diagnosis of alcohol-related liver cirrhosis, and therefore, a prior liver disease aetiology screen, liver biopsy and ultrasound to exclude any other causes of liver disease are necessary. Table 6.3 demonstrates Mr Smith's initial laboratory investigations, normal values and rationale for abnormalities.

Table 6.3 Laboratory results and normal values.

Laboratory results	Normal values	On presentation	Reason for abnormality
INR (seconds)	0.9–1.2	1.3	Decreased synthesis of clotting factors and indicative of poor hepatic function
Prothrombin (seconds)	12–16	18	Decreased synthesis of clotting factors and indicative of poor hepatic function
Platelets ($\times 10^9$/l)	150–450	47,000	Reduced due to portal hypertension and enlarged spleen (splenomegaly)
Alanine aminotransferase (ALT) (IU/l)	3–30	63	Increased enzyme release reflecting damage to hepatic cells
Aspartate transaminase (AST) (U/l)	7–40	80	Increased enzyme release reflecting damage to hepatic cells
Albumin (g/l)	35–54	28	Protein synthesised by liver and marker of poor hepatic synthesis
Total bilirubin (μmol/l)	<17	52	Decreased hepatic clearance due to cirrhosis

Endoscopic treatment of oesophageal varices

Prior to the initiation of endoscopic therapy, patients need to be cardiovascularly stable, as the process itself poses an additional risk of pulmonary aspiration of inhaled blood. This justifies the need for Mr Smith to be intubated in order to protect his airway prior to endoscopy therapy (Wong 2009).

Endoscopic variceal band ligation (EVL) is the first choice of endoscopic management therapy and should be used unless banding is difficult due to profuse bleeding or it is technically unavailable (Jalan and Hayes 2000; SIGN 2008). Meta-analysis has demonstrated that EVL is superior to sclerotherapy for the control of acute bleeding, and is associated with less adverse events and a decreased mortality (Bosch 2009). EVL uses a specialised suction chamber that is inserted onto the end of an endoscope. At endoscopy the varix is sucked into the chamber and a rubber band applied. As the side effect of EVL is the formation of oesophageal ulceration, protein pump inhibitors (in Mr Smith's case omeprazole) should be administered post-endoscopic therapy (Wong 2009).

Initial resuscitation and management of active variceal haemorrhage

Acute variceal haemorrhage can be torrential, constituting a medical emergency that may culminate in death if not promptly and properly controlled (Mihas and Sanyal 2006). Initial resuscitation and management of an active variceal haemorrhage should follow the classic ABCDE approach which is described in detail below along with the management of associated complications. There are two distinct phases in the course of variceal bleeding: the acute phase and a later phase in which there is a high risk of secondary bleeding thus necessitating the need for secondary prophylaxis. Only the management of the acute phase is reviewed in this chapter.

Airway

Mr Smith should be continually assessed and receive appropriate management of his airway. Consequently, staff involved in his care should be competent in the recognition of airway compromise and basic airway manoeuvres (SIGN 2008).

Mr Smith initially received 0.6 FiO_2 (60%) via a face mask. As his initial oxygen saturations were only 94%, this was increased to 1.0 (100%). Collins (2000) and Bench (2004) recommend that all patients receive 100% oxygen via a non-rebreathe face mask during the acute phase of shock.

Endotracheal intubation is always advocated prior to insertion of a balloon tamponade tube (Figure 6.3) due to the technical difficulties of tube insertion, the inability for patients to clear secretions and the risk of bronchial aspiration. Additional indications for intubation in patients with an acute variceal bleed are uncontrolled bleeding, severe hepatic encephalopathy, inability to maintain oxygen saturations above 90% or aspiration pneumonia (Jalan and Hayes 2000; Bosch 2009).

There are three main types of balloon tamponade tube (Sengstaken–Blakemore, Minnesota and Linton–Nachlas) which achieve haemostasis in up to 90% of cases by direct compression by the gastric balloon. However, there is no demonstrated survival benefit associated with their use, and a complication rate of 15–20% (asphyxiation, pneumonia, oesophageal tears, patients discomfort, tube migration and erosion and oesophageal necrosis). Balloon tamponade tubes should therefore only be used in cases of uncontrolled bleeding, or in the case of Mr Smith, where there is a delay in commencing endoscopic therapy (Jalan and Hayes 2000; Mihas and Sanyal 2006; SIGN 2008).

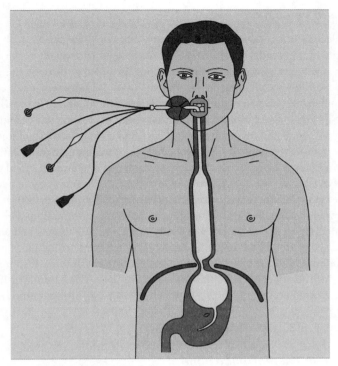

Figure 6.3 Picture of balloon tamponade tube. (McPherson 2006). Reproduced with kind permission of the BMJ.

The Sengstaken, Blakemore and Minnesota balloon tamponade tubes (Figure 6.3) all have a gastric and oesophageal balloon. Once the tube is trans-orally positioned by a skilled practitioner, it is, however, rarely necessary to inflate the oesophageal balloon (Wong 2009). After the tube position is confirmed, the gastric balloon is usually inflated with 250 ml of water or a mixture of water and 10% radio opaque contrast (Wong 2009). Using air alone for gastric balloon inflation is associated with a risk of balloon deflation and tube migration into the pharynx, causing possible airway obstruction and potential rupture of the oesophagus (Collyer 2007).

The balloon tamponade tube is then withdrawn, and the balloon held tight against the gastro-oesophageal junction by firm skin traction (Wong 2009). The use of external traction such as a 500 ml bag of crystalloid remains common practice; however, this is deemed unnecessary and increases the risk of tube migration (Collyer 2007).

In the case of Mr Smith, the balloon tamponade tube only remained *in situ* for a short duration prior to successful endoscopic therapy. Most guidelines recommend that balloon tamponade tubes should only be used for a period of up to 24 hours due to the high risk of associated complications. The risk of re-bleeding post-removal of the balloon tamponade tube is approximately 50% (Jalan and Hayes 2000; De Franchis 2005).

Breathing and ventilation

Prior to his elective intubation, Mr Smith was noted to be tachypnoeic with an increased respiratory rate of 23 breaths per minute. This increase in both respiratory rate and depth is due to a physiological response to cellular hypoxia resulting from his stage three hypovolaemic shock (Table 6.4) (Collins 2000; Bench 2004). It is also worth remembering that variceal haemorrhage is extremely distressing and patients are likely to have high levels of anxiety. Post-intubation and transfer to intensive care, Mr Smith was commenced on intravenous propofol and fentanyl to minimise stress and anxiety and to facilitate ventilation and achieve ventilator synchrony (see Chapter 11 for more in-depth information regarding the use of intravenous sedation). Both oxygen saturations and arterial blood gases need to be monitored closely to assess oxygenation levels and to detect any associated metabolic acidosis related to inadequate oxygen delivery (Collins 2000; Bench 2004).

Mr Smith was found to have tense ascites on physical examination. This fluid within the peritoneal cavity will cause both a reduction in his lung volumes and an increase on his abdominal pressure. Therefore, it is usual once the haemorrhaging is controlled for patients to undergo both a diagnostic and a therapeutic paracentesis. If more than 5 litres of ascitic fluid are removed, Mr Smith should receive 6–8 g of albumin per litre of ascites removed (for example, 100 ml 20% albumin for each 2–3 litres drained) (Moore and Aithal 2006).

Circulation with haemorrhage control

Hypovolaemic shock is associated with a greater risk of death; therefore, the primary treatment aims are prompt recognition, adequate venous/central access and early aggressive fluid resuscitation (SIGN 2008). The degree of shock and physical manifestations are dependent on the percentage of blood loss and are demonstrated in Table 6.4.

Table 6.4   Classification of hypovolaemic shock by blood loss.

	Class 1	Class II	Class III	Class IV
Volume of blood loss	<750 ml	750–1500 ml	1500–2000 ml	>2000 ml
Percentage of circulating blood loss	0–15 %	15–30%	30–40%	>40%
Systolic blood pressure	No change	Normal	Reduced	Very reduced
Diastolic blood pressure	No change	Raised	Reduced	Very reduced or unrecordable
Pulse (beats per minute)	Slightly tachycardic	100–120	120 (thread)	>120, very thready
Respiratory rate	Normal	Normal	>20/min	>20/min
Mental status	Alert, thirsty	Anxious and aggressive	Anxious, aggressive and drowsy	Drowsy, confused or unconscious

Source: Adapted from SIGN (2008).

On initial presentation Mr Smith's percentage of circulating blood loss and increases in both respiratory and heart rate would categorise him in class 3 hypovolaemic shock (Table 6.3). The body's response to hypovolaemia firstly results in a compensatory stage. During this stage the body attempts to compensate for the blood lost by vasoconstriction and diversion of blood to 'vital organs' (Adam and Osborne 2005). This can be seen in Mr Smith's haemodynamic profile on admission, whereby in response to his hypotension and low circulatory volume, he presented with tachycardia. This occurs because the catecholamines adrenaline and noradrenaline are released in an attempt to increase cardiac output. It is worth noting that because of such compensation, a significant decrease in systolic blood pressure does not usually occur until 30% of blood volume has been lost (Collins 2000; Bench 2004; Garreton and Malberti 2007).

As this case study demonstrates, the need for intravenous access for rapid fluid resuscitation is of paramount importance. Multiple wide-bore peripheral cannulae should be inserted initially into anticubical fossa for rapid access. Ideally, patients should also have central venous access, and in some cases it may be necessary to use wide-bore central access into the femoral vein for rapid fluid replacement (Wong 2009).

Red blood cell transfusion should be considered after a 30% loss of the circulatory volume (SIGN 2008). Most patients can, however, be resuscitated with appropriate plasma expanders whilst cross-matched blood is awaited. Nonetheless, in severe cases of variceal haemorrhage, the administration of group-compatible or O-negative blood may be warranted whilst cross matching is taking place (Wong 2009).

Previous Cochrane reviews (Alderson et al. 2000; Finfer et al. 2004) have failed to demonstrate any statistically significant difference between crystalloids and colloids and no studies to date have compared these two fluid types in patients with an upper gastrointestinal bleed. Current guidelines therefore advocate that either solution may be used for volume restoration prior to blood transfusion (SIGN 2008).

Although a low haemoglobin is associated with a reduction of oxygen-carrying capacity, the optimal level for red blood cell (RBC) transfusion in critically ill patients remains controversial (van Heerden et al. 2002). The pioneering Canadian multi-centre study by Hébert et al. (1999) and subsequent research and meta-analyses continue to demonstrate the link between RBC transfusions and increased morbidity and mortality (Marik and Corwin 2008). A haemoglobin (Hb) of 8 g/dl is usually considered adequate for most critical care patients, with the exception of those with chronic respiratory conditions, cerebral vascular disease, cardiac disease or elderly patients who may need a higher threshold (Adam and Osborne 2005). For patients like Mr Smith, with acute variceal haemorrhage, it has been recommended that blood should be given cautiously, supporting a transfusion threshold of 8 g/dl of Hb or a haematocrit of 0.24, unless there is rapid ongoing bleeding or the patient has ischaemic heart disease (De Franchis 2005). Furthermore, it has been suggested that blood transfusions may induce rebound increases in portal hypertension, and thus increase the risks of both re-bleeding and death (Bosch 2009). Generally in the anaemic patient, a transfusion of 4 ml/kg packed cells should raise Hb by 1 g/dl (Adam and Osborne 2005). In addition to the association of increased mortality in critical care patients and RBC transfusions, a comprehensive literature research by Gerber (2007) suggests infections, immunosuppression, impairment of microcirculatory blood flow, 2,3-diphosphoglycerate deficiency and numerous biochemical and physiological derangements, including hypocalcaemia and coagulopathy, can additionally be seen. These problems are usually caused by either storage or inherent properties of the transfused blood.

Hepatocyte cells in the liver synthesise all clotting factors apart from factor Vlll which are synthesised in the epithelial cells. As a result, patients with liver disease have impaired production of these plasma proteins, and consequently, it is common for patients like Mr Smith to have altered coagulopathy as demonstrated in his laboratory findings (elevated PT and INR – Table 6.3). Cardenas and Gines (2009) suggest that as patients with acute variceal haemorrhage have advanced liver disease, this coagulopathy may contribute to the failure to control bleeding. This view is, however, not universally supported (Lisman and Leebeek 2007).

Fresh-frozen plasma (FFP) is frequently administered to patients who have cirrhosis and a prolonged prothrombin time (PT). O'Shaughnessy et al. (2004), however, suggest patients with a PT greater than four seconds longer than control, are unlikely to show any benefit from this. However, as no clotting factors remain in transfused RBC, it is usual for patients receiving large transfusions to additionally receive transfused FFP, as each unit of FFP increases each clotting factor by 2–3%. One unit is usually administered for each 5–6 units of RBCs transfused (Adam and Osborne 2005; Low and Milne 2007).

A mild to moderately reduced platelet count, as seen in Mr Smith's data (Table 6.3), is common in patients with chronic liver disease and portal hypertension. One of the causes for thrombocytopenia is an increased platelet sequestration, as 90% of platelets are stored in the spleen. This occurs as a result of congestive splenomegaly, secondary to portal hypertension (Lisman and Leebeek 2007). Mr Smith's platelet count on presentation was 47 000 ($\times 10^9$/l). It is advocated that patients should receive a platelet transfusion, if platelets are <50 000 ($\times 10^9$/l) (Mihas and Sanyal 2006). Each unit of platelets will increase the platelet count by 5000 ($\times 10^9$/l) (Low and Milne 2007).

Studies exploring the use and safety of haemostatic agents such as intravenous factor Vll (FVll), transexamic acid and desmopressin (DDAVP) in acute variceal haemorrhage have not demonstrated any benefits and are therefore not advocated for routine usage (Lisman and Leebeek 2007; Cardenas and Gines 2009).

One of the first-line therapies for acute variceal bleeding is the intravenous administration of terlipressin. Terlipressin is a synthetic derivative of vasopressin, and works by causing vasoconstriction of the mesenteric arterioles thus decreasing portal venous blood inflow and portal venous pressures. It is the initial drug of choice as it has clinically been proven to improve survival in placebo-controlled randomised control trials and meta-analyses (Mihas and Sanyal 2006; Bosch 2009). In the United Kingdom, terlipressin remains the only licensed therapy for variceal bleeding, although octreotide and somatostatin have been demonstrated to have some benefits and are widely used in North America.

The vasoconstrictive effects of terlipressin are not isolated to the splanchnic arterial bed; therefore, it is imperative to obtain a baseline ECG, prior to commencing therapy. Additionally, Mr Smith would need to be monitored for any signs and symptoms of ischaemia, for example, abdominal pain (small bowel ischaemia), chest pain (myocardial ischaemia) or peripheral vascular ischaemia (Mihas and Sanyal 2006; Wong 2009). The optimal time for drug therapy ranges between 2 and 5 days, when secondary prophylactic beta blockers can be commenced (De Franchis 2005).

Kidney failure due to either acute kidney injury (AKI) or hepatorenal syndrome frequently occurs with variceal bleeding. Consequently, early fluid resuscitation is of paramount importance to avoid hypovolaemia and hypotension (Bosch 2009). It is imperative that Mr Smith's urine output and renal function are closely monitored, with the initiation of renal support therapies if warranted. AKI and renal replacement therapies are discussed in depth in Chapter 9.

Disability of the central nervous system

Hepatic encephalopathy is often precipitated by a gastrointestinal haemorrhage, as each 100 ml of blood within the gut will contain 15–20 g protein which when broken down will increase the ammonia production and thus potentiate or increase the level of hepatic encephalopathy. The main aim of therapy, therefore, is to clear the gut/bowel of blood to decrease ammonia production. Lactulose should be administered to Mr Smith either orally or nasogastrically at a dose of 10–30 ml three times daily with the aim of producing 2–3 semi-soft stools per day. In severe bleeds, however, this is often given alongside phosphate enemas to accelerate blood clearance (Abou-Assai and Vhahcevic 2001; Sargent 2007; Houlston and O'Neil 2009). Prior to his admission, Mr Smith had abstained from alcohol for several months. Patients who are actively drinking prior to admission, however, should be monitored for alcohol withdrawal and commenced on an appropriate alcohol withdrawal protocol (Mihas and Sanyal 2006). Patients with alcohol-related liver injury are additionally at risk of developing Wernicke's encephalopathy caused by thiamine deficiency. Mr Smith should, therefore, receive intravenous B vitamins (Pabrinex[R]) followed by a course of oral thiamine (Sargent 2006).

There are still some false assumptions that patients with liver cirrhosis need to be protein restricted to reduce the risk of hepatic encephalopathy. Protein intolerance is rare, and protein restriction has not been shown to have any major consequence on either liver function or plasma ammonia and can exacerbate protein breakdown (Cordoba et al. 2004; McCullough 2006). The incidence of protein calorie malnutrition in decompensated cirrhosis has a prevalence of 80–100%, regardless of the underlying aetiology. Nutritional requirements should therefore be met aggressively (Hamlin and Leaper 2009). The European Society of Parenteral and Enteral Nutrition (ESPEN) advocates that patients with cirrhosis should receive 35 kcal/kg/day and 1.2 g/kg/day of protein (Plauth et al. 2006). Reluctance to place a nasogastric tube due to fears of displacement or precipitating further variceal bleed is unfounded. Tubes can usually be placed 24 hours post-cessation of bleeding without risk (Plauth et al. 2006).

Insulin resistance and diabetes frequently occur in cirrhotic liver disease; therefore, Mr Smith will need his blood glucose monitored regularly (Hamlin and Leaper 2009). The management of altered blood glucose and the benefits of tight glycaemic control are discussed in greater depth in Chapter 7.

Exposure/environment

Because of the high risk of sepsis in this group of patients, and the link between infection and early re-bleeding, antibiotic therapy is considered an integral part of therapy and, as in the case of Mr Smith, should be instituted from admission (De Franchis 2005). A meta-analysis has demonstrated that antibiotic use reduces the mortality of patients who develop acute upper gastrointestinal bleeding in association with chronic liver disease (SIGN 2008). Strict asepsis of invasive lines with early removal is also paramount.

Because of the risk of spontaneous bacterial peritonitis (SBP) of his ascitic fluid, Mr Smith should undergo routine paracentesis. The diagnosis of SBP is made upon microscopic examination of the ascitic fluid. The presence of a white cell count of >250 polymorphonuclear leucocyte cells/mm^3 is usually diagnostic and indicates the need to commence broad spectrum antibiotics (Gines et al. 2004).

Conclusion

Variceal haemorrhage associated with liver cirrhosis and portal hypertension is associated with high mortality. As this scenario demonstrates the initiation of appropriate airway management, aggressive fluid resuscitation, the application of pharmacological and endoscopic therapy and recognition and prevention of any associated complications are of paramount importance.

Key learning points

- The development of portal hypertension and subsequent complications of oesophageal varices and ascites mark the transition from compensated to decompensated cirrhosis.
- Oesophageal varices can result in torrential haemorrhage which is associated with a high mortality.
- The securing of a patent airway and maintaining of haemodynamic stability with aggressive fluid resuscitation are of paramount importance and take priority over endoscopic therapy.
- Endoscopic band ligation is considered superior to sclerotherapy.
- Nutrition support with no protein restrictions, good bowel management and prophylactic antibiotic therapy are an essential part of management in patients with liver cirrhosis.

Critical appraisal of research paper

Vincent JL, Sakr Y, Sprunh C (2008) Are blood transfusions associated with greater mortality rates? Results of the sepsis occurrence in acutely ill patients study. *Anesthesiology* **108**, 31–39.

The Sepsis Occurrence in Acutely Ill Patients Study investigated the relationship between blood transfusions to mortality in 198 European intensive care units. All patients admitted during a two-week period in May 2002 were included in the study, and followed either until death or hospital discharge or for a period of 60 days. Results demonstrated that the transfused patients had both a longer length of admission and a higher mortality rate.

Reader activities

1. Read the research article written by Vincent et al. (2008).
2. Using the critical appraisal framework in Appendix I, consider the methodological quality of the paper.
3. Reflect on the use of transfused blood products in your clinical practice; consider your current haemoglobin thresholds and which groups of patients are the primary recipients of blood products.

A commentary on this paper has been provided by the author in Appendix VII.

References

Abou-Assai S, Vhahcevic ZR (2001) Hepatic encephalopathy. Metabolic Consequences of cirrhosis is often reversible. *Postgraduate Medicine* **109**(2), 52–70.

Adam SK, Osborne S (2005) *Critical Care Nursing: Science and Practice*, 2nd edn. Oxford University Press, Oxford.

Alderson P, Schierhout G, Roberts I (2000) Colloids versus crystalloids for fluid resuscitation in critically ill patients (Cochrane Review). The Cochrane Library Issue 3, 2004. Wiley, Chichester, UK.

Bacon BR, O'Grady JG, Di Bisceglie AM, Lake JR (eds) (2006) *Comprehensive Clinical Hepatology*, 2nd edn. Mosby Elsevier, Philadelphia.

Bench S (2004) Clinical skills: assessing and treating shock: a nursing perspective. *British Journal of Nursing* **13**(12), 715–721.

Bosch J (2009) Management of active variceal hemorrhage. In: *ASSLD Postgraduate Course Handbook (2009), Keeping the Patient with End Stage Cirrhosis Alive*. AASLD, Boston, USA.

Cardenas A, Gines P (2009) Portal hypertension. *Current Opinions in Gastroenterology* **25**(3), 195–201.

Cordoba J, Lopez-Hellin JI, Planas M, Sabin P, Sanpedro F, Castro F, Eseban R, Guardia J (2004) Normal protein diet for episodic hepatic encephalopathy: results of a randomised study. *Journal of Hepatology* **42**(suppl 1), S124–S133.

Collins T (2000) Understanding shock. *Nursing Standard* **14**(49), 35–39.

Collyer TC (2007) Acute upper airway obstruction due to displacement of a Sengstaken-Blakemore tube. *European Society of Anaesthesiology* **25**, 341–342.

De Franchis R (2005) Evolving consensus in portal hypertension report of the Braveno IV consensus workshop on methodology of diagnosis and therapy in portal hypertension. *Journal of Hepatology* **43**, 167–176.

Finfer S, Bellomo R, Boyce N, French J, Myburgh J, Norton R, SAFE Study Investigators (2004) A comparison of albumin and saline for fluid resuscitation in the intensive care unit. *The New England Journal of Medicine* **350**(22), 2247–2256.

Garreton S, Malberti S (2007) Understanding hypovolaemic, cardiogenic and septic shock. *Nursing Standard* **22**(21), 46–55.

Gerber DR (2007) Packed red blood cell transfusion in the intensive care unit: limitations and consequences. *American Journal of Critical Care*. Available online at: http://www.thefreelibrary.com/_/print/PrintArticle.aspx?id=157587492 accessed 12/12/09.

Gines P, Cardenas A, Arroyo V, Rhodes J (2004) Management of cirrhosis and ascites. *The New England Journal of Medicine* **350**(16), 1646–1654.

Hamlin S, Leaper J (2009) Nutrition in liver disease. In: *Liver Diseases: An Essential Guide for Nurses and Health Care Professionals*, Sargent S (ed). Wiley-Blackwell, Oxford.

Hébert P, Wells G, Martin C, Tweedale M, Marshall J, Blajchman M, Pagliarello G, Sandham D, Schweitzer I, Boiswert D, Calder L (1999) Variation in red cell transfusion practice in the intensive care unit; a multi centre study. *Critical Care* **3**, 57–63.

Houlston C, O'Neil H (2009) Hepatic encephalopathy. In: *Liver Diseases: An Essential Guide for Nurses and Health Care Professionals*, Sargent S (ed). Wiley-Blackwell, Oxford.

Jalan R, Hayes PC (2000) UK guidelines on the management of variceal haemorrhage in cirrhotic patients. *Gut* **46**(suppl lll), iii1–iii5.

Krige JE, Beckingham IJ (2001) ABC of diseases of liver, pancreas, and biliary system; portal hypertension – 1: varices. *British Medical Journal* **322**, 348–351.

Lisman T, Leebeek FWG (2007) Homostatic alterations in liver disease: a review on pathophysiology, clinical consequences, and treatment. *Digestive Surgery* **24**(4), 250–258.

Low D, Milne M (2007) Crystalloids, colloids, blood, blood products and blood substitutes. *Anaesthesia and Intensive Care Medicine* **8**(2), 56–59.

Marik PE, Corwin HL (2008) Efficacy of red blood cell transfusion in the critically ill: a systematic review of the literature. *Critical Care Medicine* **36**(9), 2667–2674.

McArdle J (1999) Understanding oesophageal varices. *Nursing Standard* **14**(9), 46–52.

McCormack PA, O'Keefe C (2001) Improving prognosis following the first variceal bleed over four decades. *Gut* **49**, 682–685.

McCullough A (2006) Malnutrition in cirrhosis. In: *Comprehensive Clinical Hepatology*, 2nd edn, Bacon BR, O'Grady JG, Di Bisceglie AM, Lake JR (eds). Mosby Elsevier, Philadelphia.

Mihas AA, Sanyal AJ (2006) Portal hypertension and gastrointestinal hemorrhage. In: *Comprehensive Clinical Hepatology*, 2nd edn, Bacon BR, O'Grady JG, DiBisceglie M, Lake JR (eds). Mosby Elsevier, Philadelphia.

Moore KP, Aithal, G.P. (2006) Guidelines on the management of ascites in cirrhosis. *Gut* **55**(suppl 6), vi1–vi12.

O'Shaughnessy DF, Atterbury C, Bolton MP, Murphy M, Thomas D, Yates S, Williamson LM (2004) Guidelines for the use of fresh-frozen plasma, cryoprecipitate and cryosupernatant. *British Journal of Haematology* **126**, 11–28.

Plauth M, Cabre E, Riggio O, Assis-Camilo M, Pirlich M, Kondrup J (2006) ESPEN guidelines on enteral feeding: liver disease. *Clinical Nutrition* **25**(2), 285–294.

Sargent S (2006) Management of the patient with advanced liver cirrhosis. *Nursing Standard* **21**(11), 48–56.

Sargent S (2007) Pathophysiology and management of hepatic encephalopathy. *British Journal of Nursing* **16**(6), 335–339.

Scottish Intercollegiate Guidelines Network (SIGN) (2008) 105: management of acute upper and lower gastrointestinal bleeding. A national clinical guideline available online at: http://www.sign.ac.uk accessed 6/11/09.

Stonesifer E (2004) Common laboratory and diagnostic testing in patients with gastrointestinal disease. *AACN Clinical Issue: Advanced Practice in Acute and Critical Care* **15**(4), 582–594.

van Heerden N, S Rau S, Groba CB (2002) Changing the practice of blood transfusion in intensive care. *Critical Care* **6**(suppl 1), 170.

Vincent JL, Sakr Y, Sprunh C (2008) Are blood transfusions associated with greater mortality rates? Results of the sepsis occurrence in acutely ill patients study. *Anesthesiology* **108**, 31–39.

Wong T (2009) Portal hypertension. In: *Liver Diseases: An Essential Guide for Nurses and Health Care Professionals*, Sargent S (ed). Wiley-Blackwell, Oxford.

Chapter 7

The patient with altered blood glucose

Danielle Fullwood

Introduction

Hyperglycaemia is a common occurrence in critically ill patients (Montori et al. 2002; Krinsley 2003; Merz and Finfer 2008). Whilst for many years this has been considered a normal response to stress, more recent studies have established a possible link between hyperglycaemia and increased morbidity and mortality (Van den Berghe et al. 2001, 2006; Krinsley 2003; Vanhorebeek et al. 2005). This chapter focuses on the need for early recognition of hyperglycaemia and discusses the possible complications of both hyper- and hypoglycaemia.

Scenario

Lilly Reynaulds is a 23-year-old woman admitted to a high dependency unit 12 hours ago with an acute exacerbation of asthma. She has been on high-flow oxygen and continuous salbutamol nebulisers. She has been eating and drinking small amounts and is also on a maintenance fluid infusion of Hartmann's solution. She has been receiving hydrocortisone intravenously every six hours. Her current clinical status can be seen in Table 7.1.

Reader activities

Having read this scenario, consider the following:

- What are the clinical manifestations of hyperglycaemia?
- What effect does hyperglycaemia have on other organs?
- Why does hyperglycaemia occur in critical illness?
- How should hyperglycaemia be managed?

Critical Care Nursing: Learning from Practice, 1st edition. Edited by Suzanne Bench and Kate Brown.
© 2011 Blackwell Publishing Ltd.

Table 7.1 Clinical data.

Cardiovascular	Blood pressure 96/50 mmHg (MABP 64 mmHg) Pulse 102 bpm
Respiratory	Self ventilating on 50% O_2 via a humidified face mask Respiratory rate 24 bpm
Arterial blood gas	pH 7.31 PaO_2 9.5 kPa PCO_2 7.0 kPa HCO_3 19 mmol/L BE −3.1 Lactate 3 mmol/L Glucose 17.8 mmol/L
Renal	Urine output 15–20 ml/h (weight 68 kg) Creatinine 120 μmol/L Urea 13 mmol/L Sodium 145 mmol/L Potassium 5.0 mmol/L

Pathophysiology

Hyperglycaemia has been varyingly defined as a blood glucose level of >6.1 mmol/L (Van den Berghe et al. 2001) to one of >10 mmol/L (Devos and Preiser 2004). In critical illness, hyperglycaemia has been thought to benefit organs by allowing them a greater energy supply during a period of stress (Parsons and Watkinson 2007). Stress experienced in critically ill patients causes an increase in cortisol, growth hormones, epinephrine and glucagon to be produced, all of which act to increase the hepatic production of glucose (Montori et al. 2002). The usual mechanism by which blood glucose is controlled relies on insulin produced by the pancreas. Insulin reduces glucose production by the liver and enhances the uptake of glucose by the skeletal muscle. This assists in the storage of glucose as glycogen or for use in the Krebs cycle for energy production (Robinson and Van Soeren 2004).

In critical illness, uptake of glucose by the peripheries (i.e. skeletal muscle) is reduced (Montori et al. 2002) possibly due to a decrease in exercise-stimulated glucose uptake, as a result of the patients' immobility (Vanhorebeek et al. 2005). This decreased utilisation by the peripheries is known as insulin resistance (Robinson and Van Soeren 2004). This increase in hepatic glucose release and reduced peripheral uptake causes hypergly-caemia despite insulin release from the pancreas. Thus, as a patient in a high-dependency area, Lilly would have raised glucose levels due to her body increasing hepatic glucose production in response to stress and due to her immobility.

Lilly's hyperglycaemia may also be exacerbated by excess calorie provision from dextrose infusions for fluid resuscitation and medication administration. Lipid-based in-fusions such as Propofol contain calories which increase blood glucose levels. Steroids and immunosuppressant drugs can also cause hyperglycaemia (Montori et al. 2002). The hydrocortisone being administered to Lilly will increase hepatic glucose production and decrease glucose utilisation (Neal 2009). Additionally, Lilly's continuous salbutamol neb-ulisers could lead to a reduced level of serum potassium as it causes potassium to shift from the plasma into the cells. This, in turn, will have an effect on glucose levels as these two positive ions exchange with each other.

Effects of hyperglycaemia

When glucose levels rise, the body tries to reduce this by excretion of glucose by the kidneys. Glucose is an osmotic force when in excess, and as it is excreted, it attracts electrolytes such as sodium and potassium to be excreted with it. This leads to a situation whereby the body becomes fluid depleted with electrolyte imbalance. In order to maintain cardiac output, the heart rate will rise and the renal arteries will constrict, attempting to increase glomerular filtration. However, over time as the hyperglycaemia persists, the glomerular filtration rate decreases and the kidneys' ability to excrete glucose and elec-trolytes is also reduced. Renal markers of dysfunction will rise and poor tissue perfusion may cause the release of lactic acid from anaerobic metabolism in the cells (Morton and Fontain 2008). Lilly's blood results are illustrative of the start of renal dysfunction with electrolyte imbalance and poor tissue perfusion, leading to a raised lactate. Acute kidney injury is explained in detail in Chapter 9.

Hyperglycaemia and outcome

Studies on specific groups of patients have found that hyperglycaemia affects outcome. DiNardo et al. (2004) reported altered fluid balance and dehydration from increased uri-nary glucose, and McCowen et al. (2001) found increased inflammation and reduced immune functioning when hyperglycaemia occurred. In patients with myocardial infarc-tion, hyperglycaemia was associated with a higher mortality rate and an increased risk of cardiogenic shock and congestive heart failure (Capes et al. 2000). The first major study looking at critical care patients was performed in 2001 by Van den Berghe et al. This is considered a landmark study. Findings appeared to be so beneficial to critical care patients that study recommendations to control blood glucose levels between 4.5–6.0 mmol/L were adopted worldwide (Wiener et al. 2008). Van den Berghe et al. (2001) found that control-ling blood glucose to within this tight range significantly reduced mortality rates, length of critical care stay, ventilator time, septicaemia and the occurrence of neuropathy. The study was, however, performed solely on surgical patients in a single centre. When the same study was recreated in a medical critical care environment by Van den Berghe et al. in 2006, findings were less conclusive, reporting that critical care stay was reduced in patients who had their blood glucose controlled between 4.5–6.0 mmol/L but no difference was seen in mortality rates or bacteraemia. In patients who stayed in the critical care area for more than five days on intensive insulin therapy, mortality rates were, however, improved.

In another study on a large sample of general critical care patients, Krinsley (2003) found that a blood glucose between 4.4–5.5 mmol/L was significantly associated with reduced mortality. Mortality rates were observed to rise as blood glucose increased until patients with blood sugars exceeding 16.5 mmol/L had a 42.5% mortality rate. The sepsis care bundle also includes tight glucose control of <8.3 mmol/L as the best practice for the treatment of severe sepsis (Dellinger et al. 2008). Despite this evidence the biggest study to date looking at glucose control in a general critical care population found no benefit of keeping glucose between 4.5–6.0 mmol/L and, therefore, could not recommend it as the best practice for critical care patients (Finfer et al. 2009).

Tight glucose control has been found to have improved outcomes in some patient populations but not in all. Falciglia et al. (2009) found that the effects of hyperglycaemia on mortality were different depending on the admission diagnosis. Patients admitted with unstable angina, myocardial infarction and heart failure were found to be more at risk of higher mortality rates in the presence of hyperglycaemia than patients with chronic obstructive airways disease or post-coronary artery bypass graft. It needs to be recognised, therefore, that hyperglycaemia may affect the mortality rates in certain patients, so controlling hyperglycaemia is necessary in order to reduce associated complications in these patient groups. Lilly is therefore started on an infusion of insulin at a concentration of 1 unit/mL, titrated against a sliding scale.

Tests and investigations

Blood glucose testing

Several methods of blood glucose testing are available in the critical care setting. Arterial blood sampling via an arterial catheter is a common procedure to measure levels of oxygen, carbon dioxide, bicarbonate, lactate and electrolytes using a blood gas analyser. Many of the studies performed to look at glucose control used this method for all glucose results (Van den Berghe 2001, 2006; Finfer et al. 2009). This method is considered to be accurate and was found to be the most reliable method of measurement when compared to laboratory testing (Kanji et al. 2005). However, frequent arterial line sampling may increase the risks of air embolus, infection and anaemia in critical care patients (Parsons and Watkinson 2007). Samples must be taken using a non-touch technique and there is some support for closed blood sampling circuits which allow the blood to be returned to the patient to reduce the occurrence of chronic anaemia.

Point-of-care testing using capillary blood sampling and a bedside glucometer (see Figures 7.1, 7.2 and 7.3) would prevent the nurse from having to leave Lilly unattended to use a blood gas analyser for glucose measurements (Parsons and Watkinson 2007). Using capillary sampling, however, has been found to be the least accurate method of measuring glucose levels when compared to laboratory results. Kanji et al. (2005) found that capillary sampling over-estimated blood glucose significantly, and in cases of hypoglycaemia, results using this method agreed with laboratory results only 26.3% of the time. The use of arterial blood for glucometer testing is therefore preferable to capillary blood sampling (Van den Berghe et al. 2006; Finfer et al. 2009), and is thus recommended for use to monitor Lilly's blood glucose levels (Dellinger et al. 2008; Finfer et al. 2009).

Point-of-care testing is commonly used in practice as it is easy to use, is quick and does not require blood to be wasted. Although Lilly's hyperglycaemia was initially discovered on an arterial sample, subsequent measurements were taken using capillary blood on point-of-care equipment at the bedside. This has implications for the accuracy of the measurements obtained.

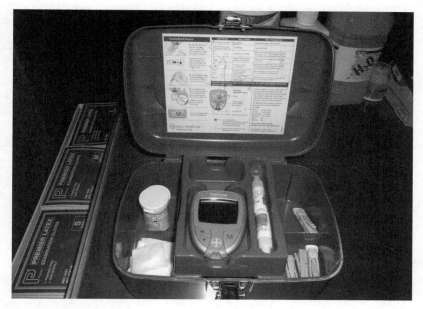

Figure 7.1   Bedside glucometer.

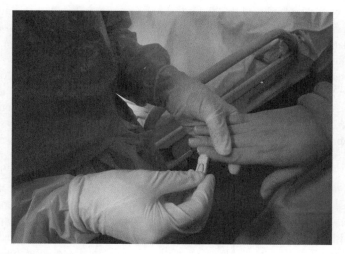

Figure 7.2   Finger pricking.

Methods of controlling blood glucose levels

Insulin infusions are recommended to achieve normoglycaemia. Soluble insulin such as Actrapid has an onset time of 30 minutes (Neal 2009) and can be infused intravenously or subcutaneously. In critical care patients like Lilly, however, the rate of absorption via a subcutaneous route is not predictable due to altered tissue perfusion (DiNardo et al.

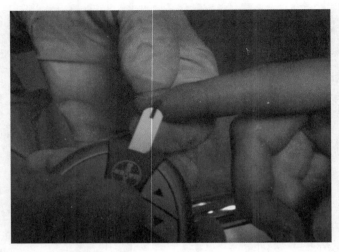

Figure 7.3   Blood glucose testing.

2004). Van den Berghe (2001, 2006) recommends use of a continuous insulin infusion starting at 1 unit/mL to achieve the set targets.

Insulin should be infused along with a glucose calorie source (Dellinger et al. 2008). Ideally, this would be achieved by feeding Lilly, via an enteral route, starting the feeding process as early as possible (Van den Berghe 2006). An intravenous glucose infusion is recommended before feeding is commenced (Van den Berghe et al. 2001) or if enteral nutrition is not being absorbed effectively.

Glucose samples should be taken regularly to achieve the target blood glucose range. A protocol may allow more consistent glucose control and the achievement of target ranges. Brown and Dodek (2001) found that blood glucose levels could be controlled much quicker with the use of a protocol or nomogram than with *ad hoc* sliding scale insulin. This is supported by Krinsley (2004), who found that glucose levels were improved without the occurrence of hypoglycaemia by using a protocol to achieve target levels of glucose.

Many protocols which have been used to control blood glucose levels are nurse led and most suggest intravenous insulin with glucose infusions as the best method to achieve target levels. Depending on the protocol chosen, insulin doses can be titrated within set ranges or with the use of complex calculations to work out the change in insulin infusion rates (see Table 7.2). It is possible that a protocol developed and validated in a specific area will not be appropriate for different patient populations, and therefore, it is important to choose a protocol which has been validated with a similar patient group to the group being treated (Wilson et al. 2007).

The role of the nurse in this process is key to the success of a protocol. Achieving and maintaining Lilly's target level of blood glucose is a time-consuming process for the critical care nurse. It is of paramount importance that they have the knowledge and skills to safely titrate infusions in order to achieve target levels, and that they are trained to use blood glucose testing equipment (Aragon 2006).

Table 7.2 Insulin infusion protocol.

To start Insulin Infusion

Glucose	11.5–14 mmol/L	14.1–17 mmol/L	17.1–20 mmol/L	20.1–24 mmol/L	>24 mmol/L
Bolus and infusion rate	Bolus 3 u and start infusion 2 u/h	Bolus 6 u and start infusion 2 u/h	Bolus 8 u and start infusion 2 u/h	Bolus 10 u and start infusion 2 u/h	Call doctor for order

Ongoing Insulin Infusion

Glucose level	Infusion rate 1–3 ml/h	Infusion rate 4–6 u/h	Infusion rate 7–9 u/h	Infusion rate 10–12 u/h	Infusion rate 13–16 u/h	Infusion rate >16 u/h
<3.5	Stop infusion and give 50% dextrose	Stop infusion and give 50% dextrose	Stop infusion and give 50% dextrose	Stop infusion and give 50% dextrose	Stop infusion and give 50% dextrose	Stop infusion and give 50% dextrose
3.5–4.5	Stop infusion, recheck glucose after 1 h. If >7 mmol/L, restart infusion but decrease rate by 1 u/h	Stop infusion, recheck glucose after 1 h. If >7 mmol/L, restart infusion but decrease rate by 1 u/h	Stop infusion, recheck glucose after 1 h. If >7 mmol/L, restart infusion but decrease rate by 2 u/h	Stop infusion, recheck glucose after 1 h. If >7 mmol/L, restart infusion but decrease rate by 2 u/h	Stop infusion, recheck glucose after 1 h. If >7 mmol/L, restart infusion but decrease rate by 3 u/h	Stop infusion, recheck glucose after 1 h. If >7 mmol/L, restart infusion but decrease rate by 3 u/h
4.6–5.5	Reduce infusion rate by 50%	Reduce infusion rate by 50%	Reduce infusion rate by 50%	Reduce infusion rate by 50%	Reduce infusion rate by 50%	Reduce infusion rate by 50%
5.6–7	Reduce infusion by 1 u/h	Reduce infusion by 2 u/h	Reduce infusion by 3 u/h	Reduce infusion by 4 u/h	Reduce infusion by 5 u/h	Reduce infusion by 6 u/h
7–11.5	No change to regime	No change to regime	No change to regime	No change to regime	No change to regime	No change to regime

Glucose level	Infusion rate 1–5 u/h	Infusion rate 6–10 u/h	Infusion rate 11–16 u/h	Infusion rate >16 u/h
11.6–14	Bolus 2 u and increase infusion by 1 u/h	Bolus 2 u and increase infusion by 2 u/h	Bolus 2 u and increase infusion by 3 u/h	Call doctor for order
14.1–17	Bolus 3 u and increase infusion by 1 u/h	Bolus 5 u and increase infusion by 2 u/h	Bolus 5 u and increase infusion by 3 u/h	Call doctor for order
17.1–20	Bolus 8 u and increase infusion by 1 u/h	Bolus 8 u and increase infusion by 2 u/h	Bolus 8 u and increase infusion by 3 u/h	Call doctor for order
20.1–24	Bolus 10 u and increase infusion by 1 u/h	Bolus 10 u and increase infusion by 2 u/h	Bolus 10 u and increase infusion by 3 u/h	Call doctor for order
>24	Call doctor for order	Call doctor for order	Call doctor for order	Call doctor for order

Source: Adapted from Brown and Dodek (2001).

Developing scenario

Four hours after the insulin infusion is commenced, Lilly complains of feeling lethargic and weak. Two hours later she is found unresponsive, requiring further assessment.

Airway/breathing

Lilly is currently maintaining her own airway but to ensure her airway is protected she is positioned on her side. This also reduces the risk of secretion aspiration (Morton and Fontaine 2008). Oxygen concentrations should be increased to prevent the risk of hypoxia and respiratory rate and saturations should be observed and documented, particularly in view of her admitting diagnosis of acute asthma.

Circulation

A full set of observations are required, looking at her heart rate, blood pressure and perfusion. Lilly is found to be tachycardic with a heart rate of 117 beats per minute and blood pressure 90/49 mmHg, and she is cold and clammy with a capillary refill time of 3 seconds.

Disability

Pupil assessment is essential as there has been a change in neurological status. Lilly is found to have dilated pupils which are reactive to light. She is not responsive to voice but has facial grimacing on painful stimuli. A blood glucose level is required to exclude hypoglycaemia (Resuscitation Council 2006). Using a bedside point of care glucometer, Lilly is found to have blood glucose of 1.9 mmol/L.

Exposure

As there is a risk of seizures when blood glucose levels fall below 2.2 mmol/L, precautions should be made to ensure that the bedside rails are up, that any hazardous objects are removed and that Lilly's safety is of paramount importance. An oral airway and suction must be available in order to ensure airway patency in the event of seizure activity (Sole et al. 2009).

Managing hypoglycaemia

Hypoglycaemia is defined as a blood glucose level of <2.2 mmol/L and is a serious adverse event (Finfer et al. 2009). Hypoglycaemia, as a result of a rapid decrease in blood glucose levels, can have symptoms of tachycardia; palpitations; pale, cool and clammy skin; and dilated pupils. The level of consciousness may decrease profoundly and seizure activity can be seen. If Lilly's hypoglycaemia is prolonged or left untreated, coma and brain damage could occur (Sole et al. 2009).

Lilly's risk of hypoglycaemia would be increased as her nutritional intake is likely to have been inadequate due to her distress. The hypoglycaemia could also be due to appropriate adjustments in her insulin infusion not being made by the nurses. Risks will be further increased if she has sepsis, inotropic support or a prior diagnosis of diabetes mellitus (Vriesendrop et al. 2006).

Treatment of Lilly's hypoglycaemia must be quickly addressed with intravenous glucose and levels should be measured 15–20 minutes after the treatment is given. Insulin infusions should be stopped at this time and observations taken regularly to assess both neurological status and vital signs (Sole et al. 2009). 20% Dextrose is recommended in a 50 mL bolus, given into a large vein through a large-bore needle. 50% Dextrose can also be used in 25 mL bolus; however, this can be more difficult to administer due to the viscosity of the solution (British National Formulary 2009).

Hypoglycaemia has been found to occur in studies looking at tight glucose control and may now be seen as an independent risk factor for death (Van den Berghe 2006). Even one episode of hypoglycaemia has been linked to increased risk of patient mortality (Krinsley and Grover 2007). Trying to maintain a glucose level within such tight limits and administering infusions of insulin increases the risk of hypoglycaemia (Brunkhorst et al. 2008). For this reason, the NICE-SUGAR study (Finfer et al. 2009) could not recommend such a tight glucose limit and extended the acceptable levels to 8–10 mmol/L to avoid these complications.

Conclusion

It is apparent that hyperglycaemia is linked to increased mortality in certain critical care patient populations. Tight blood glucose control with insulin, using a protocol, is successful at reducing blood glucose levels, and has been found in some studies to improve outcome; however, the risk of hypoglycaemia must not be overlooked. Insulin infusions must run concurrently with adequate nutrition and dextrose infusions if nutrition is not able to be commenced or if absorption is poor.

The critical care nurse has an essential role in performing blood glucose monitoring, understanding the uses and limitations of the equipment, and titrating both insulin and dextrose infusions appropriately. These significantly affect the workload of the critical care nurse, and therefore, education and teaching programmes must ensure that nurses have a full understanding of the purpose of blood glucose monitoring and its impact on the morbidity and mortality of critically ill patients. Whilst the exact range of ideal blood glucose levels is yet to be decided upon in the literature, it is evident that controlling levels between 4.5–6.0 mmol/L increases the risk of hypoglycaemic events. Equally, raised blood glucose levels of >10 mmol/L has an adverse impact on survival in some patient populations. Therefore, each critical care unit should define a blood glucose range which can be achieved for their patients without risking either extreme.

Key learning points

- Hyperglycaemia is a common occurrence in patients with critical illness.
- Hyperglycaemia of >10 mmol/L is associated with poor outcome and increased complications such as infection and increased length of critical care stay.

- Tight glucose control with intensive insulin can improve survival in some patient groups but may also increase the risk of hypoglycaemia.
- Hypoglycaemia can be considered an independent risk factor for poor survival.
- The method of glucose testing may impact on the accuracy of the results, with capillary sampling and point-of-care testing having the lowest accuracy when compared with laboratory testing.
- Protocols allow more control over blood glucose levels, although the choice of protocol must be made carefully based on the population it was designed for and validated on.
- There is no currently agreed level within which blood glucose levels should be maintained. However, the majority of research agrees that keeping blood glucose <10 mmol/L avoids both hyper- and hypoglycaemia.

Critical appraisal of a research paper

Aragon D (2006) Evaluation of nursing workload and perceptions about blood glucose testing and tight glucose control. *American Journal of Critical Care* **15**(4), 370–377.

This single-centre, observational and exploratory study uses time and motion studies to analyse the impact of blood glucose monitoring on nursing workload. It also uses a survey to identify nurses' opinions of blood glucose testing and tight glucose control. A total of 21 observations were made to ascertain the average time taken to obtain a blood glucose level and adjust insulin infusions. It was concluded that the average time needed every hour for this activity was 4.72 minutes.

The survey was completed by 66 nurses (54% response rate). Nurses agreed that glucose measurements were important, but many found that regular blood glucose measurements and point of care testing impacted on their work load and were time consuming. Most were in agreement that a continuous or automated way of measuring blood glucose was needed.

Reader activities

- Read the research article by Aragon (2006).
- Using the critical appraisal framework in Appendix I, consider the methodological quality of the paper.
- Consider the findings of this paper and reflect on the current practice in your clinical environment. What implications does it have for your own practice?

A commentary on this paper has been provided by the chapter author in Appendix VIII.

References

Aragon D (2006) Evaluation of nursing work effort and perceptions about blood glucose testing in tight glycaemic control. *American Journal of Critical Care* **15**(4), 370–377.

British National Formulary (BNF) (2009) British Medical Association and The Royal Pharmaceutical Society of Great Britain, London.

Brown G, Dodek P (2001) Intravenous insulin nomogram improves blood glucose control in the critically ill. *Critical Care Medicine* **29**(9), 1714–1719.

Brunkhorst FM, Engel C, Bloos F, Meier-Hellmann A, Ragaller M, Weiler N, Moerer O, Gruendling M, Oppert M, Grond S, Olthoff D, Jaschinski U, John S, Rossaint R, Welte T, Schaefer M, Kern P, Kuhnt E, Kiehntopf M, Hartog C, Natanson C, Loeffler M, Reinhart K (2008) Intensive insulin therapy and pentastarch. Resuscitation in severe sepsis. *The New England Journal of Medicine* **358**(2), 125–139.

Capes SE, Hunt D, Malmberg K (2000) Stress hyperglycaemia and increased risk of death after myocardial infarction in patients with and without diabetes: a systematic overview. *Lancet* **355**, 773–778.

Dellinger RP, Levy MM, Carlet JM, Bion J, Parker MM, Jaeschke R, Reinhart K, Angus DC, Brun Buisson C, Beale R, Calandra T, Dhainaut JF, Gerlach H, Harvey M, Marini JJ, Marshall J. Ranieri M, Ramsey G, Sevransky J, Thompson BT, Towbsend S, Venders JS, Zimmerman JL, Vincent JL (2008) Surviving sepsis campaign: international guidelines for management of severe sepsis and septic shock. *Intensive Care Medicine* **34**, 17–60.

Devos P, Preiser JC (2004) Tight blood glucose control: a recommendation applicable to any critically ill patient? *Critical Care* **8**, 427–429.

DiNardo MM, Korytkowski MT, Siminerio LS (2004) The importance of normoglycaemia in critically ill patients. *Critical Care Nurse Quarterly* **27**(2), 126–134.

Falciglia M, Freyberg RW, Almenoff PL, D'Alessio DA, Render ML (2009) Hyperglycaemia-related mortality in critically ill patients varies with admission diagnosis. *Critical Care Medicine* **37**(12), 3001–3009.

Finfer S, Chittock DR, YuShuo Su S, Blair D, Foster D, Dhingra V, Bellomo R, Cook D, Dodek P, Henderson WR, Herbert PC, Heritier S, Heyland DK, McArthur C, McDonald E, Mitchell I, Mybergh JA, Norton R, Potter J, Robinson BG, Ronce JJ (2009) Intensive versus conventional glucose control in critically ill patients. *The New England Journal of Medicine* **360**, 1283–1297.

Kanji S, Buffie J, Hutton B, Bunting PS, Singh A, McDonald K, Fergusson D, McIntyre LA, Herbert PC (2005) Reliability of point of care testing for glucose measurement in critically ill adults. *Critical Care Medicine* **33**(12), 2778–2785.

Krinsley JS (2003) Association between hyperglycaemia and increased hospital mortality in a heterogenous population of critically ill patients. *Mayo Clinic Proceedings* **78**, 1471–1478.

Krinsley JS (2004) Effect of an intensive glucose management protocol on the mortality of critically ill adult patients. *Mayo Clinic Proceedings* **79**(8), 992–1000.

Krinsley JS, Grover A (2007) Severe hypoglycaemia in critically ill patients: risk factors and outcomes. *Critical Care Medicine* **35**(10), 2262–2267.

McCowen KC, Malhotra A, Bistrian BR (2001) Stress induced hyperglycaemia. *Critical Care Clinics* **17**, 107–124.

Merz TM, Finfer S (2008) Pro/con debate: is intensive insulin therapy targeting tight blood glucose control of benefit in critically ill patients? *Critical Care* **12**(2), 212–217.

Montori VM, Bistrian BR, McMahon MM (2002) Hyperglycaemia in acutely ill patients. *JAMA* **288**(17), 2167–2169.

Morton PG, Fontaine D (2008) *Critical Care Nursing – A Holistic Approach*, 9th edn. Lippincott Williams and Wilkins, Philadelphia.

Neal MJ (2009) *Medical Pharmacology at a Glance*, 6th edn. Blackwell Science, Singapore.

Parsons P, Watkinson P (2007) Blood glucose control in critical care patient – a review of the literature. *Nursing in Critical Care* **12**(4), 202–210.

Resuscitation Council (2006) *Immediate Life Support*, 2nd edn. Resuscitation Council (UK), London.

Robinson LE, Van Soeren MH (2004) Insulin resistance and hyperglycaemia in critical illness – role of insulin in glycaemic control. *AACN Clinical Issues* **15**(1), 45–62.

Sole ML, Klein DB, Mosely MJ (2009) *Critical Care Nursing*, 5th edn. Saunders Elsevier, London.

Van Den Berghe G, Wouters P, Weekers F, Verwaest C, Bruyninckx F, Shetz M, Vlasselaers D, Ferdinande P, Lauwers P, Bouillon R (2001) Intensive insulin therapy in critically ill patients. *The New England Journal of Medicine* **345**(19), 1359–1367.

Van Den Berghe G, Wilmer A, Hermans G, Meersseman W, Wouters PJ, Milants I, Van Wijngaerden E, Bobbaers H, Bouillon R (2006) Intensive insulin therapy in the medical ICU. *The New England Journal of Medicine* **354**(5), 449–461.

Vanhorebeek I, Langouche L, Van den Berghe G (2005) Glycemic and nonglycaemic effects of insulin: how do they contribute to a better outcome of critical illness? *Current Opinion in Critical Care* **11**, 304–311.

Vriesendorp TM, Van Santen S, DeVries JH, De Jonge E, Rosendaal FR, Schultz MJ, Hoeskstra J (2006) Predisposing factors for hypoglycaemia in the intensive care unit. *Critical Care Medicine* **34**(1), 96–101.

Wiener RS, Wiener DC, Larson RJ (2008) Benefits and risks of tight glucose control in critically ill adults. *JAMA* **300**(8), 933–936.

Wilson M, Weiner J, Soo Hoo GW (2007) Intensive insulin therapy in critical care. *Diabetes Care* **30**(4), 1005–1011.

Chapter 8

The patient with increased abdominal pressure

Suzanne Bench

Introduction

Increased intra-abdominal pressure (IAP) can cause intra-abdominal hypertension (IAH), which can lead to life-threatening sequelae. This scenario focuses on the knowledge and skills necessary to manage a patient with suspected IAH.

Patient scenario

Ludwik Borkowski is a 58-year-old man admitted with severe pancreatitis. Initial assessment information can be seen in Table 8.1.

A decision is made to intubate and ventilate Mr Borkowski, and to institute aggressive fluid resuscitation. However, six hours later his respiratory and renal conditions significantly deteriorate. The consultant asks that an IAP measurement be taken. The initial recording is 18 mmHg. He is then taken to theatre for an emergency laparotomy.

Table 8.1 Initial assessment information.

Respiratory	Respiratory rate	32 bpm (shallow)
	On auscultation breath sounds are significantly reduced bi-basally.	
Arterial blood gas	Hypoxaemia and a mixed respiratory and metabolic acidaemia on 60% facemask oxygen	
Cardiovascular	Blood pressure	100/60 mmHg
	Heart rate (HR)	125 bpm
	Central venous pressure (CVP)	8 mmHg
	Core temperature	37.7°C
	Urine output 20–30 mL/h – dark and concentrated	
Laboratory data	Lactate	2.2 mmol/L
	Albumin	19
	Amylase	105
	WCC	21×10^9/L
	CRP	262 mg/L

Critical Care Nursing: Learning from Practice, 1st edition. Edited by Suzanne Bench and Kate Brown.
© 2011 Blackwell Publishing Ltd.

Reader activities

Having read this scenario, consider the following:

- For what reasons might the consultant have requested IAP measurements? Consider how a valid measurement might be obtained.
- Consider the rationale for an emergency laparotomy in this scenario.
- Why was it necessary to intubate and ventilate Mr Borkowski?
- What concerns might you have regarding the renal function of Mr Borkowski?

Pathophysiology related to increased intra-abdominal pressure

Normal IAP is 05 mmHg (Brush 2007b). Abdominal compartment syndrome (ACS) is a condition caused by an increase in abdominal pressure, referred to as intra-abdominal hypertension (IAH) (Walker and Criddle 2003). Physiological compromise starts when the pressure rises above 12 mmHg (Brush 2007b). Once pressures reach 20 mmHg, irreversible tissue ischemia occurs and organ function is compromised (World Society of Abdominal Compartment Syndrome (WSACS) 2009). As Mr Borkowski's IAP is already 18 mmHg, he is at significant risk. At this point the abdomen often looks distended, and can feel rigid and tense on palpation (see Figure 8.1).

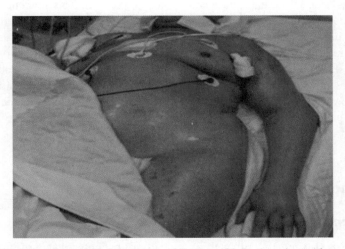

Figure 8.1   Rigid abdomen. (Photo courtesy of Dr Manu Malbrain, adapted from Deeren DH, Zachée P, Malbrain MLNG (2005) Granulocyte colony-stimulating factor-induced capillary leak syndrome confirmed by extravascular lung water measurements. *Annals of Hematology* **84**(2), 89–94.)

The main cause of IAH is reduced gut perfusion, causing capillary endothelial damage and cellular ischemia, leading to further secondary damage (Walker and Criddle 2003). Large amounts of interstitial fluid can accumulate, due to loss of integrity of the capillary membrane causing the abdominal wall to expand. As compliance reduces, the pressure within the abdominal cavity rises, causing occlusion of capillary blood flow and compromise of venous return and arterial flow (Wolfe 2009). This worsens the ischemia, triggering a vicious cycle leading to further increases in IAH.

Any patient with a severe inflammatory response can develop IAH. Patients who have suffered direct peritoneal or retroperitoneal injury from trauma, surgery or inflammation are also at risk (Wolfe 2009). Pancreatitis, the diagnosis for Mr Borkowski, is a recognised cause, as is bowel obstruction (Tiwari et al. 2006). Sepsis is also often associated with IAH due to uncontrolled inflammation. Obese patients with a body mass index >45 kg/m^2 are also at high risk, particularly when placed in the supine position (Brush 2007a).

A high IAP compromises the function of a number of other organs. The kidneys are affected by direct renal artery compression, and because of central venous compression. Once the IAP exceeds central venous pressure (CVP), preload is reduced, lowering cardiac output and arterial blood pressure, thus reducing perfusion to the kidneys (Wolfe 2009). The effects of this can be seen in Mr Borkowski's haemodynamic and renal data. This would also partly explain the metabolic acidaemia as being related to the development of acute tubular necrosis (Brush 2007a). The production of lactic acid related to cellular hypoxia would be another contributing factor explaining this metabolic picture.

The pulmonary effects of IAH are largely mechanical. As the pressure under the diaphragm increases, there is an increased work of breathing resulting in rapid shallow breathing, as seen in the data presented for Mr Borkowski. This reduction in alveolar ventilation causes atelectasis and a resultant V/Q mismatch, and this has demonstrated itself in the blood gas analysis results revealing hypoxaemia, hypercarbia and a respiratory acidaemia (Brush 2007a). This might necessitate the use of ventilatory support for Mr Borkowski. The high peak inspiratory pressures required to maintain adequate tidal volumes, however, increases the risk of barotrauma, volutrauma, biotrauma and acute lung injury (Wolfe 2009). IAH can also contribute to a rise in the intracranial pressure of susceptible patients as cerebral venous return becomes obstructed (Walker and Criddle 2003; Brush 2007a; Wolfe 2009).

Tests and investigations

Intra-abdominal pressure monitoring

Normal IAP is 0–5 mmHg, although in critically ill patients a value of up to 7 mmHg is acceptable (WSACS 2009). Mr Borkowski should be assessed for signs of IAH. The WSACS (2009) recommends that all critically ill patients should be screened for signs of IAH, and that a baseline IAP recorded when two or more of the risk factors for ACS are present. In the presence of IAH, the WSACS (2009) recommend that serial measurements should be taken throughout the period of critical illness (see Figure 8.2).

Recognising higher levels of IAP is vital to prevent the above sequelae from developing. Traditionally, this was done by clinical observation of the abdomen, monitoring for

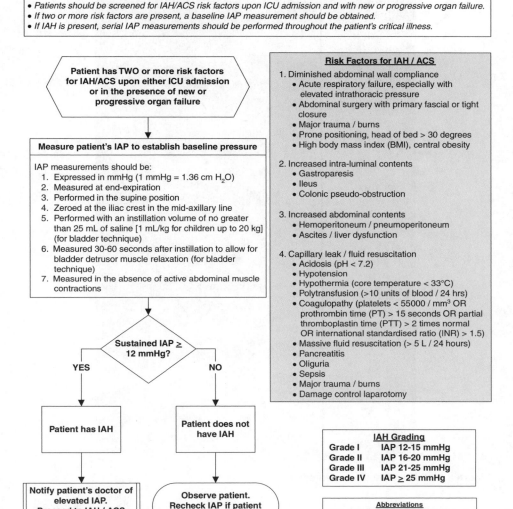

Figure 8.2　Intra-abdominal hypertension (IAH) assessment algorithm. (Algorithm courtesy of the World Society of the Abdominal Compartment Syndrome (WSACS).)

signs of tautness, often combined with girth measurements if concern was apparent. These subjective assessments have, however, more recently been shown to be unreliable determinants of IAP (Kirkpatrick et al. 2000; Sugrue et al. 2002), and more direct measurements of IAP are now available.

There are a number of different methods that can be utilised to measure IAP, but the most common approach currently in use is via an indwelling urinary catheter. This can be done using either a fluid manometer set (see Figures 8.3 and 8.4) or a transducer

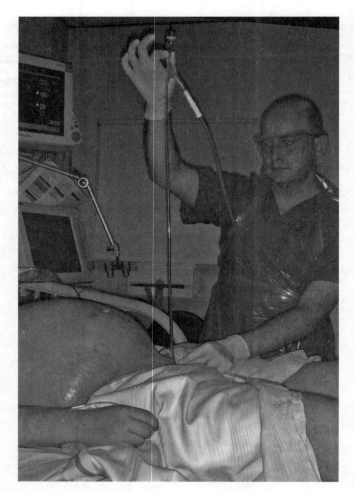

Figure 8.3   Foley catheter measurement.

system (Harrahill 1998; Brush 2007b). A good overview of the range of methods and their potential advantages and limitations can be found in Malbrain (2004).

A number of recent studies have tried to determine which method of IAP measurement is the most valid and reliable (e.g. De Waele et al. 2004; Peters et al. 2004; Kimball et al. 2009) but still no consensus has been reached. The review by Malbrain (2004) concluded that there is no gold standard, but that in critically ill patients it may be preferable to use a continuous rather than an intermittent system. Some of the problems with accurate measurement have been found to be related to human error (Wolfe and Kimball 2004a), whilst others have been linked to choosing the optimal amount of fluid for priming of the circuit (Wolfe and Kimball 2004b). Malbrain (2004) discusses the optimal amount of fluid for bladder priming prior to IAP monitoring, with reference to studies suggesting that 50–100 mL of fluid is required for optimal performance (Gudmundsson et al. 2002; Verbrugghe et al. 2003). The WSACS (2009) suggests that volumes should be no more

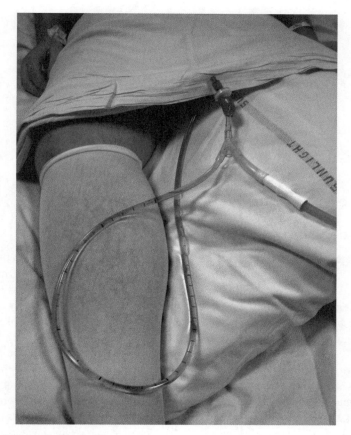

Figure 8.4   Foley catheter *in situ*.

than 25 mL, and comments that higher volumes may actually lead to overestimation of the IAP.

Developing scenario

Mr Borkowski returns from theatre three hours later. A laparotomy revealed a necrotic pancreas with peri-pancreatic involvement. His abdomen has been left open for pressure relief (Figure 8.5) and he is being ventilated on synchronised intermittent mandatory ventilation (volume control) with pressure support.

Managing the patient with an open abdomen

The WSACS (2009) has produced an algorithm to guide the management of patients with IAH (see Figure 8.6).

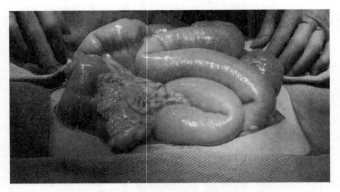

Figure 8.5   Open abdomen. (Photo courtesy of KCI Licensing Inc.)

Airway and breathing

As an intubated patient, Mr Borkowski should be nursed in accordance with the ventilator care bundle (Pruitt and Jacobs 2006). Further details of these aspects of management can be found in Chapter 1. Compliance of the chest wall can be improved by attention to positioning, with the goal being to allow the diaphragm to move freely. Raising the head of the bed to >20° can significantly increase IAP due to abdominal splinting of the diaphragm, and use of the reverse Trendelenberg position is therefore advocated by authors such as Cheatham (2009). Positioning Mr Borkowski could also be problematic for a variety of other reasons, including post-operative pain and the size of the abdomen. The nurse should ensure that his work of breathing is adequately supported by the use of appropriate ventilation settings of both mandatory and pressure supported breaths. Airway pressures should be closely monitored and should start to reduce as the pressure from the abdomen is lessened. Neuromuscular blockade (paralysing) agents may also be prescribed to improve abdominal wall compliance and thus facilitate effective ventilation if the IAP continues to be high (Cheatham 2009).

Circulation

Mr Borkowski will need close monitoring for signs of sepsis (see Chapter 4). Large fluid losses are likely due to the open abdomen and fluid management will need to be carefully planned with this in mind. In addition to fluids, early nutritional support will maximise wound-healing potential, help prevent sepsis and aid weaning from ventilation. This is best achieved by the use of the enteral route (Kreymann et al. 2006) and may require the use of prokinetic agents. A bowel protocol should be instigated to ensure abdominal pressures are not further increased by impacted faeces. If enteral feed cannot be tolerated, then parenteral nutrition should be commenced.

Disability of the nervous system

Effective analgesia and sedation are vital components of Mr Borkowski's management (see Chapters 10 and 11), and will help to reduce muscle tone and thus improve abdominal

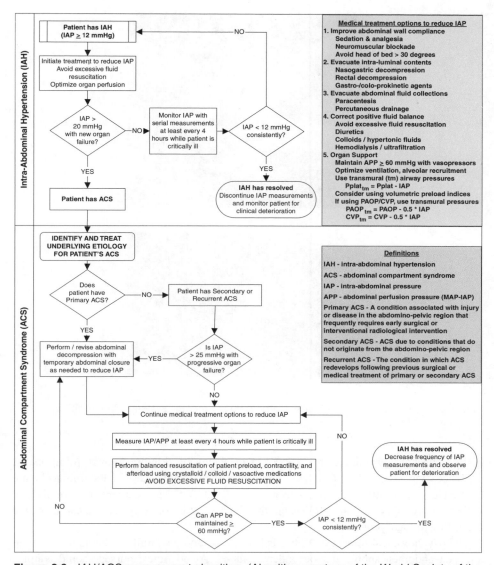

Figure 8.6 IAH/ACS management algorithm. (Algorithm courtesy of the World Society of the Abdominal Compartment Syndrome (WSACS).)

compliance (Cheatham 2009). Appropriate use, titrated against agreed targets and goals, will also aid early weaning from ventilation and help prevent the occurrence of secondary sepsis (see Chapter 4).

Exposure/environment

The use of a vacuum assisted closure (VAC$^{®}$) therapy system for managing the open abdomen will help to ensure that fluid losses can be monitored (see Figures 8.7a and

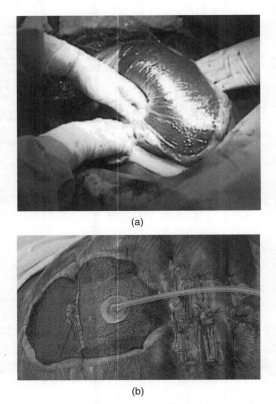

(a)

(b)

Figure 8.7 (a) VAC® dressing application. (b) VAC® therapy system. (Photos courtesy of KCI Licensing Inc.)

8.7b). Its use will also reduce the risks of exudate causing skin breakdown. Additionally, evidence suggests that the use of VAC® improves the rate of successful abdominal closure and reduces mortality (Boele van hensbrook et al. 2009). Critical care nurses should liaise with tissue viability specialists to ensure that the system is correctly applied and managed according to local protocols.

The psychological impact on both Mr Borkowski and his family of being nursed with an open abdomen should not be underestimated. At all times, nurses should adopt a sensitive approach to his management, respecting his privacy and taking active steps to help acceptance of this temporary condition. Accurate and consistent information will help them to understand the rationale for leaving the abdomen open and the plans for ongoing management.

Conclusion

This scenario has discussed the complex challenges associated with the care of a patient with IAH. The condition does not just affect the abdominal system and a holistic approach to management is imperative.

Key learning points

- IAH and ACS can occur in a variety of critically ill patients.
- All patients admitted to critical care should be screened for IAH.
- Patients with IAP >12 mmHg should have their IAP measured every 4–6 hours or continuously.
- Therapy should be aimed at keeping IAP <15 mmHg, thus reducing risks of tissue ischaemia and organ dysfunction.

Critical appraisal of research paper

Kimball E, Baragoshi G, Mone M, Hansen H, Adams D, Alder S, Jackson P, Cannon P, Horn J, Wolfe T (2009) A comparison of infusion volumes in the measurement of intra-abdominal pressure. *Journal of Intensive Care Medicine* **24**(4), 261–268.

This recent prospective cohort study investigated the effects on intra-abdominal pressure of using infusion volumes of 10–60 mL (in increments of 10 mL). These were then compared to IAP measurements using standard local practice guidelines of 50 mL. It was conducted on 18 adult surgical intensive care patients in the United States who required IAP measurement. Three to 24 sets of measurements were taken per patient using the AbViser bladder measurement system, according to a protocol, which was designed by the investigators. Results revealed a clinically insignificant increase in mean IAP as the infusion volume increased from 10–60 mL (9.3 mmHg compared to 11 mmHg). There were also a few incidences of substantial IAP rises during data collection related to patient agitation, valsalva movements or ventilator dys-synchrony. Sensitivity and specificity for the diagnosis of IAH using each of the infusion volumes were also assessed. Lower infusion volumes were shown to moderately increase sensitivity but notably decreased specificity. Higher cut-off volumes were shown to have the opposite effect. Authors concluded that volumes between 10 and 60 mL are safe and do not significantly increase IAP, but volumes between 10 and 30 mL are sufficient and may help to avoid overestimation of the IAP.

Reader activities

1. Read the research article written by Kimball et al. (2009).
2. Using the critical appraisal framework in Appendix I, consider the methodological quality of the paper.
3. Reflect on this aspect of your own practice and the implications for future practice management that this paper arises.

A commentary on this paper has been provided by the chapter author in Appendix IX.

References

Boele van Hensbroek P, Wind J, Dijkgraaf MG, Busch OR, Carel Gsolings J (2009) Temporary closure of the open abdomen: a systematic review on delayed primary fascial closure in patients with an open abdomen. *World Journal of Surgery* **33**(2), 199–207.

Brush K (2007a) Abdominal compartment syndrome. The pressure is on. *Nursing* **37**(7), 36–41.

Brush K (2007b) Measuring intra-abdominal pressure. *Nursing* **37**(7), 42–44.

Cheatham ML (2009) Nonoperative management of intraabdominal hypertension and abdominal compartment syndrome. *World Journal of Surgery* **33**(6), 1116–1122.

De Waele J, Hoste E, Blot S, Decruyenaere J (2004) Bladder compliance and intra-abdominal pressure measurement in critically ill patients. In: Surgical Research; World Congress on Abdominal Compartment Syndrome, Queensland, Australia, December 2004: selected abstracts (www.wsacs.org). *ANZ Journal of Surgery* **75**, A1–A24.

Gudmundsson F, Viste A, Gislason H, Svanes K (2002) Comparison of different methods for measuring intra-abdominal pressure. *Intensive Care Medicine* **28**, 509–514.

Harrahill M (1998) Intra-abdominal pressure monitoring. *Trauma Notebook* **24**(5), 465–466.

Kimball E, Baragoshi G, Mone M, Hansen H, Adams D, Alder S, Jackson P, Cannon P, Horn J, Wolfe T (2009) A comparison of infusion volumes in the measurement of intra-abdominal pressure. *Journal of Intensive Care Medicine* **24**(4), 261–268.

Kirkpatrick AW, Brenneman FD, McLean RF, Rapanos T, Boulanger BR (2000) Is clinical examination an accurate indicator of raised intra-abdominal pressure in critical patients? *Canadian Journal of Surgery* **43**, 207–211.

Kreymann KG, Berger MM, Deutz NEP, Hiesmayer M, Jolliet P, Kazandjiev G, Nitenberg G, Van Den Berghe G, Wernerman J, Ebner C, Hartl W, Heyman C, Spies C (2006) ESPEN guidelines on enteral nutrition-intensive care. *Clinical Nutrition* **25**(2), 210–223.

Malbrain M (2004) Different techniques to measure intra-abdominal pressure (IAP); time for a critical re-appraisal. *Intensive Care Medicine* **30**, 357–371.

Peters K, Jones F, Sugrue M, Bauman A, Parr M, Balogh Z (2004) How reliable in intra-abdominal pressure measurement in intensive care? In: Surgical Research; World Congress on Abdominal Compartment Syndrome, Queensland, Australia, December 2004: selected abstracts (www.wsacs.org). *ANZ Journal of Surgery* **75**, A1–A24.

Pruitt B, Jacobs M (2006) Best practice interventions: How can you prevent ventilator associated pneumonia? *Nursing* **36**(2), 36–41.

Sugrue M, Bauman A, Jones F *et al.* (2002) Clinical examination is an inaccurate predictor of intraabdominal pressure. *World Journal of Surgery* **26**, 1428–1431.

Tiwari A, Myint F, Hamilton G (2006) Recognition and management of abdominal compartment syndrome in the United Kingdom. *Intensive Care Medicine* **32**, 906–909.

Verbrugghe W, Van Mieghem N, Daelemans R, Lins R, Malbrain M (2003) Estimating the optimal bladder volume for intra-abdominal pressure measurement by bladder pressure volume curves. *Critical Care* **7**(Suppl. 2), 184.

Walker J, Criddle L (2003) Pathophysiology and management of abdominal compartment syndrome. *American Journal of Critical Care* **12**(4), 367–371.

Wolfe T (2009) Intra-abdominal hypertension and abdominal compartment syndrome (powerpoint presentation). Available online at: http://www.abdominalcompartmentsyndrome.com/. Accessed 9 December 2009.

Wolfe T, Kimball T (2004a) Infusion volumes between 20 and 100 ml do not affect IAP measurement accuracy in a controlled IAP/IAH model. In: Surgical Research: World Congress on Abdominal Compartment Syndrome, Queensland, Australia, December 2004: selected abstracts (www.wsacs.org). *ANZ Journal of Surgery* **75**, A1–A24.

Wolfe T, Kimball T (2004b) Bladder pressure measurement with manometry: infusion volumes and human error significantly affect IAP measurement accuracy in a controlled IAP/IAH model. In Surgical Research; World Congress on abdominal compartment syndrome, Queensland, Australia, December 2004: selected abstracts (www.wsacs.org). *ANZ Journal of Surgery* **75**, A1–A24.

WSASC (2009) World Society of the Abdominal Compartment Syndrome. Available online at: http://www.wsacs.org./. Accessed 9 December 2009.

Chapter 9

The patient with an acute kidney injury

Annette Davies and Suzanne Bench

Introduction

Acute kidney injury (AKI) is a common problem in the hospitalised patient, with an incidence of 25% and a mortality rate of up to 70% for those admitted to an intensive care unit (ICU) (Hall and Esser 2008). NCEPOD (2009) highlights the importance of early recognition and effective management of such patients. This scenario focuses on a patient presenting with AKI in a high-dependency unit (HDU) who goes on to require renal replacement therapy (RRT) in an ICU.

Scenario

Elizabeth James is a 48-year-old schoolteacher admitted to HDU 12 hours ago with community-acquired pneumonia. Past medical history includes regular migraines for which she takes ibuprofen. Despite 12 hours of intravenous (IV) antibiotics, her condition is deteriorating. Significant features of her clinical presentation can be seen in Table 9.1.

Reader activities

Having read this scenario, consider the following:

- What aspects of Elizabeth's assessment would make you think she has AKI?
- What do you think is the cause of Elizabeth's AKI?
- Considering the Acute Dialysis Quality Initiative (ADQI) AKI staging, what stage do you consider Elizabeth to have presented with and why?
- What do you consider to be the priorities for her management?

Definitions of kidney injury

Acute kidney injury (AKI) is a clinical syndrome characterised by a rapid reduction in renal excretory function underpinned by a variety of causes. It is one of the most common

Critical Care Nursing: Learning from Practice, 1st edition. Edited by Suzanne Bench and Kate Brown.
© 2011 Blackwell Publishing Ltd.

Table 9.1 Patient clinical assessment data

Cardiovascular	Blood pressure 90/40 mmHg (MABP 58 mmHg) Pulse 105 bpm Sinus rhythm Temperature 38.5°C
Respiratory	Self-ventilating on 0.35 FiO_2 (35%) via a face mask Respiratory rate 18 bpm SpO_2 97%
Arterial blood gas	pH 7.32 PaO_2 11 kPa $PaCO_2$ 5.2 kPa HCO_3^- 20 mmol/L Base excess −4
Input/output	Urine output 100 mL in last 6 h (weighs 60 kg) Oral intake 400 mL since midnight (8 h) Intravenous input 150 mL (IV antibiotics)
Drug history	Ibuprofen as required
Laboratory results	Creatinine 125 µmol/L Urea 18 mmol/L Potassium 5 mmol/L Sodium 146 mmol/L Hb 12.5 g/dL WCC 15 000 CRP 12 mg/L Lactate 2.3 mmol/L

secondary problems seen within critical care (Kellum et al. 2007). The term AKI replaces the long-standing term acute renal failure (ARF) (Ostermann and Chang 2007). The Acute Kidney Injury Network (AKIN) diagnostic criterion for AKI is an abrupt (within 48 hours) reduction in kidney function currently defined as an absolute increase in serum creatinine (SCr) of either ≥ 26.4µmol/L or a percentage increase of $\geq 50\%$ (1.5-fold from baseline) with or without oliguria (documented as <0.5 mL/kg/h for >6 hours).

The original AKI classification system known by the acronym RIFLE was proposed by the ADQI group (Bellomo et al. 2004). It was designed to be a simple and readily available tool. More recently, this classification has been updated by the AKIN group (Mehta et al. 2007) (see Table 9.2). The three new stages (1–3) map to the original first three stages of RIFLE, and define the grades of increasing severity of AKI based on changes in both SCr and urine output from a known baseline. The 'loss' and 'end-stage kidney disease' (ESKD) categories (from the original RIFLE classification) can be seen as outcomes, with 'Loss' being defined as a need for RRT for more than 4 weeks and ESKD where dialysis is required for longer than 3 months (Bellomo et al. 2004). Patients receiving RRT are automatically classified as being in AKIN stage 3 (Table 9.2).

There a number of problems related to the use of this classification system. Firstly, a significant number of patients are admitted without any baseline measurement of renal function, although Ostermann and Chang (2007) argue this can be overcome by assuming a normal baseline level. Additionally, not all patients will be catheterised thus output cannot be measured. Further, the sensitivity and specificity of the classification system

Table 9.2 AKIN AKI staging

AKIN stage	Serum creatinine (SCr)	Urine output	RIFLE criteria
1	Increase in SCr ≥ 26.4 μmol/L or increase in SCr ≥150–200% (1.5 to 2-fold) from baseline	<0.5 mL/kg/h for >6 h	Risk
2	Increase in SCr > 200–300% (2 to 3-fold) from baseline	<0.5mL/kg/h for >12 h	Injury
3	Increase in SCr >300% (>3-fold) from baseline or SCr ≥354 μmol/L with an acute rise of ≥44 μmol/L in ≤24 h	<0.3 mL/kg/h for 24 h or anuria for 12 h	Failure
			Loss End stage

Source: Adapted from Mehta et al. (2007).

will be lost when diuretics are used (Ricci et al. 2008). These factors need to be taken into account during their use.

Patients are staged based on the worst value: creatinine or urine output. As her urine output is <0.5 mL/kg/h, despite not knowing her baseline creatinine, Elizabeth can be placed at stage II (see Table 9.2).

The pathophysiology of acute kidney injury

The first priority of management is to detect early signs of kidney failure (NCEPOD 2009). Elizabeth's urine output has significantly decreased and she has passed only 100 mL in the last 6 hours (<20 mL/h). A urine output of 0.5mL/kg/h (30 mL/h) is required for Elizabeth to achieve adequate clearance of nitrogenous waste products, which, over 6 hours, would be 180 mL. Also her SCr is 125 μmol/L, a 1.5 times increase from her normal baseline (see the section 'Tests and investigations' below). Elizabeth's sodium and urea are also raised, and she has a metabolic acidaemia. This data could suggest hypovolaemia with or without kidney impairment.

The causes of AKI are classically divided into pre-kidney, intrinsic and post-kidney. The relative incidence of each of these is dependent on age, gender and clinical setting. Pre-kidney refers to a reduction in perfusion pressure. This can be due to a low cardiac output, caused by poor contractility, intravascular volume depletion or systemic vasodilation. In their multi-national study, Uchino et al. (2005) found the commonest contributing factor to ARF within the critical care environment to be hypovolaemia secondary to septic shock. Pre-kidney injury can also be caused by constriction of the afferent arteriole due to stress, drug use, for example, NSAIDs and/or the normal compensatory response initiated due to nitric oxide induced vasodilation (e.g. during sepsis) (Armitage and Thomson 2003). This leads to a kidney perfusion pressure below the auto-regulatory level required. What this level is will be determined by a number of individual factors such as age, ethnicity and pre-morbid status. However, a mean arterial blood pressure (MABP) up to 80 mmHg may be required (Bellomo et al. 2008). The most likely cause of Elizabeth's AKI is sepsis.

Her elevated temperature, white cell count and C-Reactive Protein (CRP) are evidence of infection and her poor fluid input, hypotension and tachycardia are indicative of secondary hypovolaemia. She also regularly takes non-steroidal anti-inflammatory drugs (NSAIDs) in the form of Ibuprofen, potentially affecting prostaglandin release and causing renal vasoconstriction (Huerta et al. 2005).

Intrinsic AKI refers to damage (potentially reversible) to the structures of the nephron, such as the glomeruli, tubules, vessels or interstitium; the major cause of which is acute tubular necrosis (ATN). ATN is commonly induced by ischaemic or nephrotoxic injury to the kidney and is a specific histopathological and pathophysiological entity. Nephrotoxic drugs include NSAIDs, aminoglycosides, ACE inhibitors and X-ray contrast mediums. The term ATN is considered by many authors as an inaccurate term because necrosis is rarely seen in biopsies (Armitage and Thomson 2003). Tubular cells do, however, actually die, and fall into the filtrate where they form casts that then block the lumen. Although these cells have the ability to regenerate, this can take a number of weeks. During this period kidney function is severely decreased and some form of renal support therapy may be required. Pre-kidney or ischaemic ATN often occurs as a continuum of the same pathophysiological process and together they account for the majority of AKI cases. Elizabeth's potassium is already 5mmol/L and she has an associated metabolic acidaemia indicating a reduction in normal tubular function. If her hypovolaemia and sepsis are not resolved swiftly, then she will develop ATN.

Finally post-kidney relates to outflow obstruction in the lower urinary tract. Examples include prostatic hypertrophy and bilateral ureteric strictures. Obstructions generate a backpressure into the kidney raising the hydrostatic pressure in the Bowman's capsule and reducing the glomerular filtration rate (GFR). Although post-kidney obstruction is an unlikely primary cause of AKI in Elizabeth, critical care nurses should be aware of the potential obstructions which could be induced by blocked indwelling urinary catheters or other unrelated conditions that Elizabeth might suffer from. For example, fibroids or other gynaecological problems can obstruct urinary flow. If there is no obvious cause, an ultrasound scan of the kidney and renal tract would be indicated to aid diagnosis.

Further details of normal kidney physiology and AKI can be found in Perkins and Kisiel (2005).

Tests and investigations

Serum creatinine (SCr)

Creatinine is produced by muscle cell breakdown, and is filtered out of the bloodstream by the kidneys. The serum level of creatinine therefore depends on a balance between the amount produced and the efficiency of filtration in the kidneys (National Kidney Federation 2008).

Daily production of creatinine depends on how much muscle the person has. Normal SCr can range between 60 and 120 μmol/L (National Kidney Federation 2008). A 48-year-old white female such as Elizabeth would be expected to have a SCr of approximately 64 μmol/L (Renal Association 2008). Assuming that she has a normal GFR for her age, sex and ethnic grouping, Elizabeth's SCr, measured at 125 μmol/L, is an increase of >1.5 times from baseline.

Glomerular filtration rate (GFR)

This is considered to be the best index to measure kidney function. It is the sum of the filtering capacity of all individual 'healthy' nephrons. A normal GFR is approximately 120 mL/min. GFR declines naturally with age by about 1mL/min per year. The majority of GFRs are now calculated by estimation (eGFR) as this only requires knowledge of the SCr, gender, age and ethnicity (black or other) (Renal Association 2008). Elizabeth's eGFR can therefore be calculated as 42 mL/min per 1.73 m^2 or approximately 42% of her kidney function. It should, however, be noted that eGFR may not be reliable in AKI as there is no steady state from which to calculate it.

Urea

Urea is a product of protein metabolism, usually cleared by the kidney, and therefore serum levels are usually raised in kidney injury (normal 3.5–5 mmol/L). Urea can, however, also be raised for other reasons, for example dehydration, red cell breakdown and/or liver impairment making it a less reliable indicator of kidney function (Perkins and Kisiel 2005).

Urinalysis

Urinalysis must be performed on all patients who can produce urine (NCEPOD 2009). The urine should be observed both for volume and colour. A dark colour commonly indicates increased concentration due to hypovolaemia, which can be confirmed by noting the specific gravity. Renal tubular epithelial cells and casts may also be seen in the form of 'sediment' during ATN as these cells have been sheared off from the inside of the tubule. Urinalysis is therefore a mandatory tool to assist in investigation of the underlying pathology. The presence of significant protein further suggests intrinsic glomerular disease, while haematuria in the presence of proteinuria may indicate a glomerular aetiology for AKI. Haematuria may also be found in lower urinary tract obstruction (post-kidney AKI). It is often associated with tumours, and also less commonly with calculi, infection or severe renal ischaemia. Red blood cells (RBC) may also be seen in cases of AKI. Myoglobinuria, a protein released from the muscle in conditions such as rhabdomyolysis, will also cause a positive reaction for blood without evidence of red cells on urine microscopy (Renal Association 2008). Any abnormalities detected on the urinalysis strip should be followed up by sending a sample to the laboratory to assess for microscopy, culture and sensitivity.

New biochemical markers of kidney injury

Waiker and Bonventre (2008) suggest the change from the term kidney failure to injury is a paradigm shift as failure refers to the kidneys' inability to perform glomerular filtration, while injury does not. Such a shift is in line with new biochemical markers of kidney injury, which it is hoped will enable a diagnosis to be made before changes are seen in either the SCr or the urine output. SCr and urine output, although considered the best markers of kidney function at present, do not provide any information on the type or site of injury to the kidney.

New potential markers should enable an earlier diagnosis as they will be measured in the urine as a result of injury and not cellular death. The epithelial cells that line the tubules contain numerous microvilli, which contain proteins with enzymatic functions, and it is these enzymes that it is hoped can be isolated and measured to detect early damage (Waiker and Bonventre 2008). Markers that are currently being researched and that hold promise are urine biomarkers; N-acetyl-β-D-glucosaminidase (NAG), neutrophil gelatinase-associated lipocalin (NGAL), kidney injury molecule – 1 (KIM-1) and serum cystatin C. It is hoped that these future markers will aid the diagnosis of the disorder before any functional decline is measured (Kellum 2008).

Developing scenario

Twenty-four hours later, Elizabeth's condition has deteriorated further. She has received two colloid fluid challenges (each of 500 mL). She is, however, increasingly tachycardic (128 bpm), hypotensive (MABP 58 mmHg), and acidaemic (metabolic) and she has become anuric. Her Central Venous Pressure (CVP) is 12 mmHg and she has widespread crackles on auscultation, with a respiratory rate of 20 breaths per minute. Laboratory results reveal the following:

Creatinine: 300 µmol/L
Urea: 25 mmol/L
Potassium: 5.8 mmol/L
Sodium: 147 mmol/L
Hb: 10.5 g/dL

A decision is made to transfer her to the ICU for further management.

Managing the patient with AKI

Airway/breathing

Elizabeth will require administration of supplemental oxygen titrated against regular arterial blood gases to help ensure adequate pulmonary gas exchange and maintenance of renal cell oxygenation (Perkins and Kisiel 2005). The crackles heard on auscultation of Elizabeth's lung fields are likely to indicate pulmonary oedema. If this is significantly affecting her oxygenation then a loop diuretic such as frusemide might be prescribed to offload the fluid and restore gas exchange. The nurse should also be alert for signs of a chest infection, which could be indicated by the increase in respiratory rate and widespread crackles, particularly as Elizabeth was admitted with community-acquired pneumonia. Assistance with positioning, coughing and suctioning, in conjunction with physiotherapy input, should therefore be provided as required. Elizabeth may also require non-invasive or invasive ventilation to maintain adequate oxygenation and ventilation if the fluid overload combined with the pneumonia and an attempt to breathe off the metabolic acid (Kussmual respirations), excessively increases her work of breathing, and worsens her blood gases.

Circulation

Fluid resuscitation

Optimal intravascular volume is vital to ensure adequate renal perfusion. Fluid resuscitation should be initiated as soon as hypoperfusion is recognised. The majority of cases of AKI can be effectively treated and resolved by adequate volume replacement and treatment of the underlying medical condition. Vincent and Weil (2006) suggest there are four phases of decision making in relation to fluid administration: type of fluid, either crystalloid or colloids; rate of infusion; goal to be achieved, for example MABP and CVP targets and safety limits. The type of fluid required is, according to Bellomo et al. (2004), controversial. Bagshaw and Bellomo (2007), for example, argue that synthetic colloids such as hydroxyethyl starch (HES) may increase the risk of AKI. They also state that the timing and amount of fluid therapy may also affect outcome (Bagshaw and Bellomo 2007). Fluid replacement may best be achieved through the rapid infusion of repeated small volumes (250 mL of crystalloid or colloid) of fluid alongside close monitoring of CVP, urinary output and other end points. Fluid challenges should be administered and repeated based on response (Vincent and Gerlach 2004), and administration of fluid should continue until identified targets have been reached (Vincent and Weil 2006).

Fluid challenges and resuscitation targets (early goal-directed therapy)

A fluid challenge is quite distinct from fluid administration, the purpose being to ascertain the intravascular fluid status of a patient. Dellinger et al. (2008) describe it as a technique in which large amounts of fluids are administered over a defined time period with the patients' response to the challenge being closely observed. For a fluid challenge, Dellinger et al. (2008) recommend 20 mL/kg of crystalloid over 5–10 minutes titrated to haemodynamic goals.

Nurses should have an understanding of the optimal CVP target and other fluid resuscitation goals. In 1979, Weil and Henning argued that it was necessary to achieve a sustained CVP rise of at least 2 mmHg to confirm adequate circulating volume (Weil and Henning 1979). Much has been written since regarding the improvement in survival by patients with the introduction of early goal-directed therapy, whereby end goals are set to determine success of the determined intervention (e.g. Rivers et al. 2001). Recently, the surviving sepsis guidelines have advocated a CVP target of 8–12 mmHg for septic patients (Dellinger et al. 2008). Other fluid resuscitation goals include lactate < 4 mmol, MABP >65 mmHg, central venous oxygen saturations >70% and a urine output >0.5mL/kg/min (Dellinger et al. 2008). In some critical care areas, more sophisticated tools might also be available to aid fluid assessment. These include, for example, measurement of pulmonary artery occlusion pressure (PAOP) using a pulmonary artery catheter; extra-vascular lung water (EVLW) using the PiCCO system (Pulsion medical) and stroke volume variation (SVV) and/or pulse pressure variation (PPV) using the LiDCO system. The value of non-invasive assessment should also be remembered, and clinical examination should therefore include measurement of jugular venous pressure (JVP), capillary refill time (CRT) and assessment of peripheral warmth and perfusion wherever possible.

Although Elizabeth has received 1 L of colloid, there has been no improvement in her kidney function. She also has a worsening metabolic acidaemia, which is likely to be of a mixed cause (both lactic and renal). This could suggest that more fluid may be required to improve oxygen delivery, especially as she has signs of sepsis, which requires administration of large volumes of fluid (Dellinger et al. 2008). She already has a CVP of 12 mmHg and signs of pulmonary oedema, however, suggesting that other treatments also now need consideration.

Optimal management of both fluids and electrolytes can be challenging during AKI, and will require different strategies during each phase of the illness (anuric/oliguric, diuretic, recovery). During the anuric/oliguric phase, once adequate intravascular filling has been established, Elizabeth may require a strategy of fluid restriction to prevent fluid volume overload (Hall and Esser 2008). It is first important, however, to ensure that the anuria is not caused by a blocked indwelling urinary catheter. If fluid volume overload is suspected, then frusemide may be prescribed to reduce clinical symptoms (Small and McMullen 2005). Frusemide is a loop diuretic which works to maintain renal blood flow and urine output, preventing further tubule obstruction. However, inappropriate administration risks a further reduction in renal perfusion worsening the AKI (Small and McMullen 2005). It should therefore be used with caution, and only when a thorough assessment to ensure adequate intravascular volume has been established. Dopamine has also been used for this purpose, but current research evidence does not support its continued use (Kellum and Decker 2001). If Elizabeth enters the diuretic phase, additional fluids may again be necessary to prevent dehydration. As the urine may still be of poor quality, electrolyte dysfunction can continue to be problematic during this period. Strict attention to monitoring and recording all input, output and electrolyte values will be vital throughout all phases.

Red blood cells (RBC) might be prescribed for Elizabeth if she becomes anaemic. Anaemia can be due to decreased erythropoietin production and a shortened RBC life span (Ward 2005). In AKI, however, it is more likely to be due to frequent blood sampling and/or haemodilution. In septic patients, the usually accepted strategy is to aim for an Hb >7 g/dL (Hébert et al. 1999). Red cell administration will assist in optimising her intravascular filling, but may also contribute to further total body fluid overload. Multiple units could also exacerbate the risk of infection, and could worsen the already evident hyperkalaemia. Hyperkalaemia is of concern as it may cause cardiac dysrhythmias, and thus requires vigilant cardiac monitoring and potential pharmacological treatment. It can be treated by correcting the metabolic acidaemia, and/or by the use of hypertonic glucose and insulin or nebulised salbutamol to force potassium back into the cells. Intravenous (IV) calcium might also be used to decrease the effect of potassium on the cardiac membrane (Hall and Esser 2008). Alternatively, a rectal or oral calcium resonium preparation might be prescribed which allows the exchange of sodium ions for potassium ions, thus excreting potassium into the stool (Hall and Esser 2008). Renal replacement therapy (RRT) might also be considered if the hyperkalaemia becomes life threatening.

Elizabeth's nutritional status needs consideration as patients with AKI tend to have high energy and protein requirements, which are further increased during mechanical ventilation and sepsis (Hall and Esser 2008). Perkins and Kisiel (2005) note, however, that a diet should be offered that has sufficient calorific content to meet the increased metabolic demand (higher in fat and carbohydrates), whilst being low in phosphate and protein to prevent further protein metabolism, and low in sodium to prevent further water retention. The type of nutritional input will also depend on whether or not Elizabeth is receiving RRT. Enteral feeding should be continued where possible as this will assist in preventing secondary sepsis from occurring and reduce the risk of gastrointestinal bleeding. Optimal nutritional management will require dietetic advice. Specialist enteral nutrition formulas such as Nepro® are available for use, but should be stopped during RRT. They are also expensive and should not be used without consideration to their relative benefits. Concentrated feed formulas can also help in the oliguric patient who is not receiving RRT. Detailed guidance for use of enteral nutrition in AKI is available from the European Society for Clinical Nutrition and Metabolism (ESPEN) (Cano et al. 2006).

Disability of the central nervous system

A close watch on the neurological status of Elizabeth is vital during her treatment for AKI. Rising urea and haemodynamic instability alongside an increased tendency for anaemia and bleeding and the potential for toxicity may cause symptoms of drowsiness, coma, psychosis and possible seizure activity (Hall and Esser 2008). Accurate neurological assessment may be more challenging, however, if Elizabeth requires intubation with associated sedation. Blood glucose levels should also be monitored regularly as insulin resistance can develop, leading to hyperglycaemia (Hall and Esser 2008).

Exposure/environment

Whilst in critical care, the risk of Elizabeth contracting an infection will be high, not least due to the large number of invasive cannulae she is likely to have. She may also be immunocompromised due to uraemia (Perkins and Kisiel 2005). Infection is an important contributor to poor mortality in this patient group (Hall and Esser 2008). Unnecessary lines should be removed whenever possible to reduce this risk, and universal precautions and guidelines for maintaining asepsis should be adhered to at all times (see Chapter 4 for more information on sepsis). If Elizabeth is anuric, removal of the urinary catheter during RRT should be considered. Assistance with personal hygiene and good skin care is vital for Elizabeth, particularly as she may have itchy, dry flaky skin coupled with areas of dependent oedema (Redmond et al. 2004).

Owing to the increasing inability of her kidneys to excrete metabolic waste products, a review of all Elizabeth's medication, in particular the use of antibiotics and NSAIDs, should be undertaken in order to identify any potential alterations to drugs or doses that might be required (Perkins and Kisiel 2005). Involvement of the pharmacist will be vital, both during RRT when normal drug doses may be possible and when not receiving RRT, as doses may then need to be reduced to prevent higher than acceptable serum drug levels.

Renal replacement therapy (RRT)

The best way to control Elizabeth's worsening metabolic acidosis, increasing urea abnormal electrolytes, in particular the hyperkalaemia, and fluid overload is to commence RRT. The AKIN classification does not indicate when RRT should be initiated. In their retrospective review of >41 000 patients, however, Ostermann and Chang (2007) noted that the mean GFR at the time of initiation of RRT was 23.8mL/min/1.73m^{2} There are, however, large variations in practice between units and within departments (Ostermann and Chang 2007). In their guidelines on septic shock, Dellinger et al. (2008) suggest that continuous renal replacement therapies (CRRTs) can be used over intermittent haemodialysis in patients with severe sepsis and AKI, despite the lack of randomised studies. The majority of ICUs (78%) in the United Kingdom use continuous veno-venous haemofiltration (CVVH) for this purpose (Gatward et al. 2008).

What is CVVH?

Helen Dickie, a critical care renal nurse specialist at Guys and St Thomas NHS Foundation Trust in London, describes CVVH in the following way:

The patient is attached to an extracorporeal blood circuit in which blood is pumped through a haemofilter (see Figures 9.1 and Figures 9.2, for examples, of haemofiltration machines). It is a veno-venous circuit, connected either to two separate central venous catheters or, more commonly, to one dual lumen central venous catheter.

Haemofilters are constructed of synthetic and biocompatible porous hollow fibres, made of semi-permeable material. The fibres in the filter are bundled together in a cylindrical tube and are encapsulated so that they are free at either end to allow blood to enter and exit the hollow lumens (see Figure 9.3). As the blood flows through the filter, the pressure within the hollow fibres is higher than in the outer compartment and this hydrostatic pressure difference (trans-membrane pressure (TMP)) causes water to pass through the fibre walls into the outer compartment. This process, known as ultra-filtration, or simply filtration, is analogous to what happens in the glomerulus. The water and solutes removed from the patient through the filter are known as ultra-filtrate or filtrate. To enable adequate clearance of waste products and correction of electrolyte balance, more ultra-filtrate has to be removed than the volume of fluid required to achieve the patients' fluid balance. This excess volume is replaced by infusing 'replacement fluid' administered into the circuit either before the filter (pre-dilution) or after the filter (post-dilution), or as a combination. A warming device controls the temperature of the replacement fluid prior to its entry into the circuit to prevent patient cooling.

As water is filtered out of the blood, solutes which are dissolved in it, and are small enough to pass through the fibre material, are swept through with it by convection (also

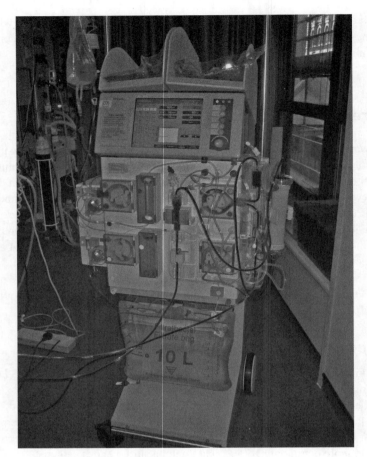

Figure 9.1   Haemofiltration machine type 1.

called solvent drag). The volume of ultra-filtrate removed (and so the solute clearance rate) is regulated by the filtrate pump. The size of the pores in the membrane, along with the pressure exerted, further determines the type of solutes filtered out and the volume of filtrate. Larger filters have more fibres, and so a greater surface area across which filtration can occur. They should be used when higher filtration rates are required. Small solutes such as amino acids, glucose, vitamins, small plasma proteins, ammonia, urea and electrolytes are able to move through the semi-permeable membrane easily. Some larger solutes may also be removed dependent on the pore size of the filter fibre membrane.

Before CVVH can be started, access to Elizabeth's bloodstream is required. Vascular access in the form of a long, 15 cm dual lumen catheter inserted into the right internal jugular vein is preferred for a temporary catheter (Oliver et al. 2000) as it is associated with a lower incidence of accidental pneumothorax and long-term venous stenosis compared with subclavian access (Uldall 1996). A femoral catheter may also be considered, although risks of infection and femoral vein thrombosis are increased.

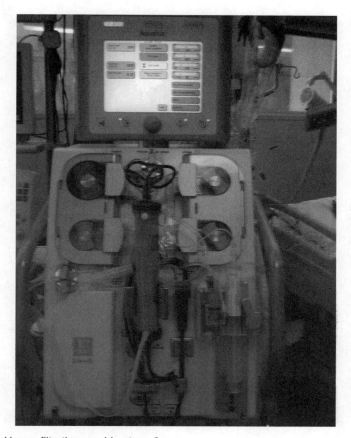

Figure 9.2 Haemofiltration machine type 2.

Prescription

Clinical evidence from a study undertaken by Ronco et al. in 2000 suggested that the optimal dose for CVVH is 35 mL/kg/h which equates to a rate of 2.1 L/h for Elizabeth. During continuous therapy, a clearance rate of less than 2 L/h will almost definitely be insufficient in an adult patient (Ricci et al. 2006). According to Ronco et al. (2000), there is experimental and clinical data to suggest that early high-volume haemofiltration may be effective in critically ill patients with sepsis like Elizabeth and may even limit her need for invasive ventilation. Research by Piccini et al. (2006) further supports this view. They undertook a study in which patients received early haemofiltration at 45 mL/kg/h for 6 hours followed by conventional CVVH of 35 mL/kg/h. Benefits were shown as improved gas exchange and urine production, earlier weaning from mechanical ventilation, shortened duration of ICU stay, and increased survival (Piccini et al. 2006). The VA/NIH Acute Renal Failure Trial Network (2008), however, failed to demonstrate any mortality benefit or reduction in rate of non-renal organ failure with the use of a more intense (20 mL/kg versus 35 mL/kg) strategy.

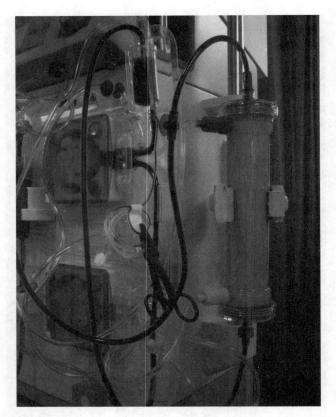

Figure 9.3 Haemofilter.

Blood flow rates should be set according to the exchange rate required; the desired filtration fraction (FF) and patient tolerance. If the blood flow rate is too slow, there is greater risk of the filter clotting. Blood flow rates <150 mL/min should generally be avoided. Increasing the blood flow may extend circuit life, but will be limited by the quality of flow through the catheter lumens.

Filtration fraction (FF) refers to the portion of plasma water that is removed from the blood during haemofiltration, and so is a measure of haemoconcentration. A high FF increases the risk of filter clotting. To minimise the risk of clotting, the FF should be kept below 25%. The formula in Box 9.1 can be used to calculate the FF. Using this formula, Elizabeth's FF is calculated to be 14% (Box 9.2).

Box 9.1 Calculation of filtration fraction

Filtration fraction (FF) = QUf/Qb × 100
where QUf = total ultrafiltration rate (post-dilution and net loss only)
Qb = blood flow rate

Box 9.2   Calculation of Elizabeth's filtration fraction

QUf (2100: ultrafiltration rate) divided by Qb (250 × 60: blood flow rate) × 100
= FF of 14

Fluid replacement

Replacement fluid can join the blood circuit either pre-dilution (before the filter) or post-dilution (after the filter). In pre-dilution the risk of filter clotting is reduced as the blood is less concentrated. However, solute clearance is also reduced. On the other hand, post-dilution increases the risk of filter clotting as the blood becomes concentrated. The higher the rate of post-dilution, the greater the haemoconcentration (and FF), limiting the proportion of replacement fluid which can be given post-dilution at any given blood flow rate. Only by increasing the blood flow rate can a higher post-dilution rate be used without exceeding the recommended FF limit. A possible way to deliver higher replacement rates is to divide the total flow, simultaneously infusing fluid both pre- and post-filter. According to Feliciana et al. (2007), a mixed strategy allows the maximum convection while preserving the filter membrane permeability. Mixed replacement has been shown to be efficient in removing both small and middle-sized solutes (Feliciana et al. 2007), and would therefore be the recommended strategy for Elizabeth.

Lactate is often used as a buffer in prepared replacement fluid, as the solution is very stable. Yet, Elizabeth may have difficulty clearing the lactate as it has to be broken down by the liver into bicarbonate, and sepsis may have affected her liver function. This could worsen her metabolic acidaemia. A bicarbonate-based solution may therefore be better tolerated. Bicarbonate is, however, unstable when mixed with calcium and magnesium chloride, and so these components have to be mixed just prior to use. A number of companies now manufacture solutions with bicarbonate in a separate sealed compartment, which can be broken and mixed with the other compartment just prior to treatment.

The appropriate concentration of potassium in the replacement fluid will vary depending on Elizabeth's serum potassium level. In AKI patients often develop hyperkalaemia and if this is this case, replacement fluid without potassium should be used initially for CVVH.

Alarms

A range of information about the RRT is available to the nurse, an example of which can be seen in Figure 9.4. Alarms are a key feature of RRT machines, not only for the safety of the patient but also for the longevity of the circuit and the filter. Any alarm related to blood flow should be rectified immediately as static blood is more likely to clot. Alarms can alert the practitioner to either high or low pressures within the circuit, empty fluid bags, presence of air in the circuit or incorrect weight loss (fluid replacement) (see Table 9.3).

Table 9.3 Alarm troubleshooting

Alarm	Possible causes	Possible remedy
Venous pressure too high	Clot in return line of circuit, drip chamber or central venous catheter Line kinked or clamped or against vessel wall	Relieve obstruction. Ensure all clamps open. Check lines not kinked or clamped. Change patient position.
Access pressure too negative	Inadequate blood flow from access port Obstruction Line kinked or clamped or against vessel wall	Access and return may be temporarily switched but this can reduce clearance and should be avoided. Discontinue, wash back if possible. Reposition vascular access.
Access pressure not negative enough	Additional infusions pre-blood pump	Stop or reduce infusion rate of pre-blood pump fluids.
Return pressure too low	Disconnection or loose connection Low pump speed	Tighten all connections. Check line – keep visible. Increase pump speed.
High pre-filter pressure	Filter clotting (gradual increase)	Reduce post-dilution and increase pre-dilution. Alter blood flow rate to reduce FF.
High TMP	Blood flow to exchange ratio too high	Alter blood flow rate and/or replacement fluid/exchange rate.
Air detected	Disconnection Air chamber not correctly positioned Blood level too low Turbulence in chamber	Check line. Clamp access and return lumens. Reposition drip chamber. Raise fluid level in chamber. Gently 'knock chamber' to push air to the surface. If a large amount of air, disconnect and re-prime new circuit.
Fluid balance	Bag swing Obstruction to flow	Try to ensure bags are not knocked. Ensure all connections are open. Relieve any obstruction. Avoid repeatedly over-riding this alarm as can lead to incorrect volumes of fluid removal.
Blood leak detected	Damaged filter (ultrafiltration pink coloured)	Discontinue and reset up with new lines.

Note: Troubleshooting guides provided by each machine manufacturer should be referred to for more specific advice.

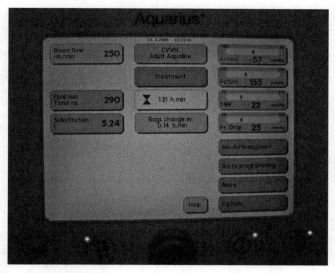

Figure 9.4   Example of screen.

Complications

Clotting

Probably the most common complication during CVVH is clotting. It is the nurses' responsibility to continually monitor Elizabeth's circuit for signs of clotting, and aim to reduce the risk. The chances of the filter clotting can be reduced by use of a mixed replacement fluid (pre- and post-dilution) strategy, maintaining a blood flow rate of greater than 200 mL/min, a FF of <25% and preventing the 'stopping and starting' of the blood flow pump.

As CVVH utilises an extracorporeal circuit, without any anticoagulation blood passing through it will activate platelets and coagulation resulting in clot formation, and a significantly reduced filter life. In contrast, excessive anticoagulation can lead to systemic bleeding complications (Davenport and Mehta 2009). Choosing the most appropriate anticoagulation strategy for Elizabeth therefore needs to take into account a number of factors. Elizabeth is likely to have sepsis which alters the homeostatic balance between coagulation and fibrinolysis (Dellinger et al. 2008). This could mean that she already has extended clotting times and an increased presence of micro-thrombi in her circulation. Ensuring that there is sufficient anticoagulation for the extracorporeal circuit without further increasing the risk of systemic bleeding is of paramount importance. The ideal would be to use a method of anticoagulating the circuit, not Elizabeth. ('regional anticoagulation') If she has extended clotting times, it is worth trying a no-anticoagulation strategy.

Making the best decision regarding the choice of anticoagulation strategy for Elizabeth will depend on having a good understanding of the effects of the anticoagulants available in the critical care department, on local expertise with each of the agents discussed, and on the availability of equipment and monitoring.

Table 9.4   Comparison of commonly used anticoagulants

	UFH	LMWH	Prostacyclin (flolan)	Citrate
Advantages	• Short half-life • Antagonized with protamine • Large clinical experience • Cheap • Effects measurable with APTT and bedside clotting assay	• Stable pharmacokinetics • Less impact on platelets • Stable anticoagulation	• Platelet inhibition • Synergistic effects with UFH and LMWH • Can be used with HITS • Improved filter patency and circuit life	• Improved filter patency and circuit life • Can be used with HITS
Disadvantages	• Systemic bleeding risk • Prolonged half-life in critical illness • Unpredictable effects • Risk of HIT	• Systemic bleeding risk • Only partially antagonized with protamine • More difficult to measure effects • Risk of HIT	• Systemic bleeding risk (but less than UFH) • Vasodilation	• Complex metabolic effects • Specialized equipment

Source: Data extracted from Oudemans-van Straaten et al. (2006) and Davenport and Mehta (2009).

There is no consensus regarding which anticoagulant should be first choice for patients receiving CVVH (Davenport and Mehta 2009). Continuous administration of unfractionated heparin (UFH) is, however, the most common agent used (Davenport and Mehta 2009), and acts by potentiating the effect of anti-thrombin and inhibiting factors Xa and thrombin (Oudemans-van Straaten et al. 2006). Low molecular weight heparin (LMWH), for example, enoxaparin, may be used as an alternative, and has some potential advantages over UFH as it has more predictable effects (see Table 9.4). Neither agent has, however, been demonstrated to have overall superiority (Oudemans-van Straaten et al. 2006). Both drugs have been associated with heparin-induced thrombocytopaenia (HIT), although this is less commonly reported in LMWH preparations (Martel et al. 2005). An alternative or additional anticoagulant choice may be the use of pre-filter prostacyclin, which inhibits platelet activation, and has been shown to work synergistically with both UFH and LMWH (Oudemans-van Straaten et al. 2006). The associated vasodilatory effects need to be accounted for however, and close monitoring of Elizabeth's blood pressure would be necessary if this were to be commenced. The potential for systemic bleeding with all agents also needs consideration.

Regional anticoagulation using citrate has recently come into vogue within critical care, and has been shown, in one study, to reduce mortality, when compared to heparin due to a reduced risk of systemic bleeding (Oudemans-van Straaten et al. 2009). Pre-filter infused sodium citrate chelates calcium, resulting in a decrease of ionised calcium (iCa). Once below 0.35 mmol/L coagulation is inhibited (Oudemans-van Straaten et al. 2006). Calcium is then infused at the end of the circuit to restore the iCa level to normal and so reverse the anticoagulation. Citrate anticoagulation requires use of specialised solutions and equipment, and competence in the setting up and use of this method is still being developed in many critical care units. Additionally, it has complex metabolic effects which require close monitoring (Oudemans-van Straaten et al. 2006), potentially limiting the value of widespread use. In the conclusion of a review of studies comparing the use of heparin to citrate, Tillman (2009) notes that the use of citrate; as with all treatments in clinical practice, should be used with caution and assessed on an individual patient basis.

Monitoring levels of anticoagulation

The most common sites for circuit clotting are the haemofilter, the venous drip chamber and the vascular access site (Davenport and Mehta 2009). In order to reduce the clotting risk whilst preventing systemic complications, UFH is commonly titrated using activated partial thromboplastin time (APTT) with a usual systemic target aim of 1–1.4 times normal. Alternatively, post-filter activated clotting time (ACT) can be used. Both methods can, however, be unreliable in critically ill patients (Oudemans-van Straaten et al. 2006). Platelet levels should also be monitored for signs of HIT, which would necessitate stopping any heparin currently being used for Elizabeth. Doses of citrate anticoagulation should be titrated to iCa concentration in the circuit blood to keep this below 0.35 mmol/L. This must be done alongside careful monitoring of systemic iCa, base excess and total systemic calcium concentration. Anticoagulation monitoring is more challenging with prostacyclin, which does not affect the APTT, and therefore cannot be easily measured by simple laboratory analysis (Davenport and Mehta 2009).

Other mechanisms for monitoring clot formation must be used alongside any anticoagulation strategy. These include evaluation of circuit life, monitoring pre-filter pressure and TMP, and visual observation of clot formation. Filter life can also be promoted by increasing the rate of pre-dilution, use of intermittent saline flushes and/or reducing the FF. It is also important to remember that mechanical obstruction might be the cause of high-pressure alarms and close attention should therefore be paid to ensure all access lines remain patent (Chrysochoou et al. 2008).

Elizabeth should be observed closely for signs of haemorrhage and/or air embolus, both of which could occur if lines are not connected tightly. All lines must be visible and safely secured. If an air embolus occurs Elizabeth may complain of dyspnoea, mid-chest and shoulder pain, be pale, nauseated and light headed. Prompt action is required. She must be laid on her left side in the Trendelenburg position with high concentration oxygen administered. This position aims to move the air embolus away from the pulmonary valve, and the oxygen causes the nitrogen in the air bubble to dissolve (Hadaway 2002).

Hypothermia

Hypothermia is common during CVVH as up to 200 mL or more of the patients' blood is in the extracorporeal circuit and is cooled to room temperature. The temperature of the replacement fluid can also contribute to this cooling (Chrysochoou et al. 2008). Most modern CVVH machines have the capability to warm therapy fluids to body temperature. Hypothermia can cause dysfunction of clotting factors and platelets, activation of fibrinolysis and cardiac dysrhythmias (Dirkes and Hodge 2007). Elizabeth's temperature should be monitored regularly and the replacement fluid temperature adjusted as necessary.

Cardiac arrest

AKI causes both electrolyte and fluid imbalances, which can cause cardiac arrest requiring immediate resuscitation. In the event of a cardiac arrest, the CVVH will need to be discontinued. The pump needs to be stopped and both the lines clamped. After the resuscitation period, lines should be disconnected and the central venous catheter lumens should then be flushed with 0.9% Normal Saline.

Conclusion

An understanding of the pathophysiology, clinical course and management strategies required for patients with AKI is vital to the improvement of mortality for this population group. The nurse at the bedside plays a key role in ensuring patient safety at this time.

Key learning points

- Early recognition of the clinical symptoms associated with AKI can prevent or minimise its progression.
- Pre-renal kidney injury is the most common problem found in critically ill patients, often secondary to hypovolaemia and/or sepsis.
- Adequate intravascular filling can prevent development of ATN and should always be the first-line management goal.
- Caring for a patient undergoing RRT requires a good technical understanding of the machinery involved, local protocols and the physiological and psychological effects of the therapy on the patient.
- Alterations in a number of associated interventions (e.g. nutritional and pharmacological support) may be required during RRT, necessitating effective communication and collaboration with the inter professional team.

Critical appraisal of research paper

Rickard et al. (2004) Preventing hypothermia during continuous veno-venous haemodiafiltration: a randomized controlled trial. *Journal of Advanced Nursing* **47**(4), 393–400.

This single centre prospective RCT conducted in Australia examined the effect of an IV fluid warmer on the incidence of hypothermia in patients undergoing haemodiafiltration (CVVHD), a form of RRT. Fifty-one CVVHD circuits from 24 patients were analysed, 26 in the intervention group (fluid warmed to 38.5°C using integral fluid warmer) and

25 in the control. Core temperature was measured using either a rectal or oesophageal probe. Following data analysis, no significant difference was demonstrated between the two groups in baseline, minimum or temperature loss. Instead, baseline temperature and being of the female gender were shown to be stronger predictors for hypothermia. Authors concluded that together with the associated costs, risks of contamination and additional nursing time, findings suggest that the practice of using fluid warmers should be abandoned.

Reader activities

1. Read the research article written by Rickard et al. (2004).
2. Using the critical appraisal framework in Appendix I, consider the methodological quality of the paper.
3. Reflect on this aspect of your own practice and the implications for future practice management that this paper arises.

A commentary on this paper has been provided by the chapter author in Appendix X.

References

Armitage AJ, Thomson C (2003) Acute renal failure. *Medicine* **31**(6), 43–48.

Bagshaw S, Bellomo R (2007) The influence of volume management on outcome. *Current Opinion in Critical Care* **13**(5), 541–548.

Bellomo R, Wan L, May C (2008) Vasoactive drugs and acute kidney injury. *Critical Care Medicine* **36**(4) (Suppl), S179–S186.

Bellomo R, Ronco C, Kellum JA, Mehta RL, Palevsky P and the ADQI workgroup (2004) Acute renal failure – definition, outcome measures, animal models, fluid therapy and information technology needs: The Second International Consensus Conference of the Acute Dialysis Quality Initiative (ADQI) Group. *Critical Care* 8. R204–R212.

Cano N, Fiaccadori E, Tesinky P, Toigo, Druml W, Kuhlmann M, Mann H, Hörl WH (2006) ESPEN guidelines on enteral nutrition: adult renal failure. *Clinical Nutrition* **25**, 295–310.

Chrysochoou G, Marcus R, Sureshkumar K, McGill RL, Carlin BW (2008) Renal replacement therapy in the critical care unit. *Critical Care Nursing Quarterly* **31**(4), 282–290.

Davenport A, Mehta S (2009) *Acute Dialysis Quality Initiative (ADQI) Workgroup 6. Access and Anticoagulation.* Available online at: www.ccm.upmc.edu/adqi/ADQIg6.pdf. Accessed 20 May 2009.

Dellinger P, Levy M, Carlet J *et al.* (2008) Surviving Sepsis Campaign: International guidelines for management of severe sepsis and septic shock: 2008. *Critical Care Medicine* **36**(1), 296–327.

Dirkes S, Hodge K (2007) Continuous renal replacement therapy in the adult intensive care unit: history and current trends. *Critical Care Nurse* **27**(2), 61–77.

Feliciana A, Riva MA, Zerbi S, Ruggiero P, Plati AR, Cozzi G, Pedrini LA (2007) New strategies in haemofiltration (HDF): prospective comparative analysis between on-line mixed HDF and mid-dilution HDF. *Nephrology Dialysis Transplantation* **22**(6), 1672–1679.

Gatward JJ, Gibbon GJ, Wrathall G, Padkin A (2008) Renal replacement for acute renal failure: a survey of practice in adult intensive care units in the United Kingdom. *Anaesthesia* **65**, 959–966.

Hadaway lC (2002) Action stat: Air embolus. *Nursing 2000* **32**(10), 104.

Hall G, Esser E (2008) Challenges of care for the patient with acute kidney injury. *Journal of Infusion Nursing* **31**(3), 150–156.

Hébert P, Wells G, Blajchman M, Marshall J, Martin C, Pagliarello G, Tweeddale M, Schweitzer I, Yetisir E for the Transfusion Requirements in Critical Care Investigators for the Canadian Critical Care Trials Group (1999) A multicentred randomized controlled clinical trial of transfusion requirements in critical care. *New England Journal of Medicine* **340**(6), 409–417.

Huerta C, Castellsague J, Varas-Lorenzo C, Rodriguez LAG (2005) Non-steroidal anti- inflammatory drugs and risk of ARF in the general population. *American Journal of Kidney Diseases* **45**(3), 531–539.

Kellum J (2008) Acute kidney injury. *Critical Care Medicine* **36**(4) Suppl, S141–S145.

Kellum J, Bellomo R, Ronco C (2007) Classification of acute kidney injury using RIFLE: what's the purpose? *Critical Care Medicine* **35**(8), 1983–1984.

Kellum JA, Decker JM (2001) Use of dopamine in acute renal failure: a meta-analysis. *Critical Care Medicine* **29**(8), 1526–1531.

Martel N, Lee J, Wells P (2005) Risk of heparin induced thrombocytopaenia with unfractionated and low molecular weight heparin thromboprophylaxis: a meta analysis. *Blood* **106**, 2710–2715.

Mehta RL, Kellum JA, Shah SV, Molitoris BA, Ronco C, Warnock DG, Levin A (2007) Acute injury network: report of an initiative to improve outcomes in acute kidney injury. *Critical Care* **11**(2), R31.

National Kidney Federation (2008) *About Creatinine*. Available online at: http://www.kidney.org. uk/Medical-Info/ckd-info/creatinine.html Accessed 30 June 2009.

NCEPOD (2009) *Adding Insult to Injury: A Review of the Care of Patients Who Sied in Hospital with a Primary Diagnosis of Acute Kidney Injury (Acute Renal Failure)*. National Confidential Enquiry into Patient Outcome and Death (NCEPOD), London.

Oliver MJ, Callery SM, Thorpe KE, Shcwab SJ, Churchill DN (2000) Risk of bacteraemia from temporary hemodialysis catheters by site of insertion and duration of use: a prospective study. *Kidney International* **8**, 2543–2545.

Ostermann M, Chang R (2007) Acute kidney injury in the intensive care unit according to RIFLE. *Critical Care Medicine* **35**(8), 1837–1843.

Oudemans-van Straaten H, Bosman R, Koopmans M, van der Voort PHJ, Wester JPJ, van der Spoel JI, Dijksman LM, Zandstra DF (2009) Citrate anticoagulation for continuous venovenous hemofiltration. *Critical Care Medicine* **37**(2), 545–552.

Oudemans-van Straaten H, Wester J, dePont A, Schetz MR (2006) Anticoagulation strategies in continuous renal replacement therapy: can the choice be evidenced based? *Intensive Care Medicine* **32**(2), 188–202.

Perkins C, Kisiel M (2005) Utilizing physiological knowledge to care for acute renal failure. *British Journal of Nursing* **14**(14), 768–773.

Piccini P, Dan M, Barbacini S, Carraro R, Lieta E, Marafon S, Zam-peretti N, Brendolan A, D'Intini V, Tetta C, Bellomo R, Ronco C (2006) Early isovolaemic haemofiltration in oliguric patients with septic shock. *Intensive Care Medicine* **32**(1), 80–86.

Redmond A, McDevitt M, Barnes S (2004) Acute renal failure: recognition and treatment in ward patients. *Nursing Standard* **18**(22), 46–53.

Renal Association (2008) *Clinical Practice Guidelines*. Available online at: http://www.renal.org/ pages/pages/guidelines.php. Accessed 5 January 2010.

Rickard C, Couchman B, Hughes M, McGrail MR (2004) Preventing hypothermia during continuous veno-venous haemodiafiltration: a randomized controlled trial. *Journal of Advanced Nursing* **47**(4), 393–400.

Ricci Z, Bellomo R, Ronco C (2006) Dose of dialysis in renal failure. *Clinical Journal of the American Society of Nephrology* **1**, 380–388.

Ricci Z, Cruz D, Ronco C (2008) The RIFLE criteria and mortality in acute kidney injury; a systematic review. *Kidney International* **73**(5), 538–546.

Rivers E, Nguyen B, Havstad S, Ressler J, Muzzin A, Knoblich B, Peterson E, Tomlanovich M for the Early Goal-Directed Therapy Collaborative Group (2001) Early goal directed therapy in the treatment of severe sepsis and septic shock. *New England Journal of Medicine* **345**(19), 1368–1377.

Ronco C, Bellomo R, Homel P, Brendolan A, Dan M, Piccinni P, La Greca G (2000) Effects of different doses in continuous veno-venous haemofiltration on outcomes of acute renal failure: a prospective randomised trial. *Lancet* **356**(9223), 26–30.

Small K, McMullen M (2005) When clear becomes cloudy: a review of acute tubular necrosis, a form of renal failure. Critical Care Extra. *American Journal of Nursing* **105**(1), 72AA–72GG.

Tillman J (2009) Heparin versus citrate for anticoagulation in critically ill patients treated with continuous renal replacement therapy. *Nursing in Critical Care* **14**(4), 191–199.

Uchino S, Kellum J, Bellomo R, Doig GS, Morimatsu H, Morgera S, Schetz M, Tan I, Bouman C, Macedo E, Gibney N, Tolwani A, Ronco C for the Beginning and Ending Supportive Therapy for the Kidney (BEST Kidney) Investigators (2005) Acute renal failure in critically ill patients: a multinational study. *The Journal of the American Medical Association* **294**(7), 813–818.

Uldall R (1996) Vascular access for continuous renal replacement therapy. *Seminars in Dialysis* **9**, 93–97.

VA/NIH Acute renal failure trial network (2008) Intensity of renal support in critically ill patients with acute kidney injury. *New England Journal of Medicine* **359**(1), 7–20.

Vincent JL, Weil MH (2006) Fluid challenge revisited. *Critical Care Medicine* **34**(5), 1333–1337.

Vincent JL, Gerlach H (2004) Fluid resuscitation in severe sepsis and septic shock: an evidence-based review. *Critical Care Medicine* **32**(11) Supplement, S451–S454.

Waiker S, Bonventre J (2008) Biomarkers for the diagnosis of acute kidney injury. *Nephron Clinical Practice* **109**, 192–197.

Ward K (2005) Kidneys, don't fail me now. *Nursing Made Incredibly Easy* **3**, 18–27.

Weil MH, Henning RJ (1979) New concepts in the diagnosis and fluid treatment of circulatory shock. *Anesthesia and Analgesia* **58**, 124–132.

Chapter 10

The patient in acute pain

Dr. Sinead Mehigan

Introduction

This scenario looks at the challenge of managing the critically ill patient in pain. Pain has been defined within nursing as whatever the person experiencing it says it is (Mc-Caffery 1972). It is an unpleasant sensory and emotional experience and is always subjective (IASP 1994), thus requiring an individual and holistic approach to its assessment and effective management. It has been acknowledged that pain is not managed well by nurses and other health care professionals (Shannon and Bucknall 2003). Using a patient case, this scenario will therefore discuss relevant pathophysiology, before considering how pain assessment and management might be optimised within a critical care setting.

Scenario

Meena is a 72-year-old lady, with a long history of osteoarthritis, who is in post-operative recovery, awaiting transfer to the high-dependency unit (HDU). She has undergone a total hip replacement, and has two wound drains *in situ*, both draining large amounts of blood. She received intravenous (IV) fentanyl during theatre, and has been given incremental doses of IV morphine up to a total of 10 mg since her admission to the recovery unit, as she stated that she had a lot of pain. She is becoming increasingly hypotensive, and her current vital signs are as follows:

Blood pressure:	90/47 mmHg
Pulse rate:	124bpm
Respirations:	26bpm
Temprature:	36.5°C

She looks pale, and her skin is clammy to touch. She drifts off to sleep easily, but when awake is restless and agitated.

Critical Care Nursing: Learning from Practice, 1st edition. Edited by Suzanne Bench and Kate Brown.
© 2011 Blackwell Publishing Ltd.

Reader activities

- What factors need to be considered when assessing Meena's pain? How should this be done?
- What are the possible options for the management of Meena's pain? Which might be more effective? Why?
- What are the particular challenges in the optimal management of Meena's pain?

One of the biggest challenges with post-operative pain management in critical care is that potential problems such as shock, respiratory or cardiac insufficiency are more likely to be seen as priorities of care. It is possible, therefore, that pain management may not be considered further until such priorities have been addressed. However, poorly managed pain has been shown to compromise recovery, and leads to untoward physiological (circulatory, respiratory, gastrointestinal) and psychological (stress, anxiety, depression) complications (Ferguson 1995; Shannon and Bucknall 2003). In order to adequately manage Meena's pain, a sound knowledge base of the pathophysiology, assessment and treatment options is required. It might also be useful to reflect on some of the current issues surrounding pain management in the critical care setting and your own attitudes to acute pain management.

The physiology of pain

From a physiological perspective, pain can be seen as a response to noxious stimuli – whether physical (mechanical or thermal) or chemical in nature (McHugh and McHugh 2000). For Meena, physical stimuli, such as her surgical incision and hip replacement, will have produced immediate mechanical pain. In addition to this, chemicals released as a result of tissue damage will cause further pain. Meena may have surgical inflammation, nerve damage, or tissue ischaemia and resultant tissue hypoxia. Pain might also be related to positioning during surgery, and could be further compounded by her history of osteoarthritis.

There are four basic processes involved in the process of nociception (processing of pain): transduction, transmission, perception and modulation (Wood 2008).

Transduction

Meena will feel physical pain through any painful stimuli, such as pressure on damaged tissue around her wound site. These stimuli will be detected and converted into nerve impulses by the actions of nociceptors (specialised free nerve endings at the distal end of pain sensing neurones), located in skin, muscle, joints, arterial walls and visceral organs (Godfrey 2005a). These are in proximity to mast cells and small blood vessels and all three act together in response to injury. Chemicals released from nearby sympathetic fibres will also contribute to Meena's pain and inflammation (Alexander 2006). What this means is that as a result of surgery, the area around Meena's surgical site will have suffered inflammation and cellular damage, increasing the concentration of chemical mediators, such as histamine and prostaglandins in the area surrounding the nociceptors, mast cells and small blood vessels. These mediators act together to enhance the transmission of pain along sensory nerve fibres (McHugh and McHugh 2000).

Transmission

This is where pain becomes a conscious experience. Painful stimuli are transmitted to the brain stem and thalamus. The reticular system, somatosensory cortex and limbic system are then activated and emotional, behavioural, autonomic and motor responses are elicited (Wood 2008).

Two types of nerve fibres are involved in conducting pain impulses from the nociceptors. Myelinated A-delta fibres conduct impulses quickly, and connect with high threshold mechanical receptors, whereas the slower conducting unmyelinated C-fibres connect with polymodal receptors (Julius and Basbaum 2001). Both A-delta and C-fibres (first-order neurones) carry impulses from the nociceptors to the dorsal horn, within the spinal cord. Most terminate in the substantia gelatinosa. From there, they synapse with second-order nociceptive neurones, which cross over in the spinal cord and transmit the pain signals to the brain. The second-order nociceptive neurones cross over in the spinal cord from grey to white matter and rise up to the brain along a number of different ascending pathways.

The second-order neurones synapse with third-order neurones either at the level of the thalamus or reticular formation in the brainstem. Both the reticular formation and hypothalamus are thought to play a role in integrating the autonomic responses observed when someone is in pain (Godfrey 2005a). This could account for the alteration of heart rate, blood pressure and respiratory rate, and the sweating seen in Meena's clinical data.

From the reticular formation, third-order neurones send pain information to the cerebral cortex of the brain. From the thalamus, third-order neurones send information to the frontal cortex and others to the somatosensory cortex (Cross (1994) in Godfrey 2005a), specialised areas of the cortex that represent the sense of touch. This region is seen to form the core of a 'neuromatrix' distributed over the entire forebrain that interprets pain from the pattern of activity across all of the convergent sensory neurons. This suggests that different feelings of pain may have their own specially adapted pathways, and that within the brain itself, there are specific pain centres (Craig 2005).

Modulation

Descending pathways originating in the cortex of the brain, the thalamus and brain stem, will also contribute to Meena's pain perception by modulating pain in one of two ways – inhibition or facilitation. This is done through the release of specialised neurotransmitters at the dorsal horn. The main neurotransmitters associated with these pathways are noradrenaline and serotonin (5-HT) (Alexander 2006); when released, these stimulate the inhibitory neurone, which secretes natural opioids such as enkephalins and endorphins. These inhibit the second-order neurones from sending further pain signals (Barasi 1991). Modulation helps explain the wide variations in individual pain perception (Wood 2008).

The gate control theory

The gate control theory of pain, developed by Melzack and Wall (1965), explains how Meena's pain might be modulated at the level of the spinal cord. They proposed that the transmission of information from a potentially painful stimulus can be modified by a gating mechanism situated in the dorsal horn of the spinal cord. This mechanism can increase or decrease the flow of nerve impulses from the periphery to the brain. If the gate is open, impulses pass through; if it is partially open, some pass through and if shut, no impulses get through and pain is not experienced. Melzack and Wall (1965) proposed that the substantia gelatinosa is activated by large A-beta fibres (carrying sensory information such as pressure, touch or temperature) that shut the gate. It is inhibited by small A-delta and C-fibres that open the gate. This then influences the information sent to the brain, which, in turn, sets up descending inhibitory controls depending on the information from other areas such as the cortex.

Sensitisation and 'wind up' of pain response

Although the kind of acute post-operative pain experienced by Meena could be seen as relatively short term, recent neurobiological research suggests that the neural pathways involved in the perception and modulation of pain can be modified – with neurones used to carrying pain information becoming sensitised (Godfrey 2005a; Woolf 2005; Carr 2007). What this means, when caring for Meena, is that if the decision is taken to relieve her pain only after meeting other priorities, such as treating her hypovolaemia, it is possible that leaving her in pain for prolonged periods has the potential to leave an imprint, or send her central nervous system into a state of hyperactivity. Thus, as a result of sustained peripheral neuronal activity, it is possible that there might be a change in the way it responds to stimuli. If sensitised, ordinary sensory information, such as light touch, could become transformed into pain information (allodynia). This may help to explain how reports of a patient's pain might seem out of proportion to the tissue damage. If Meena's pain is not controlled, and her body is subject to sustained pain stimuli, particularly tissue inflammation, then C-fibres might respond by progressively increasing (or winding up) the response rate of second-order neurones. Such sensitisation can contribute to the development of chronic pain (Carr 2007).

   Reflecting on the relevance of the sections above to Meena, a key message is that in order to manage her pain successfully, it is really important that a multi-modal approach is taken. Although much of the discussion of the pathophysiology of pain suggests that it is the physical aspects that need to be focused on, the gate theory and sensitisation, in particular, should alert the reader to the importance of needing to deal with the emotional and psychological aspects of pain. This is discussed further below.

Tests and Investigations Assessing pain

Meena's description is the most reliable indicator of her pain. There is also an implied assumption that through such description and a pain assessment tool, the nurse will be able to estimate the severity of the pain. However, Sloman et al. (2005) compared nurses' and patients' ratings of pain intensity, in adult surgical patients using the same pain assessment tool, and found that nurses underestimated all dimensions of their patients' pain, Clabo (2008) discusses a series of studies carried out by Sjöström and colleagues who have attempted to explore the actual approaches used by nurses to assess patients' post-operative pain. They describe four criteria used by the nurses in their studies – how the patient looks, what the patient says, the way the patient talks and the nurses' experience in similar circumstances. Other studies show that patients wait for nurses to ask about their pain before reporting it (Carr 1990; Gélinas 2007).

Meena has verbalised that she is in pain. However, she may not report her true level of pain, even if asked specifically due to a fear of being thought of as difficult, or a perception that health care professionals are too busy, or a greater fear of injections. Meena may also assume that the nurses and doctors caring for her have a better knowledge about her pain than herself (Carr 2007).

It is important that, along with monitoring Meena's pulse, blood pressure, temperature and respiratory status, pain assessment is carried out regularly. It should be seen as the 'fifth vital sign' (Winslow 1998; Lynch 2001). One way of encouraging this is to utilise a pain assessment tool and ensure a specific place on observation charts for documentation of pain assessment. This will provide visible cues to prompt nurses to undertake regular pain assessments. Use of such documentation additionally means that information about her level of pain and the effects of any intervention can be relayed to members of the multi-disciplinary team. Within a critical care setting, this is particularly important as many patients will be unable to communicate such information themselves.

If Meena is conscious enough to be capable of explaining her level of pain, then a pain assessment tool should be used as part of a holistic assessment of her pain. Several tools are available for acute pain. These commonly include either a verbal or numerical rating scale (Lynch 2001). It is important that the method chosen is used consistently as, for example, a score of 4 on a scoring system ranging from 0 to 10 will have a different meaning to one where the scoring system ranges from 0 to 5.

Many of these scales focus on measuring the intensity of pain only (Dougherty and Lister 2008), and should therefore be used alongside the collection of other information to get a fuller picture of Meena's pain experience. This should include assessment of the duration of pain, and whether it is exacerbated by activity (such as movement, breathing or coughing). It would also be important to note the location of her pain. Although this is likely to be centred on her wound site, any change in location or radiation of the pain might be indicative of a new pathology. Other features of pain that need assessment include its characteristics; whether it is sharp, tingling, burning or shooting in nature, for example, and whether or not there are any relieving factors, such as being positioned in a particular way. It is also worth noting if it is associated with any other symptoms, such as nausea, or if it is affecting her ability to sleep. Meena's past medical history, particularly of osteoarthritis, would also be significant, in that it is likely that the surgical position required to perform her hip replacement will have aggravated this. Knowledge of past medical history could also give an indication as to how she might respond to being turned or positioned post-operatively. Research indicates that turning can be one of the most painful procedures for the critically ill patient (Puntillo et al. 2001). Other common causes of pain in the critically ill patient are endotracheal suctioning, physiotherapy and invasive procedures (Woodrow 2006). Heightened stress and anxiety caused by the technological environment, feelings of disempowerment and lack of control, and a fear of death can further exacerbate perceptions of pain for those in critical care.

For the critical care nurse, a particular problem in accurate pain assessment is that the patient may be unable to communicate verbally. Meena appears drowsy, and so may have difficulty in responding to direct questioning about her level of pain. Rakel and Herr (2004) identified that post-operative pain is often under-assessed in the older person. Other common barriers to communication for patients in the critical care setting include endotracheal intubation, metabolic disorders, sedation and fatigue, all of which will have an impact not only on verbal communication but also on a range of physiological or behavioural responses (such as restlessness, tachycardia, sweating, hypertension, pupil dilation and facial grimacing), which are often used as proxy measures of pain (Puntillo et al. 1997, 2002). It becomes difficult therefore to separate out the causes of these physiological and/or behavioural responses in order to provide an accurate pain assessment.

Few pain assessment tools have been specifically designed for critical care settings (Shannon and Bucknall 2003). However, recent work has resulted in the development of the critical-care pain observation tool (CPOT) for patients who cannot communicate verbally (Gélinas et al. 2006). Despite its validity and reliability only being tested on cardiac patients in one ICU (Gélinas et al. 2006), it would appear to provide a viable option for those working in a general critical care setting. Indices of pain used in this tool include facial expressions, body movements, muscle tension and either compliance with the ventilator or vocalisation, with a total score range between 0 and 8 (Gélinas et al. 2006). The reader is encouraged to review this tool and consider whether it would enhance pain assessment practices within their own unit. A few other tools have also been tested for validity and reliability within critical care, which are worthy of consideration. For example, the behavioural pain scale (BPS) (Payen et al. 2001; Aissaoui et al. 2005; Young et al. 2006) and the non-verbal pain scale (NVPS) (Odhner et al. 2003).

Discussion of interventions: methods of pain management

A holistic approach to management of Meena's pain is essential, which involves more than the administration of analgesics. This includes consideration of non-pharmacological interventions, such as physiotherapy, careful positioning, pressure area care, good communication, a reduction in noise and the establishment of a day/night routine to promote sleep.

The use of heat or cold, massage, transcutaneous electrical nerve stimulation (TENS) (Figure 10.1) or other complementary therapies could also be considered. Many of these methods have been used for those with chronic pain, although there is limited research evidence to support their effectiveness (Godfrey 2005b). The use of massage and application of heat pads are two examples of the application of the gate theory (see 'Pathophysiology' section above) to nursing practice (Carr and Mann 2000). If touch was used to stimulate Meena's skin, the theory proposes that this would increase large fibre A-beta fibres, thereby closing the gate at the level of the spinal cord and relieving some of Meena's

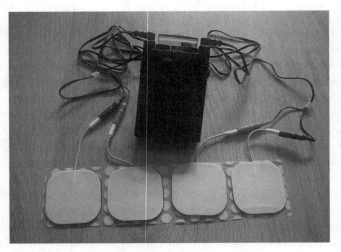

Figure 10.1   TENS. (Courtesy of Wikipedia Commons.)

pain. Another application of this theory would be to use either distraction or imagery with Meena as this might lead to the gate being closed at the level of the brain stem. Similarly, at the level of the cortex and thalamus, the gate could be closed by reducing Meena's anxiety – for example, by providing pre-operative information about the cause, likely course and relief of post-operative pain, thereby increasing Meena's confidence and sense of control (Alexander 2006).

Perhaps one of the most important methods of pain control for Meena is through the use of drugs. The three main groups of analgesics used are opioids, non-opioids and adjuvants (drugs shown to enhance the effect of analgesics) (Godfrey 2005b). A combination of these can often produce synergistic effects in the critically ill patient.

The main non-opioid analgesics include paracetamol and non-steroidal anti-inflammatory drugs (NSAIDs) such as aspirin. The pharmacokinetics of paracetamol are not clearly understood, but may be related to COX-3 inhibition and inhibition of prostaglandin E_2 (Godfrey 2005b). NSAIDs inhibit the production of cyclo-oxygenase, an enzyme involved in the production of prostaglandins. Given that prostaglandins are involved in activating and enhancing the pain response in the nociceptors, any reduction in their synthesis will help reduce pain. They could therefore be effective for Meena in helping to control any pain caused by inflammation due to surgery and for the chronic pain caused by her osteoarthritis. However, as NSAIDs commonly cause renal impairment and gastrointestinal disturbances such as gastric bleeding their use may be contraindicated in many critically ill patients.

Opioids work by binding with opioid receptors within the CNS, mimicking the effects of naturally occurring opioids, endorphins and enkephalins. Three types of opioid receptors are involved in producing an analgesic effect: mu (μ) – which is most involved, kappa (k) and delta (∂). Opioids such as fentanyl and morphine exert full agonist effect at these receptors. Other opioids, such as buprenorphine, act as partial agonists, and as such do not have as much effect (Godfrey 2005b). Side effects of opioids include nausea,

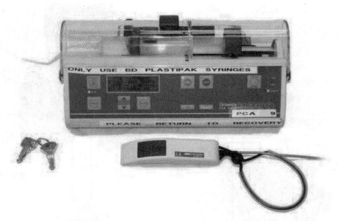

Figure 10.2   PCA pump. (Adapted from: Flinders Biomedical Engineering. Available online at: http://www.flinders.edu.au/medicine/sites/biomedical-engineering/biomedical-engineering_home.cfm. Used with permission.

vomiting, respiratory depression, itching and constipation. Common routes of administration include oral, intramuscular, IV, transdermal (fentanyl patches, for example) and via epidurals. The use of patient-controlled analgesia (PCA) devices (see Figure 10.2) where the patient self-administers medication using an electronic pump device has been shown to be more effective than reliance on intramuscular analgesics, but not as effective as epidural administration (Dolin et al. 2002). Intramuscular injections are further contraindicated in the critically ill patient due to risks of bleeding and difficulty in accessing the muscle layer due to the common presence of systemic peripheral oedema.

One drug that has both opioid and non-opioid analgesic effects is tramadol, which acts by binding with opioid receptors and inhibiting the re-uptake of two neurotransmitters within the dorsal horn of the spinal cord. This has the effect of inhibiting the pain response (Godfrey 2005a). Other groups of drugs can also be considered, and in some instances, can reduce the dosage of opioids required. For example, low doses of tricyclic antidepressants are thought to inhibit the re-uptake of serotonin and noradrenaline in a similar way to tramadol, thus reducing pain perception at the level of the dorsal horn in the spinal cord (Godfrey 2005a). See Figure 10.3 for a summary of the location of drug actions along the pain pathway.

Ideally, administration of analgesics should be titrated against reported levels of pain, until an optimal level is achieved. If given at regular intervals, large fluctuations in blood plasma levels are avoided, and there is less chance of breakthrough pain, and less likelihood of side effects (Lynch 2001). It has also been shown that the use of opioids in adequate amounts will help prevent sensitisation and wind up (McHugh and McHugh 2000). Some authors suggest that another way of helping to avoid wind up would be to explain how it might occur and stressing to Meena the importance of seeking pain relief as soon as she feels she needs it (Carr 2007). The analgesic ladder, originally described by the World Health Organisation in 1996 (WHO 2010) would provide a useful framework for managing Meena's analgesic requirements

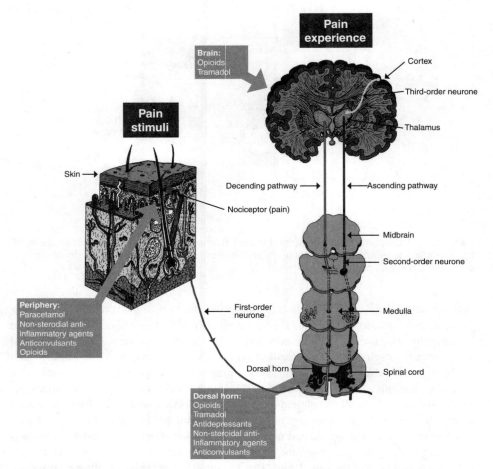

Figure 10.3   Pain pathway. (Adapted from: King's College, London.)

As Meena is in severe pain, it is likely that opioids would be the analgesics of choice. As well as diminishing her perception of pain, opioids may also have a euphoric or anxiolytic effect. However, they can also result in sedation and respiratory depression. Given that Meena has already had a total of 10 mg intravenously, it would be worth assessing whether her drowsiness is due to the sedative effects of morphine. Keeping Meena informed of what the team were doing to relieve her pain, or using distraction, might also be useful.

Although pain is a common experience, particularly in surgical patients, research suggests that it is not well managed (Watt-Watson et al 2001; Puntillo et al 2002; Seers et al 2006; Gélinas 2007). Some of the reasons given for less than optimal pain control include nurses' lack of knowledge of both the pathophysiology of pain and misconceptions surrounding the use of analgesics for treatment. Despite research indicating that the likelihood of addiction as a result of opioid analgesia for pain relief is less than 1%, many nurses believe that it is easy for a patient to become addicted (Ferrell et al. 1992). It has also been shown that many nurses fail to increase the dose of analgesia despite previous doses neither relieving the patients' pain nor producing any side effects (Ferrell et al. 1992). Further, it has been demonstrated that nurses' pain relief practices are influenced by the social contexts in which they work (Clabo 2008). Access to a wide range of information does not guarantee, however, that good decisions are made about pain management.

Conclusion

Managing pain is complex and made even more challenging by its subjective nature and the fact that it can be difficult to communicate with patients in the critical care setting. As patients deteriorate and require more complex care and management, time available to make adequate pain assessment and management decisions is reduced, and this important aspect of care can be compromised. As well as inadequate knowledge and information about how to treat pain, other variables that might compromise effective pain management include personal values and beliefs, staffing levels, the physical environment, the complexity of the patient and the interrelationships between members of the multi-disciplinary team and the patient and their families (Seers et al. 2006). Yet, allowing a patient to experience continuing pain has been shown to affect morbidity (Shannon and Bucknall 2003), and is a human rights issue. Somehow, pain assessment has to be included as the 'fifth vital sign', and managed accordingly. The whole multi-disciplinary team needs to work together to help ensure that a patient's pain is well managed (Seers et al. 2006; Carr 2007). Nurses can play a central role. However, if they are to make informed clinical decisions, they need to be knowledgeable about pain processes and understand the effects of the range of drugs; opioids, non-opioids and adjuvants used to treat pain. They also need to take responsibility for managing pain, and do so competently (Seers et al. 2006).

Key learning points

- Pain is a common experience, yet because of the complex nature of critical care, it is not always adequately assessed or managed.
- The key to managing pain effectively is timely and continual assessment and re-assessment of a patient's pain. It is important to ensure that the assessment of pain is considered as a 'fifth vital sign'.
- Nurses must understand the underlying physiology of pain, and the effects of the range of drugs and other approaches used in its treatment.
- Although pharmacological methods of pain relief may be the treatment of choice within the critical care setting, other, non-pharmacological methods should also be considered.

Critical appraisal of research paper on pain

Clabo L (2008) An ethnography of pain assessment and the role of social context on two postoperative units. *Journal of Advanced Nursing* **16**(5), 531–539.

This study was carried out in the United States of America on two post-operative units of one teaching hospital. The aim of the study was to examine pain assessment practices in both units in order to assess in what ways and to what extent the peri-operative pain assessment varied across the two units. The researcher also wanted to assess what the impact of the social context of each unit was on pain assessment practices.

Reader activities

1. Read the research article written by Clabo (2008).
2. Using the critical appraisal framework in Appendix I. consider the methodological quality of the paper.
3. Reflect on this aspect of your own practice and the implications for pain management in your unit that this paper raises.

A commentary on this paper has been provided by the chapter author in Appendix XI.

References

Alexander M (2006) *Nursing Practice: Hospital and Home – The Adult*, 3rd edn. Churchill Livingstone, Edinburgh.

Aissaoui Y, Zeggwagh A, Zekraoui A, Abidi K, Abouqal R (2005) Validation of a behavioural pain scale in critically ill sedated, and mechanically ventilated patients. *Anesthesia and Analgesia* **101**, 1470–1476.

Barasi S (1991) The physiology of pain. *Surgical Nurse* **4**(5), 14–20.

Carr E (1990) Postoperative pain: patients' expectations and experiences. *Journal of Advanced Nursing* **15**, 89–100.

Carr E, Mann E (2000) *Pain: Creative Approaches to Effective Pain Management*. Palgrave, Basingstoke.

Carr E (2007) Barriers to effective pain management. *Journal of Perioperative Practice* **17**(5), 200–208.

Clabo L (2008) An ethnography of pain assessment and the role of social context on two postoperative units. *Journal of Advanced Nursing* **16**(5), 531–539.

Craig AD (2005) *Mapping Pain in the Brain*. The Wellcome Trust, London. Available online at: http://www.wellcome.ac.uk/en/pain/microsite/science2.html. Accessed 10 December 2009.

Dolin D, Cashman J, Bland J (2002) Effectiveness of acute postoperative pain management: 1. Evidence from published data. *British Journal of Anaesthesiology* **89**, 409–423.

Dougherty L, Lister S (2008) *The Royal Marsden Hospital Manual of Clinical Nursing Procedures, Student Edition*, 7th edn. Wiley-Blackwell, London.

Ferguson J (1995) The development of a post-operative pain service (1): an overview. *British Journal of Theatre Nursing* **5**(7), 28–31.

Ferrell B, McCaffery M, Robchan R (1992) Pain management as a clinical challenge for nursing administration. *Nursing Outlook* **40**(6), 263–268.

Gélinas C, Fillion L, Puntillo K, Viens C, Fortier M (2006) Validation of the critical-care pain observation tool in adult patients. *American Journal of Critical Care* **15**(4), 420–427.

Gélinas C (2007) Management of pain in cardiac surgery ICU patients: have we improved over time? *Intensive and Critical Care Nursing* **23**, 298–303.

Godfrey H (2005a) Understanding pain, part 1: physiology of pain. *British Journal of Nursing* **14**(16), 846–852.

Godfrey H (2005b) Understanding pain, part 2: pain management. *British Journal of Nursing* **14**(17), 904–909.

International Association for the Study of Pain (IASP) Task Force on Taxonomy (1994) IASP pain terminology. In: *Classification of Chronic Pain*, 2nd edn, Merksey H, Bogduk N (eds). IASP Press, Seattle, pp. 209–214.

Julius D, Basbaum AL (2001) Molecular mechanisms of nociception. *Nature* **413**(6852), 203–210.

Lynch M (2001) Pain as the fifth vital sign. *Journal of Intravenous Nursing* **24**(2), 85–94.

McCaffery M (1972) *Nursing Management of the Patient in Pain*. Lippincott, Philadelphia.

McHugh J, McHugh W. (2000) Pain: neuroanatomy, chemical mediators, and clinical implications. *AACN Clinical Issues Advanced Practice Acute Critical Care* **11**(2), 168–178.

Melzack R, Wall P (1965) Pain mechanisms: a new theory. Science **150**, 971–979.

Odhner M, Wegman D, Freeland N, Steinmetz A, Ingersoll G (2003) Assessing pain control in non verbal critically ill adults. *Dimensions of Critical Care Nursing* **22**(6), 260–267.

Payen J, Bru O, Bosson J, Lagrasta E, Novel E, Descheux I, Lavagne P, Jacquot C (2001) Assessing pain in critically ill sedated patients by using a behavioural pain scale. *Critical Care Medicine* **29**, 2258–2263.

Puntillo K, Miaslowski C, Kehrle K, Stannard D, Gleeson S, Nye, P (1997) Relationship between behavioural and physiological indicators of pain, critical care patients' self-reports of pain, and opioid administration. *Critical Care Medicine* **25**(7), 1159–1166.

Puntillo K, White C, Morris A, Perdue S, Stanik-Hutt J, Thompson C, Wild L (2001) Patients' perceptions and responses to procedural pain: results from Thunder Project II. *American Journal of Critical Care* **10**(4), 238–251.

Puntillo K, Stannard D, Miaslowski C, Kehrle K, Gleeson S (2002) Use of a pain assessment and intervention notation (P. *A.I.N.) tool in critical care nursing practice: nurses' evaluations*. Heart and Lung **31**(4), 303–314.

Rakel B, Herr K (2004) Assessment and treatment of postoperative pain in older adults. *Journal of PeriAnesthesia Nursing* **19**(3), 194–208.

Seers K, Watt-Watson J, Bucknall T (2006) 30th Anniversary Invited Editorial reflecting on: Copp LA (1993) An ethical responsibility for pain management. *Journal of Advanced Nursing* **18**, 1–3. The Author, Journal Compilation. Blackwell Publishing Ltd, pp. 4–6.

Shannon K, Bucknall T (2003) Pain assessment in critical care: what have we learnt from research? *Intensive and Critical Care Nursing* **19**, 154–162.

Sloman R, Rosen G, Rom M, Shir Y (2005) Nurses' assessment of pain in surgical patients. *Journal of Advanced Nursing* **52**(2), 125–132.

Watt-Watson J, Stevens B, Garfinkel P, Streiner D, Gallop, R (2001) Relationship between nurses' pain knowledge and pain management outcomes for their postoperative cardiac patients. *Journal of Advanced Nursing* **36**(4), 535–545.

Winslow, E (1998) Critical care extra. Effective pain management. *American Journal of Nursing* **98**(7), 16HH–16II.

Wood S (2008) *Anatomy and Physiology of Pain*. Nursing Times.net. Available online at: www.nursing times.net. Accessed 20 April 2009.

Woodrow P (2006) *Intensive Care Nursing: A Framework for Practice*, 2nd edn. Routledge, London.

Woolf, C (2005) *Pain Hypersensitivity*. The Wellcome Trust. Available online at: www.wellcome.ac.uk/en/pain/microsite/science4.html. Accessed 10 December 2009.

World Health Organisation (WHO) (1996) Who's pain relief ladder. Available online at: http://whqlibdoc.who.int/publications/9241544821.pdf. Accessed 1st December 2010.

Young J, Siffleet J, Nikoletti S, Shaw (2006) Use of a behavioural pain scale to assess pain in ventilated, unconscious and/or sedated patients. *Intensive and Critical Care Nursing* **22**, 32–39.

Chapter 11

The patient requiring sedation

Tina Moore

Introduction

The noisy intensive care unit (ICU) environment with its unfamiliar monitoring and support equipment, medical jargon, loss of day-night cycle and painful invasive procedures is associated with a high incidence of psychological trauma and sleep deprivation. To patients, this type of environment can appear hostile and threatening. Patients' experiences whilst in an ICU include feelings of frustration with the inability to communicate during mechanical ventilation, painful procedures and anxiety caused by incomprehension of their illness (Szokol and Vender 2001). Experiences like these lead to an increase in the incidence of post-traumatic stress disorder (PTSD) after critical care discharge lasting from weeks to months (Nasraway 2001; Weiener-Kronish 2001).

Sedation has become an integral part of treatment for patients requiring intubation. Sedation goals include facilitation of mechanical ventilation relief of anxiety, agitation, delirium and pain, ensuring safety, and promoting comfort. (Weinert et al. 2001; Egerod 2002). Sadly, more hidden reasons for sedation include its use as a form of 'chemical restraint' (Leith 1998) and compensation for shortage of nursing staff (Happ 2000). It is well documented that sedation may prolong mechanical ventilation by increasing the risk of complications (Ostermann et al. 2000; Egerod 2002). Hence, there is a need to manage the administration of sedation appropriately and effectively. This scenario will explore the usage of sedation therapy and discuss current best practice.

Patient scenario

Mrs Betty Attoh, a frail 73-year-old lady, is admitted to the ICU. She is emaciated and cachectic, and has developed a respiratory infection resulting in type 1 respiratory failure and sepsis. She was admitted in an unconscious state with a Glasgow Coma Score (GCS) of 3, requiring immediate intubation, sedation and ventilation. Assessment data can be seen in Table 11.1

Critical Care Nursing: Learning from Practice, 1st edition. Edited by Suzanne Bench and Kate Brown.
© 2011 Blackwell Publishing Ltd.

Table 11.1   Initial assessment data.

Arterial blood gas results	pH	7.35
	PaCO$_2$	5.7 kPa
	PaO$_2$	7.6 kPa
	HCO$_3^-$	21 mmol/L
	Base excess	−3.1
Cardiovascular	Blood pressure	161/89 mmHg
	Temperature	38.1°C
	Heart rate	89 bpm (sinus rhythm)

An infusion of propofol 100 mg/h has been commenced, with the intention to gradually reduce the dosage over the next 24 hours. The plan is to wake Betty as quickly as possible to allow for neurological assessment, once her condition has stabilised.

Reader activities

Having read this scenario, consider the following:

- Why does Betty need sedation?
- What criteria should be used to select the type of sedation and the dosage to be administered?
- What information is required for monitoring the effects of sedation?
- What is best practice for appropriate management of Betty's sedation therapy?
- What assessments would you undertake to ensure appropriate use of sedation?

Pathophysiology and pharmacology

Pain and agitation are common in critically ill patients. This is, in part, due to activation of the stress response causing neurohormonal elevation of plasma catecholamines (Blanchard 2002), and sympathetic over-activity, with an associated increase in heart rate, myocardial oxygen consumption and respiratory rate (Ferguson and Mehta 2002). As well as untreated or intractable pain, the stress response can be attributed to a vast array of other factors including the critical care environment; medications; invasive procedures; uncomfortable positioning; an inability to communicate; fear; sleep deprivation and the vast array of monitoring and technology with which they are surrounded. The resulting anxiety and agitation can lead to dyspnoea, patient ventilator asynchrony, elevated blood pressure and heart rate and possible aggressive behaviour and PTSD. Pain, delirium, anxiety and agitation can manifest with similar signs but each may have different causes requiring different management.

Sedation is important for Betty to ensure comfort from both a psychological and physiological perspective. She currently appears mildly hypertensive possibly due to anxiety and/or pain. Sedation may be used to help control this stress response and reduce her oxygen requirements, particularly as she is already hypoxaemic, possibly due to sepsis evidenced by her pyrexia and mild metabolic acidaemia. It can also be used to reduce any patient-ventilator dys-synchrony (Ferguson and Mehta 2002). Betty needs to be awoken quickly for neurological assessment purposes. It is currently unclear if she has sustained a neurological injury. This could also be compromising her blood gases and haemodynamic status. Short-term sedation which allows for neurological assessment is therefore desirable. However, continued sedation may be necessary to facilitate other interventions and ongoing management.

In order to optimise sedation management, it is essential that nurses understand the basic pharmacological and clinical uses of the most commonly used sedative agents.

Sedatives

Benzodiazepines

Benzodiazepines (lorazepam, midazolam, diazepam) work by enhancing the effects of GABA (γ-aminobutyric acid), a potent inhibitory neurotransmitter, making neurons resistant to excitation and producing sedatory and amnesic effects (Pun and Dunn 2007). They also have anticonvulsant effects. However, they do not have analgesic properties and should therefore be used in conjunction with an appropriate analgesic agent (see Chapter 10).

The use of lorazepam has recently been reported to be an independent risk factor for the development of delirium in critically ill patients, particularly as the dosage increases (Pandharipande et al. 2006). Generally, midazolam is the preferred benzodiazepine for use (Jacobi et al. 2002) as it has a rapid onset (2–5 minutes) and has a short half-life. The intravenous (IV) route is the most reliable and effective because of absorption and administration difficulties associated with oral and/or intramuscular administration.

Midazolam may produce adverse effects, including respiratory and cardiovascular depression, physical dependence and agitation as well as unpredictable awakening (with prolonged sedation) (Nasraway 2001; Fullwood and Sargent 2010). These adverse effects result from either an accumulation of the drug or its active metabolites (Hassan et al. 1998; Jacobi et al. 2002). When associated with alcohol, used in an elderly patient such as Betty, or in patients with cirrhosis of the liver, it can also depress respiration.

Respiratory depression and hypotension are dose-dependent. Hypotension occurs primarily in hypovolaemic patients and is potentiated by the associated use of opioids (Blanchard 2002), infection and hypoxaemia. Despite the relatively short half-life, extensive re-distribution can cause prolonged sedation. Recovery time is proportional to duration; therefore, midazolam infusions generally should not exceed 48 hours (Jacobi et al. 2002).

Midazolam would not be the most appropriate agent of choice for Betty initially due to the desire to wake and neurologically assess. However, if agitation were to become problematic then small IV boluses may be considered. It is also likely that Betty may not wean easily from ventilation due to her poor physical state and respiratory failure. She may therefore require benzodiazepines as part of her ongoing management.

Propofol

Propofol (Diprovan®) a sedative–hypnotic agent has a very rapid onset (1–2 minutes) and a short half-life, making it attractive to use for Betty. How propofol works is not completely understood (Fullwood and Sargent 2010), but it is believed to enhance GABA's affinity for its receptors, much like the benzodiazepines. Propofol concentration in plasma falls quickly once the drug is discontinued.

Propofol is a useful drug for patients with neurologic injury. It decreases intracranial pressure, cerebral blood flow and cerebral metabolism (Rhoney and Parker 2001; Jacobi et al. 2002). For Betty this drug could be considered to be the safest option because currently the reason for her low GCS is unknown.

Vigilance is important when using prolonged or high doses of propofol (more than 48 hours at doses higher than 5 mg/kg/h), particularly in patients with acute neurological or inflammatory illnesses (Jacobi et al. 2002) such as Betty. Caution is also required in cases of hypovolaemia or poor cardiovascular system function due to its vasodilator and potent negative inotropic properties, which can potentially cause large decreases in blood pressure. In addition, high-dose propofol use has been linked to 'Propofol infusion syndrome', a potentially fatal syndrome characterised by cardiac failure, rhabdomyolysis (the breakdown of muscle fibres, resulting in the release of muscle fibre content (myoglobin) into the bloodstream), severe metabolic acidosis and renal failure (Ostermann et al. 2000; Jacobi et al. 2002; Vasile et al. 2003; Marik 2004) and painful peripheral administration (Ostermann et al. 2000; Jacobi et al. 2002).

This drug is prepared in a lipid emulsion, so long-term or high dose infusion may lead to elevated triglyceride levels. Serum triglyceride levels should be monitored and the emulsion considered a calorific source (Ostermann et al. 2000; Jacobi et al. 2002). Additionally, because the lipid emulsion can promote bacterial growth, strict aseptic technique and a dedicated IV catheter are also essential to help prevent the development of further sepsis in Betty.

Propofol is metabolised at least partially by the liver to inactive metabolites and excreted by the kidneys. However, the presence of renal or hepatic dysfunction does not significantly affect clearance (Sang Ko and Gwak 2008). It can also accumulate in peripheral tissues, prolonging its effects.

Neuromuscular blocking (paralysing) agents

These drugs block transmission at the neuromuscular junction causing paralysis of the affected skeletal muscles. Neuromuscular blocking agents, for example, suxamethonium, atracurium, vecuronium or pancuronium are useful to facilitate mechanical ventilation but can also be harmful. These agents should not be avoided in Betty as neurological assessment, and the ability to monitor for any seizure activity would be compromised.

If patients are adequately sedated, neuromuscular blockade is usually un-necessary. It should be used as a last resort for patients resisting or fighting the ventilator or those who are at risk of harm. It should not be used as a form of chemical restraint.

Tests and investigations

Assessment of sedation

A comprehensive assessment of Betty's sedation needs and level of sedation is required. However, the nurse must first rule out or treat any pain that Betty has as this could be influencing any agitation (see Chapters 10 and 13 for more information on pain and agitation). Although Betty should not be agitated, nervous or experiencing pain, at the same time she should not be over-sedated as this can lead to complications of its own. This balance can be difficult to achieve.

The ability to assess sedation levels may be affected by patient variables such as age, language (including aphasia), disease pathology and pain (Weinert et al. 2001). Older patients like Betty can also appear adequately sedated, but actually be under-sedated. Disruptions to communication can further decrease the reliability of any sedation assessment. For example, in the non-communicative patient it may be difficult to differentiate whether movement is a symptom of pain or inadequate sedation (Frazier et al. 2002).

Because of the limitations of the subjective assessment tools available, over- and under-sedation remain major challenges to critical care nurses. In general, there appears to be a tendency to over-sedate. This, can lead to avoidable prolongation of mechanical ventilation and ICU and hospital stay (Kress et al. 2000). Excessive sedation can cause an increased risk of venous thrombosis, decreased intestinal motility, hypotension and reduced tissue oxygen extraction capabilities. Cardiopulmonary dysfunction including restlessness, tachypnoea, irritability and hypertension may also occur secondarily to subsequent withdrawal. Equally, under-sedation may instigate psychological consequences, leading to extreme agitation, potentially associated with the accidental removal of the artificial airway or invasive lines and monitoring equipment. Evidence from follow-up of former critically ill patients suggests that unpleasant experiences may have potentially serious implications for psychological and emotional recovery (Jones et al. 2001), including the development of delirium see chapter 13 for further details on delirium. Physiological insults include myocardial ischemia, hypoxia and increased myocardial oxygen consumption (White et al. 2001), resulting in catecholamine release (tachycardia) and increased irritability, prolonging recovery and overall hospital stay. Many of these problems can, in part, be related to difficulty in accurately judging patients' medication requirements (Egerod 2002).

Titration of sedative agents continues to be reliant upon methods of assessment that are influenced by a variety of subjective factors including family presence and preconditioned social, personal and professional norms of the nurse performing the assessment. Various sedation scoring tools have been developed in order to facilitate the assessment process. However, many units continue to rely on nursing staff to assess sedation rather than routinely employing any scoring system (Soliman et al. 2001). Even when scoring systems are in place, some nurses continue to avoid their use as part of their assessment. Additionally, there is, on occasion, disagreement amongst multi-disciplinary team members about the goals of sedation, which potentially originates from miscommunication (Slomka et al. 2000).

Standardised sedation-assessment scales provide health care professionals with a common language. They can be used to judge the level of sedation through indicators such as movement and response to physical or verbal stimuli. A variety of such scales exist, although not all have been validated. These include the Ramsay sedation scale (Ramsay et al. 1974), Richmond agitation–sedation scale (Sessler et al. 2002), motor activity assessment scale (Devlin et al. 1999), the Vancouver interactive and calmness scale (de Lemos et al. 2000) and the Nursing Instrument for the Communication of Sedation (NICS) (Mirski et al. 2010).

The Ramsay scale (Ramsay et al. 1974) is still one of the most widely used tools for evaluating sedation in the United Kingdom. Sedation levels range from one (patient awake and anxious, agitated or both) to six (patient asleep and unresponsive to both light touch and loud noise). Despite its popularity, limitations of the Ramsay scoring system have resulted in some units adapting the tool, and one author comments that nurses perceive no advantages in its use (Elliott et al. 2006). Behavioural responses cannot be used to classify patients who are quietly disorientated and distressed (Elliott et al. 2006). In addition, the tool incorporates three very different constructs (agitation, anxiety and conscious level) in the same scale making classification difficult. It has also been criticised as not adequately reflecting states of consciousness in the brain-injured patient (Hansen-Flaschen et al. 1994), an important consideration for Betty. However, the assessment of consciousness and the assessment of sedation, although interlinked, should not be considered interchangeable elements of assessment. Thus, although assessment of Betty's conscious level is difficult whilst receiving sedation, an attempt to assess her neurology should be made using a recognised tool designed for such purpose (see Chapter 12 for more information on neurological issues). Further, as might be a criticism of many sedation assessment tools, observation is limited to a short, discrete period of time and does not account for changes in response that may occur between assessments. Therefore, despite the plethora of tools available, there exists little practical difference between the majority.

Objective sedation assessment tools may prove beneficial as an adjunct to subjective scales, particularly in patients receiving neuromuscular blockade. Bispectral index (BIS) monitoring (see Figures 11.1 and Figures 11.2) has been advocated to be a reliable form of sedation assessment and monitoring (Olson et al. 2004). However, this research was conducted in a neurological critical care unit with staff adept in EEG monitoring. They may be less reliable in general ICUs, with staff less familiar with such monitoring. Although BIS is used in some general units, there is currently a lack of adequate research to support its use in such areas and some studies suggest that BIS is not reliable for routine monitoring (Frenzel et al. 2002; Riess et al. 2002).

Jacobi et al. (2002) and De Jonghe et al. (2000) suggest that sedation assessment scales should do all of the following:

• Provide data that are simple to compute and record
• Describe the degree of sedation or arousal with well-defined categories
• Demonstrate validity and reliability in critically ill patients
• Enhance communication, guide dosage adjustment, help improve consistency in drug administration
• Measure changes in sedation level over time.

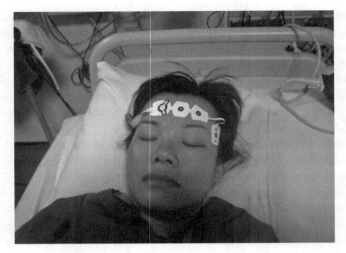

Figure 11.1   BIS *in situ* on patient.

Currently no one tool matches these criteria, reinforcing the complexity of the process. A good evaluation of currently available tools and their relative benefits and limitations can be found in Sessler et al. (2008).

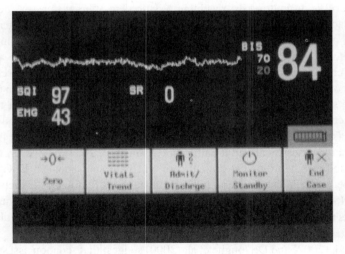

Figure 11.2   BIS data on screen.

Assessment of paralysis, i.e. testing reflexes

If neuromuscular blocking agents are being used, the extent of neuromuscular blockade (paralysis) should be assessed to ensure full therapeutic benefit, without over paralysis, which has been associated with long-term problems (Murray et al. 2002). In view of the potential risks and complications (e.g. difficulties in assessment of sedation, peripheral

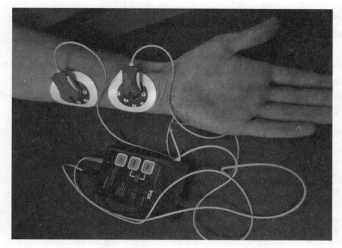

Figure 11.3   Peripheral nerve stimulator.

neuropathies and myopathies), neuromuscular blocking (paralysing) agents should be used at the lowest possible dosage for the shortest possible time (Marini and Wheeler 2006). Monitoring of the depth of paralysis can be achieved both clinically (looking for signs of movement and dys-synchrony with the ventilator) and by the use of a peripheral nerve stimulator (see Figure 11.3) using 'train of four', with an aim to achieve 1–2 twitches (Murray et al. 2002). A useful algorithm to guide nurses' assessment and management of neuromuscular blockade is available in Jones (2003).

Assessment of delirium

The confusion assessment method for ICU (CAM-ICU) is a recently designed tool for the assessment of delirium in critically ill patients (Ely et al. 2001). The aim of the CAM-ICU tool kit is to assist practitioners at the bedside to clinically assess both intubated and self-ventilating patients for compromised cognitive function (see Chapter 13 for more information on assessment of delirium).

'Other'

Monitoring pharmacologic therapy for potential adverse events is imperative for the improvement of patient outcomes. Laboratory analysis of renal and liver function with consequent titration of medication enables clinicians to achieve sedation goals whilst reducing costly complications associated with renal failure, hepatic insufficiency and neurological impairment. At the bedside, Betty's vital signs should be closely monitored as hypotension and respiratory alterations are common side effects of sedation therapy. Betty should also be observed for signs of delirium and, drug side effects such as weakness related to the use of neuromuscular blocking agents.

Discussion of sedation and the evidence base of management

Betty requires sedation in order to facilitate an artificial airway due to her decreased level of consciousness, and to facilitate effective support via the ventilator. However, sedation carries its own risks, for example, an increase in the frequency of ventilator-associated pneumonia (Kress et al. 2000).

Anecdotal observations suggest that patients who are restless or aggressive are often treated too quickly with sedatives, which can cause or worsen delirium. The goal for Betty should be to induce a calm, easily arousable state whilst minimising anxiety and agitation. It is acknowledged, however, that some situations may require deeper levels of sedation. Despite this, sedation should maintain competent patient communication where possible.

Consideration and selection of the most appropriate agents for sedation must focus on Betty's individual needs. However, although the use of sedation may be common practice in critical care units, the methodology of adjusting such medication is less well defined (De Jonghe et al. 2000; Egerod 2002).

Sedative agents are commonly prescribed by a physician and administered by a nurse, often with a wide margin of discretion (Weinert et al. 2001). Factors that may influence non-compliance with protocols include personal experiences, differences in values between the authors of protocols and those implementing them, ignorance about aspects of a protocol, personal preferences for specific medications (Bair et al. 2000; Slomka et al. 2000; Weinert et al. 2001) and practitioner knowledge and experience (Egerod 2002; Elliott et al. 2006). Where guidelines do exist, nurses and physicians have a tendency to overrate themselves in terms of compliance (Slomka et al. 2000), and where compliance exists there has been shown to be a decline over a period of time (Bair et al. 2000).

The success of any sedation management protocol seems to be achieved, in part, by allowing rapid clinical decision making at the patients' bedside. Clinical practice guidelines, which incorporate measurement of sedation levels, are one method of addressing consistency and providing clear goals for treatment. They standardise the delivery of sedation and improve patient outcomes (Brook et al. 1999; Baratteb et al. 2002). Reported benefits include a reduction in the duration of ventilation, the number of tracheostomies, the length of stay in ICU and associated costs.

Further, studies have illustrated how protocol-based practice guidelines for sedation management lead to improved patient outcomes (Kollef et al. 1998; Kress et al. 2000; Nasraway 2001). These include reductions in mortality (Kollef et al. 1998; Brook et al. 1999) and earlier ICU discharge (Kollef et al. 1998; Brook et al. 1999; Kress et al. 2000). Additional benefits of protocol use include enhanced patient comfort, the promotion of ventilator-patient synchrony, optimal oxygenation, earlier weaning from mechanical ventilation and reduced hospital costs (Jacobi et al. 2002). Goal-oriented sedation further complies with the establishment of a modern ventilation regimen to allow early spontaneous breathing (Putensen et al. 2001).

Sedation is typically provided by a continuous infusion of drugs. However, this can be associated with an increased period of mechanical ventilation, and an increase in re-intubation rates and length of ICU stay (Kollef et al. 1998). In addition, the accumulation of sedatives with a long half-life in patients with altered hepatic and/or renal function remains a problem. Nurses continually face tension between the conflicting safety aspects of sedation and administration.

Current evidence suggests that Betty should undergo a daily awakening trial (sedation hold), which involves stopping her sedation and allowing her to regain consciousness. When she reaches a certain degree of awareness (e.g. can respond to simple commands or shows signs of distress and/or agitation), sedation should be restarted at half the previous doses and further titrated as necessary (Kress et al. 2000). This practice permits doses to be fine tuned daily and should result in less medication being given to Betty over the course of her ICU stay, thus helping to prevent drug accumulation (Brooke et al. 1999; Kress et al. 2002). This strategy has been shown to reduce the length of time required on mechanical ventilation (Kress et al. 2000), reduce the length of stay in the ICU (Schweickert et al. 2004) and decrease the incidence of complications, including PTSD (Kress et al. 2003; Misak 2004). A sedation hold will also allow for reassessment of Betty's neurological status and pain level, and provide an opportunity for enhanced communication with family and staff.

Daily awakenings are contraindicated in patients' receiving neuromuscular blocking agents. Sedation should be discontinued in these patients only after paralysis has been discontinued and a reversal of its effects is evident. Additionally, the clinical team may decide that a sedation hold is undesirable in patients who are unstable as risks might outweigh any potential advantages. Even if a sedation hold is not possible, regular attempts to reduce sedation should be made in order to avoid the complications described above. Consideration should also be given to the multiple actions of many agents used for sedation. In particular, the team must consider whether or not to stop analgesic agents such as fentanyl or morphine, which also have sedative properties.

As mechanisms of action of sedatives vary widely, nurses must understand each drug category to ensure that drugs are administered safely. It is important to establish a dosage end point, and frequently reassess Betty's sedation needs, adjusting the dosage accordingly. For the same reason, when such drugs are given to the older patient (like Betty) and patients with renal and hepatic insufficiency, the lowest possible starting dose should be given and then adjusted upwards.

Finally, it is important to consider the many other ways that Betty's comfort can be improved, thus enabling the minimum level of sedation to be utilised. In addition to effective analgesia, this could include the use of effective communication strategies, complementary therapies, positioning, prevention and management of constipation or diarrhoea and manipulation of those aspects of the critical care environment conducive to alteration (e.g. levels of light and noise).

Conclusion

Sedation management is complex and made even more challenging by its subjective nature. It is, however, of special importance since it directly affects the comfort and safety of patients. Mechanically ventilated patients are exposed to intrusive stimuli, invasive procedures and unfamiliar routines. They are often unable to communicate and may experience high levels of discomfort and anxiety. The growing body of knowledge about sedation management has not been consistently applied in practice (Soliman et al. 2001), leading to inadequate or over-sedation of many mechanically ventilated patients, and associated complications adversely affecting critical illness recovery.

Nurses play a central role in effective sedation management within the critical care setting. However, if they are to make informed clinical decisions, they need to be knowledgeable about drug pharmacology and current evidenced based practice.

Key learning points from scenario

- Sedated patients are not exempt from the experience of pain.
- Sedation needs vary over the course of a critical illness.
- Sedation should be carefully titrated following comprehensive assessment and monitored in relation to agreed goals.

Critical appraisal of research paper

Egerod I (2002) Uncertain terms of sedation in ICU. How nurses and physicians manage and describe sedation for mechanically ventilated patients. *Journal of Clinical Nursing* **11**(6), 831–840.

The data presented in this paper is extracted from a larger piece of research which investigated nurses' decisions and interventions in relation to mechanical ventilation and weaning. This particular paper explores how nurses and physicians describe sedation and how the level of nursing skill relates to the level of sedation.

Reader activities

1. Read the research article written by Egerod (2002).
2. Using the critical appraisal framework in Appendix I, consider the methodological quality of the paper.
3. Reflect on this aspect of your own practice and the implications for sedation management in your unit that this paper raises.

A commentary on this paper has been provided by the chapter author in Appendix XII.

References

Bair N, Bobek MB, Hoffman-Hogg L, Mion LC, Slomka J, Arroliga A (2000) Introduction of sedative, analgesic and neuromuscular blocking agent guidelines in a medical intensive care unit: physician and nurse adherence. *Critical Care Medicine.* **28**(3), 707–713.

Barattebø G, Hofoss D, Flaatten H, Muri AK, Gjerde S, Plsek P (2002) Quality improvement report: effect of a scoring system and protocol for sedation on duration of patients' need for ventilator support in a surgical intensive care unit. *BMJ* **324**, 1386–1389.

Blanchard AR (2002) Sedation and analgesia in intensive care; medications attenuate stress response in critical illness. *Postgraduate Medicine Online* **111**(2). Available online at: http://www.postgradmed.com/issues/2002/02_02/blanchard.htm. Accessed 22 November 2009.

Brook AD, Ahrens TS, Schaiff R, Prentice D, Sherman G, Shannon W (1999) Effect of a nursing-implemented sedation protocol on the duration of mechanical ventilation. *Critical Care Medicine* **27**(12), 2609–2615.

De Jonghe B, Cook. D, Appere-De-Vecchi C, Guyatt G, Meade M, Outin H (2000) Using and understanding sedation scoring systems: a systematic review. *Intensive Care Medicine* **26**(3), 275–285.

De Lemos J, Tweeddale M, Chittock D (2000) Measuring quality of sedation in adult mechanically ventilated critically ill patients. The Vancouver Interaction and Calmness Scale. Sedation Focus Group. *Journal of Clinical Epidemiology* **53**, 908–919.

Devlin J, Boleski G, Mlynarek M, Nerenz D, Peterson E, Jankowski M, Horst H, Barowitz B (1999) Motor Activity Assessment Scale: a valid and reliable sedation scale for use with mechanically ventilated patients in an adult surgical intensive care unit. *Critical Care Medicine* **27**(7), 1271–1275.

Egerod I (2002) Uncertain terms of sedation in ICU. How nurses and physicians manage and describe sedation for mechanically ventilated patients. *Journal of Clinical Nursing* **11**(6), 831–840.

Elliott R, McKinley S, Aitken L (2006) Adoption of a sedation scoring system and sedation guideline in an intensive care unit. *Journal of Advanced Nursing* **54**(2), 208–216.

Ely EW, Inouye SK, Bernard GR, Gordon S, Francis J, May L, Truman B, Speroff T, Gautam S, Margolin R, Cook DJ (2001) Caring for the critically ill patient. Delirium in mechanically ventilated patients: validity and reliability of the Confusion Assessment Method for the Intensive Care Unit (CAM-ICU). *JAMA: Journal of the American Medical Association* **286**(21), 2703–2710, 2745–2746.

Ferguson ND, Mehta S (2002) Optimizing sedative use in the intensive care unit. *Intensive care Medicine* **28**(1), 44–47.

Frazier SK, Moser DK, Riegel B, McKinley S, Blakely W, Kim KA, Garvin BJ (2002) Critical care nurses' assessment of patients anxiety: reliance of physiological and behavioural parameters. *American Journal of Critical Care* **11**, 57–64.

Frenzel D, Greim CA, Sommer C, Bauerle K, Roewer N (2002) Is the bispectral index appropriate for monitoring the sedation level of mechanically ventilated surgical ICU patients? *Intensive Care Medicine* **28**, 178–183.

Fullwood D, Sargent S (2010) An overview of sedation for adult patients in hospital. *Nursing Standard* **24**(39), 48–56.

Hansen-Flaschen J, Cowen. J, Polomano RC (1994) Beyond the Ramsay scale: need for a validated measure of sedating drug efficacy in the intensive care unit. *Critical Care Medicine* **22**, 732–733.

Happ MB (2000) Preventing treatment interference: the nurse's role in maintaining technological devices. *Heart Lung* **29**(1), 60–69.

Hassan E, Fontaine DK, Nearman HS (1998) Therapeutic considerations in the management of agitated or delirious critically ill patients. *Pharmacotherapy* **18**(1), 113–129.

Jacobi J, Fraser GL, Coursin DB (2002) Clinical practice guidelines for the sustained use of sedatives and analgesics in the critically ill adult. *Critical Care Medicine* **30**(1), 119–141.

Jones S (2003) An algorithm for train-of-four monitoring in patients receiving continuous neuromuscular blocking agents. *Dimensions of Critical Care Nursing* **22**(2), 50–59.

Jones C, Griffiths RD, Humphries G, Skirrow PM (2001) Memory, delusions and the development of acute post-traumatic stress disorder-related symptoms after intensive care. *Critical Care Medicine* **29**, 573–80.

Kollef MH, Levy NT, Ahrens TS, Schaiff R, Prentice D, Sherman G (1998) The use of continuous I.V. sedation is associated with prolongation of mechanical ventilation. *Chest* **114**, 541–548.

Kress JP, Pohlman A, O'Connor MF (2000) Daily interruption of sedative infusions in critically ill patients undergoing mechanical ventilation. *The New England Journal of Medicine* **342**(20), 1471–1477.

Kress JP, Pohlman AS, Hall JB (2002) Sedation and analgesia in the intensive care unit. *American Journal of Respiratory Critical Care Medicine* **166**(8), 1024–1028.

Kress JP, Gehlbach B, Lacy M, Pliskin N, Pohlman AS, Hall JB (2003) The long-term psychological effects of daily sedative interruption on critically ill patients. *American Journal of Respiratory Critical Care Medicine* **168**(12), 1457–1461.

Leith B (1998) The use of restraints in critical care. *Official Journal of the Canadian Association of Critical Care Nurses* **9**, 24–28.

Marik PE (2004) Propofol: therapeutic indications and side-effects. *Current pharmaceutical design* **10**(29), 3639–3649.

Marini JJ, Wheeler AP (2006) *Critical care Medicine: The Essentials*, 3rd edn. Lippincott Williams & Wilkins, Philadelphia.

Misak CJ (2004) The critical care experiences: a patients' view. *American Journal of Respiratory Critical Care Medicine* **170**(4), 357–359.

Mirski M, Shannon N, LeDroux BS, Lewin J, Thompson C, Mirski K, Griswold M (2010) Validity and reliability of an intuitive conscious sedation scoring tool: the nursing instrument for the communication of sedation. *Critical Care Medicine* **38**(8), 1674–1684.

Murray M, Cowen J, DeBlock H, Erstad B, Gray A, Tescher A, McGee W, Prielipp R, Susla G, Jacobi J, Nasraway S, Lumb P (2002) Clinical practice guidelines for sustained neuromuscular blockade in the adult critically ill patient. *Critical Care Medicine* **30**(1), 142–156.

Nasraway S (2001) Use of sedative medications in the intensive care unit. *Seminars in Respiratory Critical Care Medicine* **22**(2), 165–174.

Olson D, Cheek D, Morgenlander J (2004) The impact of bispectral index monitoring on rates of Propofol administration. *AACN Clinical Issues: Advanced Practice in Acute and Critical Care* **15**(1), 63–73.

Ostermann ME, Keenan SP, Seiferling RA, Sibbald WJ (2000) Sedation in the intensive care unit: a systematic review. *JAMA* **283**(11), 1451–1459.

Pandharipande P, Ely E, Maze M (2006) Dexmedetomidine for sedation and perioperative management of critically ill patients. *Seminars in Anaesthesia, Perioperative Medicine and Pain* **25**(2): 43–50.

Pun BT, Dunn J (2007) The sedation of critically ill adults: part 1: assessment. *AJN* **107**(7), 20–28.

Putensen C, Zech S, Wrigge H, Zinserling J, Stuber F, Von Spiegal T, Mutz N (2001) Long term effects of spontaneous breathing during ventilatory support in patients with acute lung injury. *American Journal of Respiratory Critical Care Medicine* **164**, 43–49.

Ramsay MA, Savege TM, Simpson BR, Goodwin R (1974) Controlled sedation with alphaxalone-alphadolone. *BMJ* **2**(920), 656–659.

Rhoney DH, Parker D Jr (2001) Use of sedative and analgesic agents in neurotrauma patients: effects on cerebral physiology. *Neurological research* **23**(2), 237–259.

Riess ML, Graefe UA, Goeters C, Van AH, Bone HG (2002) Sedation assessment in critically ill patients with bispectral index. *European Journal of Anaesthesiology* **19**, 18–22.

Sang Ko J, Gwak, MS (2008) The effects of desflurane and propofol-remifentanil on postoperative hepatic and renal functions after right hepatectomy in liver donors. *Liver Transplantation* **14**(8), 1150–1158.

Schweickert WD, Gehlbach BK, Pohlman AS, Hall JB, Kress JP (2004) Daily interruption of sedative infusions and complications of critical illness in mechanically ventilated patients. *Critical Care Medicine* **32**(6), 1272–1276.

Sessler C, Grap M, Ramsay M (2008) Evaluating and monitoring analgesia and sedation in the intensive care unit. *Critical Care* **12**(Supp 3), S2.

Sessler C, Gosnell M, Grap M, Brophy G, O'Neal P, Keane K, Tesoro E, Elswick R (2002) The Richmond Agitation–Sedation Scale: validity and reliability in adult intensive care unit patients. *American Journal of Respiratory and Critical Care Medicine* **166**, 1338–1344.

Slomka J, Hoffman-Hogg L, Mion LC, Bair N, Bobek MB, Arroliga AC (2000) Influence of clinicians' values and perceptions on use of clinical practice guidelines for sedation and neuromuscular blockade in patients receiving mechanical ventilation. *American Journal of Critical Care* **9**(6), 412–418.

Soliman HM, Melot C, Vincent JL (2001) Sedative and analgesic practice in the intensive care unit: the results of a European survey. *British Journal of Anaesthesia* **87**(2), 186–192.

Szokol JW, Vender JS (2001) Anxiety, delirium and pain in the intensive care unit. *Critical Care Clinic* **17**(4), 821–842.

Vasile B, Rasulo F, Candiani A, Latronico N (2003) The pathophysiology of Propofol infusion syndrome: a simple name for a complex syndrome. *Intensive Care Medicine* **29**(9), 1417–1425.

Weinert CR, Chlan L, Gross C (2001) Sedating critically ill patients: factors affecting nurses' delivery of sedative therapy. *American Journal of Critical Care* **10**(3), 156–165.

Weiener-Kronish J (2001) Problems with sedation and analgesia in the ICU. *Pulmonary Perspectives* **18**(1), 1–3.

White S, Hollett JK, Kress JP, Zellinger M (2001) A renaissance in critical care nursing: technological advances and sedation strategies. *Critical Care Nurse* **21**, S1–16.

Chapter 12

The patient with raised intracranial pressure

Deborah Slade

Introduction

In order to provide protection to the soft matter of the brain, it is enclosed within the rigid cavity of the skull. Any increase in brain size due to bleeding, loss of compensatory mechanisms or the presence of solid tumours can give rise to life- threatening elevations in intracranial pressure (ICP). A raised ICP, if untreated, will lead to compression of brain matter and potential damage to vital brain structures that may result in the death of the patient. This scenario focuses on the knowledge and skills necessary to manage the critically ill patient with a raised ICP.

Patient scenario

Paul Rawlings is a 26-year-old man who is usually fit and well. Whilst out cycling he is involved in a collision with a car. He is taken by ambulance to the nearest emergency department. On arrival there Paul's Glasgow Coma Score (GCS) (Teasdale and Jennett 1976) has deteriorated to 9/15. The 15-point GCS should be used to assess Paul as recommended by the National Institute for Health and Clinical Excellence (NICE) in their head injury guidelines (NICE 2007). The findings of the initial physical examination are shown in Tables 12.1 and 12.2.

To secure his airway, Paul is intubated and ventilated and stabilised haemodynamically. Paul fulfils the NICE (2007) criteria for an urgent computerised tomography (CT) scan and he is transferred to the radiology department for a CT scan of his head and cervical spine (NICE 2007) and a chest X-ray. Paul's C-spine is cleared of injury and his chest X-ray is unremarkable; however, the CT scan identifies a left temporal depressed skull fracture and evidence of a subdural haematoma with diffuse cerebral contusions. Paul's present condition and investigation results are communicated to the Neurosurgical Centre 5 miles away where the consultant on-call confirms that Paul requires surgical intervention.

Critical Care Nursing: Learning from Practice, 1st edition. Edited by Suzanne Bench and Kate Brown.
© 2011 Blackwell Publishing Ltd.

Table 12.1 Paul's Glasgow Coma Score.

GCS	Paul's score
Eye opening Verbal response Motor response Total score = 9	Eyes opening to pain (E2) Making incomprehensible sounds (V2) Localising to pain with his left arm (M5) Score = E2, V2, M5 = 9

Table 12.2 Initial physical assessment using ABCDE framework.

Airway	Clear, but at risk of compromise due to Paul's reduced conscious level. Preparations are made to intubate and ventilate him.
Breathing	Respiratory rate 9/min, regular
	FiO$_2$ 0.5 via a non re-breathe reservoir bag/mask
	Arterial blood gas (ABG) analysis: pH 7.3 PaO$_2$ 11 kPa PaCO$_2$ 6.9 kPa Base Excess $^-$4
Circulation	Blood pressure 145/75 mmHg
	Heart rate 69 beats per minute, sinus rhythm
	Capillary refill < 2 seconds
Disability	GCS = 9/15; E2, V2, M5 – with evident right-arm weakness Pupils are unequal – left = 5 mm, right = 3 m. The right pupil reacts during testing of direct and consensual light reflexes; the left pupil remains fixed. Blood glucose 4.9 mmol/L
Exposure	Tympanic temperature 36.9°C Large scalp laceration over the left-temporal region and bruising over the left side of his face
	No other apparent injuries, although a cervical collar is *in situ* as a precaution for spinal injury.

Reader activities

Having read the scenario, consider the following:

- What is the cause of Paul's rapid neurological deterioration?
- What are the physiological mechanisms that maintain normal cerebral blood flow (CBF) and ICP?
- What are the implications for Paul of a raised ICP?
- What physiological changes would be evident with a rising ICP?

Pathophysiology related to increased ICP

The skull is a rigid box structure with incompressible contents of brain tissue, cerebral spinal fluid (CSF) and blood, which exist in a state of volume equilibrium. An increase in the volume of one constituent must be compensated by a decrease in the volume of another – the 'Monro-Kellie doctrine' (Lindsay et al. 2004; Lettieri 2006). Compromises in intracranial compliance or an expanding mass within the skull will consequently increase ICP (Lettieri 2006). Usually increases in ICP are controlled by autoregulatory mechanisms such as the displacement of blood via venous drainage or CSF into the spinal compartment/lumbar theca. These compensatory mechanisms will maintain ICP within physiological parameters (0–15 mmHg) up to a physiological limit (Lettieri 2006).

Maintenance of CBF is dependent on cerebral vascular resistance and cerebral perfusion pressure (CPP). CPP is calculated by subtracting mean ICP from mean arterial blood pressure (MABP) (Arbour 2004). An adequate CPP is vital in the maintenance of global cerebral perfusion and prevention of cerebral ischaemia. A CPP of above 70 mmHg is generally viewed as desirable to maintain adequate perfusion, but in TBI levels of between 60 and 70 mmHg may be acceptable (Arbour 2004). CBF is also coupled to the metabolic and energy requirements of brain tissue (Lindsay et al. 2004); essentially the rate is approximately 50 mL/100 mg/min (Ridley et al. 2003).

Following severe traumatic brain injury (TBI) autoregulation of CBF is impaired (Lindsay et al. 2004). Initially, cerebral blood volume (CBV) increases due to cerebral vasodilatation caused by raised carbon dioxide levels ($PaCO_2$), which decreases extracellular pH provoking a rise in ICP. Sustained raised ICP reduces CPP compromising CBF, and decreasing CBV. Reduced cerebral perfusion of oxygen sensitive cells in the cortex causes anaerobic cell metabolism leading to ischaemia and a build-up of metabolic by-products that lower extracellular pH (Layton et al. 2004). When CBF is < 25 mL/100 mg/min electrical activity is severely compromised and if the rate decreases below 10 mL/100 mg/min cell death occurs (Ridley et al. 2003). Hypoxia, ischaemia, low extracellular pH and blood hypo-osmolality lead to cytotoxic oedema – intracellular fluid accumulation. This compounds vasogenic oedema, which is believed to occur soon after injury and results from disruption of the blood–brain barrier (BBB), causing increased permeability of capillary walls and leakage of protein- rich fluid into the extracellular space (Ridley et al. 2003). Development of oedema increases ICP, and eventually compensatory mechanisms are exhausted. In a congested brain, CBF becomes compromised and increased pressure on the vascular bed leads to distortion and increased vascular resistance, which restricts cerebral perfusion perpetuating a vicious cycle of oedema formation and raised ICP (Lindsay et al. 2004). Raised ICP can also be caused by an expanding haematoma, restricted venous outflow and obstruction to CSF flow and /or absorption (Singh and Stock 2006). Any expanding mass causes brain tissue to shift risking herniation across fixed dural structures within the brain, leading to irreversible and potentially fatal damage (Arbour 2004; Shepard 2004).

Paul's increasing ICP and initial hypoxia would cause loss of consciousness, which compromises the airway (Lettieri 2006). Raised ICP causes pressure on the respiratory centres of the medulla oblongata in the brainstem altering breathing rate and pattern – often hypoventilation or an irregular breathing with apnoeic episodes (Mayer and Chong 2002). Inadequate ventilation may lead to a raised $PaCO_2$, which causes cerebral vasodilatation, further increasing the ICP (Mayer and Chong 2002).

Paul was diagnosed with a sub-dural haematoma. An expanding lesion on one side of the brain may cause haemiparesis/haemiplegia due to direct injury or pressure on the motor cortex (Shepard 2004). Nerve impulses for voluntary movement originate in the motor cortex of the frontal lobe (Tortora and Grabowski 2000). Upper motor neurones travel via pyramidal pathways, most 'cross over' or decussate at the level of the medulla oblongata in the brainstem, before descending the spinal cord to synapse with lower motor neurones that innervate skeletal muscle of the trunk and limbs (Tortora and Grabowski 2000). Hence, Paul's injury to the left motor cortex will cause a contralateral (right-sided) haemiparesis/haemiplegia (Lindsay et al. 2004).

As Paul's ICP increases, assessment of his pupils reveals altered size and reaction to light, which is due to medial temporal lobe pressure on the oculomotor nerve (cranial nerve III) (Lindsay et al. 2004). Initially oculomotor nerve damage is ipsilateral but may become bilateral with increasing ICP. On fundoscopy, papilloedema may be evident if increased CSF pressure in the optic nerve (cranial nerve II) sheath has impeded venous drainage, leading to retinal and optic disc haemorrhages (Lindsay et al. 2004). Generally, raised ICP causes a persistent headache due to stretching of the arteries in the brainstem and displacement of CSF. Vomiting is a frequent side effect due to pressure on the 'vomit' centre of the brainstem (Singh and Stock. 2006).

Factors that instigate changes in ICP cannot be considered separately because they each contribute to complex inter-relationships or feedback pathways that can actually exacerbate further brain injury (Lindsay et al. 2004).

In TBI, intracranial bleeding can be extradural, subdural or intracerebral; sometimes sub-arachnoid bleeding may also occur (Lettieri 2006). Secondary brain injury such as haematomas, ischaemia, infection, brain swelling and shift occur after the initial primary injury (Shepard 2004). Restricting the impact of secondary causes on ICP is the focus for management of patients with TBI.

Developing scenario

Paul arrives at the Neurosurgical Centre and immediately undergoes surgery to remove the subdural haematoma. He is transferred to the intensive care unit post-surgery.

Reader activities

Consider the following:

- What would be the main aims of treatment to limit the impact of Paul's raised ICP? (Consider the relationship between CBF, CPP and ICP. Review other monitoring modalities and their value in managing TBI).
- Paul is sedated and ventilated: What would be the optimal parameters for arterial blood gases for a patient with a raised ICP?
- How might you assess Paul's neurological function whilst he is sedated?
- What other nursing considerations will there be during the first 48 hours post-surgery?

Assessment tools

The injured brain is exceptionally susceptible to secondary ischaemic insults such as hypoxia and hypotension, which are associated with poor neurological outcome after severe TBI (Hlatky et al. 2003). Management of patients with TBI is therefore frequently dominated by techniques based on maintaining cerebral perfusion and adequacy of CBF with concomitant limitation of increases in ICP (Hlatky et al. 2003; Young et al. 2003).

Maintenance of Paul's CPP is important because of the significant physiological role it represents in a patient with TBI. CPP indicates the pressure gradient acting across the cerebrovascular bed, and therefore it is an important factor in the regulation of CBF (Hlatky et al. 2003). CPP contributes to the hydrostatic pressure within intracerebral vessels, so it has the potential to affect oedema formation in the injured brain (Hlatky et al. 2003).

Monitoring of Paul's ICP to determine his CPP warrants insertion of both an arterial line and ICP monitoring device. Monitoring of ICP has been shown to be useful in predicting outcome from TBI and in guiding therapy for raised ICP, which may lead to improved outcome for those patients who respond to ICP lowering interventions (Brain Trauma Foundation (BTF) 2007). A number of devices are currently available for the monitoring of ICP, including insertion of an intraventricular catheter, subarachnoid bolt or screw, or a subdural or epidural catheter and intraparenchymal insertion of a fiber-optic transducer tipped catheter (see Figure 12.1). A good overview of the range of ICP assessment methods and their advantages and disadvantages can be found in Arbour (2004).

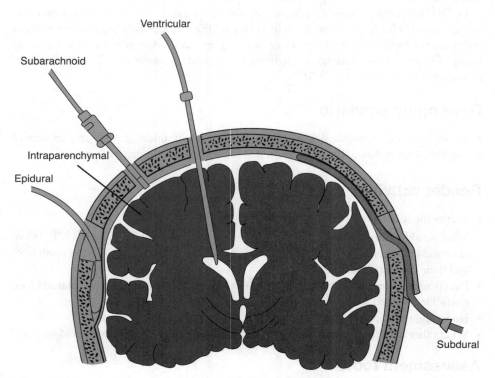

Figure 12.1   Major types of intracranial pressure monitoring. Coronal section of the brain shows potential sites for placement of the monitoring devices. (Adapted from Kerr and Crago, with permission from Elsevier.)

Intraventricular devices are currently viewed as the gold standard for accurate ICP monitoring (Arbour 2004; BTF 2007). There is a therapeutic advantage to inserting an intraventricular catheter because it allows for highly accurate measurement of ICP and also allows for the drainage of CSF if necessary (Lettieri 2006; BTF 2007). Intraventricular devices are, however, associated with a higher incidence of infection compared to an intraparenchymal microtransducer device (e.g. Codman® ICP probes) (Lane et al. 2000). Less invasive devices provide less accurate measurements and may require frequent recalibrations (Arbour 2004).

In patients with TBI, the CPP should be maintained above 60 mmHg (Juul et al. 2000; Arbour 2004). A CPP of 55 mmHg is considered a probable critical threshold for poor neurological outcome in adults and a CPP of < 50 mmHg should be avoided (BTF 2007); however, it is important to remember that CPP may be non-uniform with variable CBF to areas of injury (Lettieri 2006). Mindful of this and allowing for variations in MABP, most clinicians prefer to maintain CPP within a target range of 50–70 mmHg (BTF 2007). Aggressive attempts to maintain CPP above 70 mmHg with fluids and vasoactive drugs should be avoided because of the risk of adult respiratory distress syndrome (ARDS) (BTF 2007).

Measurements of cerebral oxygenation are also recommended in the patient with TBI (BTF 2007), and evidence supports the use of either jugular venous saturations ($SjvO_2$) or brain tissue oxygen levels ($P_{bt}O_2$) Measurements indicate the adequacy of CBF relative to metabolic requirements; for example, with rising ICP, resultant hypoperfusion will increase oxygen extraction and $SJvO_2$ will be decreased <50% (normal $SJvO_2$ 55 – 75%) (Hlatky et al. 2003). The major limitation of using $SJvO_2$ as a monitor of CBF adequacy is that regional ischaemia will not be identified (Hlatky et al. 2003; Layton et al. 2004). In TBI, where regional differences in CBF may occur, monitoring of brain tissue $P_{bt}O_2$ may be beneficial. Normal values are approximately 20–40 mmHg with a range of 8–10 mmHg representing a probable critical threshold (Hoffman et al. 1996; Kiening et al. 1996; Valadka et al. 1998, 2000; BTF 2007).

Managing the patient with raised ICP

Nursing considerations for critically ill brain injured patients aim to optimise systemic and cerebral oxygenation and CBF and minimise factors that may aggravate neuronal injury or contribute to intracranial hypertension (Mayer and Chong 2002).

Airway/breathing

If the GCS is ≤8 intubation and ventilation are required to protect the airway, allow for deep sedation, and to facilitate optimal gas exchange in the lungs. In patients with TBI, optimal oxygenation and prevention of hypoxaemia are paramount. Ventilation manipulation should aim to maintain arterial oxygen (PaO_2) levels above 12 kPa, with strenuous avoidance of PaO_2 <8.0 mmHg or O_2 saturation <90% (BTF 2007). Arterial CO_2 ($PaCO_2$) levels should be maintained at between 4.5 and 5.0 kPa. Hypercarbia ($PaCO_2$ >6 kPa) is avoided because it can cause cerebral vasodilatation and hyperaemia, which increase ICP (Lettieri 2006). Therapeutic hyperventilation, however, produces hypocarbia, which causes cerebral vasoconstriction, decreasing CBV and hence ICP (Yanko and Mitcho 2001). Even so, CBF generally decreases during the initial 24 hours following severe TBI and vasoresponsivity to carbon dioxide may therefore be reduced negating the positive effects of vasoconstriction; coupled with a loss of autoregulation, ICP may not actually decrease (Lettieri 2006). Increasing the rate of CO_2 removal from the blood will decrease hydrogen ion concentration in CSF, which precipitates chemical and ionic imbalances, such as alkalosis and hypokaleamia (Yanko and Mitcho 2001). Mayer and Chong (2002) note that prophylactic hyperventilation is associated with a poorer outcome; so traditional chronic hyperventilation should, therefore, be avoided. Transient episodes of hyperventilation, however, can be a rapid and useful method to limit the duration of acute and damaging increases in ICP (Iacono 2000; Mayer and Chong 2002; Lettieri 2006; BTF 2007).

Customary beliefs that the use of positive end-expiratory pressure (PEEP) will provoke a rise in ICP is no longer appropriate as hypoxaemia often fails to correct without the addition of PEEP and, with an adequate intravascular volume, a PEEP of 10 cmH_2O does not elevate ICP and may even decrease it due to improved cerebral oxygenation (Huynh et al. 2002).

To maintain Paul's endotracheal tube patency, mobilisation and removal of lung secretions is required. Unfortunately, chest physiotherapy and tracheal stimulation during suctioning could cause Paul adverse cerebrovascular and systemic vascular effects and may elevate his ICP (Yanko and Mitcho 2001). Endotracheal suctioning should be performed based on a Paul's clinical signs and where benefits are considered to outweigh risks. Pre-oxygenation with FiO_2 1.0 and minimising the number of catheter passes may avoid the cumulative effects that raise ICP (Yanko and Mitcho 2001).

Patient positioning is important and the head of the bed should be elevated to 30 degrees with Paul's head and neck maintained in a straight and forward (neutral) alignment (Lee 1989; Feldman et al. 1992; Simmons 1997; Patterson et al. 2005). This position should reduce cerebral and jugular venous pressure, and promote venous drainage, without severely compromising CPP, CBF or cardiac output and may help protect against ventilator acquired pneumonia (Mayer and Chong 2002; Patterson et al. 2005; DH 2007).

Extreme flexion of Paul's hips and knees should be avoided as it increases intra-abdominal pressure and hence intrathoracic pressure, which compromises venous drainage, increasing ICP (Yanko and Mitcho 2001). When turning Paul, a 'log roll' technique allows the head and neck to be kept in neutral alignment (Yanko and Mitcho 2001) (see Figures 12.2 and 12.3). If, as a precaution, Paul's cervical spine is immobilised with a rigid collar, this can elevate ICP by approximately 4–6 mmHg due to compression of the jugular vein (Ho et al. 2002; Arbour 2004). The nurse should also be mindful when tying/securing Paul's endotracheal tube tapes that jugular venous drainage is not impeded (Yanko and Mitcho 2001).

Circulation

A sizeable proportion of TBI patients develop significant hypotension resulting in hypoxia, and sustained hypotension significantly increases morbidity and mortality (BTF 2007).

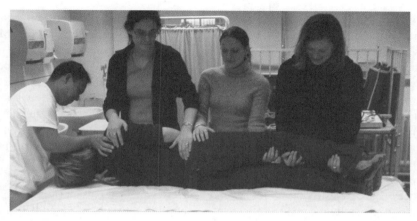

Figure 12.2   Example a of log rolling technique. Photo by the author.

Currently the defining level of significant hypotension remains unclear, but a single observation of a systolic blood pressure less than 90 mmHg should be avoided if possible or rapidly corrected (BTF 2007). Consequently accurate and continuous monitoring of blood pressure and attainment of blood pressure targets are important. Attention to systolic and MABP levels are of increased significance when caring for patients with TBI who do not have ICP monitoring *in situ* (BTF 2007).

To achieve haemodynamic stability, judicial use of isotonic fluid, such as intravenous saline 0.9%, is suggested to maintain normovolaemia and normotension, that is, Paul's blood pressure and central venous pressure (Yanko and Mitcho 2001; Mayer and Chong 2002). Serum sodium (Na$^+$) levels should be monitored and maintained approximately 140 mmol/L because hyponatraemia or hypernatraemia will exacerbate oedema formation and cerebral cell damage, respectively (Lettieri 2006). Likewise, hypotonic intravenous 5% dextrose solution should be avoided because glucose is metabolised to lactic acid

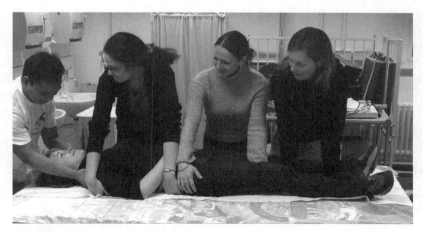

Figure 12.3   Example b of log rolling technique. Photo by the author.

in hypoxic tissue, which provokes neurotoxic acidosis causing oedema formation, and the free water contained in the solution increases cerebral oedema and ICP (Menon 1999; Yanko and Mitcho 2001). In addition to crystalloid, it may be necessary to administer blood products to optimise cerebral oxygen extraction, ensuring haematocrit is approximately 0.32 and haemoglobin (Hb) >8 g/dL (Yanko and Mitcho 2001). Once normovolaemia is achieved maintenance of MABP and consequently CPP may require administration of vasopressor drugs, such as noradrenaline, to enhance systemic vaso-constriction (Yanko and Mitcho 2001). Owing to a lack of adrenergic receptors on cerebral blood vessels, vasopressor agents do not affect cerebral vascular resistance (Iacono 2000).

Interventions aimed at decreasing ICP are controversial as there is a lack of any high-quality evidence to justify the use of any individual treatment at present (Ker et al. 2008). Mannitol is generally regarded as effective in controlling episodes of raised ICP at doses of 0.25 g/kg to 1 g/kg body weight (BTF 2007). The overall effects of Mannitol use on factors such as patient survival are unclear; however, its use is currently recommended for the treatment of dangerous elevations in ICP (Maas et al. 1997; BTF 2007). Hypotension (systolic blood pressure <90 mmHg) is a risk following Mannitol administration, and this should be avoided (BTF 2007). Mannitol has a plasma expansion effect that decreases haematocrit and blood viscosity, increasing CBF and cerebral oxygen delivery (Yanko and Mitcho 2001). Subsequent generation of an altered osmotic gradient between neural cells and plasma then facilitates fluid shifts reducing both vasogenic and cytotoxic oedema, decreasing ICP by approximately 30% after a single bolus (Yanko and Mitcho 2001; Lettieri 2006). Mannitol also scavenges free radicals associated with cerebral oedema formation (Yanko and Mitcho 2001).

Frusemide is synergistic with Mannitol and can be used to increase intravascular oncotic pressure by hypo-osmolar diuresis, which reduces cerebral oedema and CSF production (Lettieri 2006). Both agents are administered with caution to avoid hypo-volaemia and hypotension, which compromise CPP. Urine output should be replaced with crystalloid administration to maintain intravascular volume (Lettieri 2006). Repeated doses of Mannitol can cause an accumulation and result in a reverse osmotic shift exacerbating cerebral oedema. Evaluation for kidney injury and electrolyte imbalances is essential, as is observation for pulmonary congestion and compromised cardiac function (Yanko and Mitcho 2001). Some preliminary research has been undertaken to establish whether the administration of hypertonic saline would provide a more effective means of reducing cerebral oedema; however, the BTF (2007) states that, at present, the evidence is insufficient to allow recommendations on the use, concentration or administration of hypertonic saline for the treatment of traumatic intracranial hypertension.

Disability of the central nervous system

In addition to monitoring ICP, neurological assessment in the sedated and ventilated patient should include cranial nerve assessment (Lindsay et al. 2004). Nurses should note the presence of brainstem activity, for example, the protective reflexes – gag, cough, or blinking; observation of facial grimacing for noticeable weakness. Patients with TBI, however, often require deep sedation to reduce the risk of elevations in ICP thus making assessment of neurological function difficult. Paul's pupils should be assessed regularly for both direct and consensual responses to light and abnormal eye movements, such as divergent gaze or nystagmus (Arbour 2004; Patterson et al. 2005). Pupil size, shape and reactivity provide a useful indication of the presence of raised ICP.

When appropriate, the GCS is used, for example, during sedation holds; otherwise sedation scores should be performed (Roundtable meeting 2002). Normally in patients with a raised ICP sedation holds would be contra-indicated and if Paul was coughing, gagging or grimacing, this would be an indication to increase sedation. A sedation hold would only be appropriate when there is no longer concern about his ICP or when he has sufficiently recovered to allow waking and weaning from sedation (see Chapter 11 for more information on sedation holds).

Pain and agitation increase ICP and should be avoided (Lettieri 2006). Sedatives, narcotics and muscle relaxants can be administered to prevent elevations in ICP and to facilitate mechanical ventilation (Yanko and Mitcho 2001). Benzodiazepines and propofol are advantageous because they also increase seizure threshold (Lettieri 2006) (see Chapter 14 for information on seizure management). Propofol is a preferred agent because it is highly lipid soluble and crosses the BBB quickly. Its rapid onset and short half-life (<1 hour) allow for fast titration for clinical effect and intermittent neurological assessment (Patterson et al. 2005; BTF 2007). Propofol also scavenges free radicals and is a potent antioxidant, which may help to reduce episodes of raised ICP. Oxygen and glucose consumption are reduced through suppression of cerebral metabolism, which thereby reduces CBF and ICP (Yanko and Mitcho 2001).

Neuromuscular blockade may be incorporated to attenuate a cough reflex or noxious stimuli in a patient with compromised intracranial compliance that results in acute elevations in ICP (Arbour 2004). Therapeutic muscle relaxation can, however, mask seizure activity and prevents physical assessment that might disclose early signs of deterioration. It can also prolong the need for mechanical ventilation, which would put Paul at risk of developing nosocomial pneumonia, pressure ulcers and venothromboemboli. Deep sedation affords similar benefits and probably provides a safer option than neuromuscular blockade (Lettieri 2006) (see Chapters 10 and 11 for more information on pain and sedation).

Exposure/environment

The Guideline for the Management of Severe Head Injury advises that nutritional support is commenced within 72 hours of injury (Yanko and Mitcho 2001). Patients with severe TBI are frequently hypermetabolic or catabolic, and can require long periods of mechanical ventilation and often require prolonged hospitalisation (Lettieri 2006). Critical illness, in general, predisposes patients to polyneuropathy and neuromuscular weakness. It is therefore imperative to instigate adequate nutrition at an early stage, preferably via the enteral route to maintain integrity of the gut and optimal pH in the stomach, which minimises possible risk of infection (especially ventilator-associated pneumonia), sepsis, and hyperglycaemia and close monitoring of glycaemic control is essential (Vogelzang et al. 2006). Most importantly, Paul's muscular strength must be restored to facilitate timely weaning from ventilator dependence (Lettieri 2006).

A recurrent trend in management of patients with TBI is the induction of mild hypothermia (central temperature $\sim 34^{\circ}C$) to decrease ICP and CBF and stabilise cell membranes protecting the brain from ischaemia (Yanko and Mitcho 2001; Gunnarsson and Fehlings 2003). To achieve hypothermia, a patient with severe TBI admitted to the emergency department should not be re-warmed, as active cooling has to occur within 90 minutes of injury (Clifton et al. 2001). Mild hypothermia causes a left shift in the oxygen (O_2) dissociation curve, so Hb affinity for O_2 is increased, and since hypothermia also slows cerebral metabolism, O_2 supply and demand implications should be closely monitored (Clifton 2004). Complications of induced hypothermia include increased incidence of bacterial infection, myocardial suppression, cardiac arrhythmias, renal dysfunction, re-warming shock and a rebound increase in ICP (Yanko and Mitcho 2001).

Psychological care and communication with a patient who is ventilated is of paramount importance (Liao and So 2002; Geraghty 2005). Patients with TBI can often exhibit elevations in ICP in response to noxious stimuli (Arbour 2004). The multi-professional team should therefore be mindful that such noxious stimuli include sudden touch, unfamiliar environmental noise, and painful procedures. Paul's general hygiene needs should be managed according to how tolerant he is of such interventions. Clustering care is not advisable; however, a patient's response is unique and the nurse should discover the best approach in accordance with Paul's clinical signs (Eisenhart 1994). It is worth exploring what effect 'family' presence and therapeutic touch, such as stroking the hand or cheek, has on Paul (Liao and So 2002; Azoulay et al. 2003) as this may have a beneficial effect on ICP.

Conclusion

TBI is associated with significant risk of long-term neurological damage and disability (Arbour 2004). The initial 72 hours post-TBI is recognised as a crucial period in the patient's management. Close monitoring and skilled medical and nursing interventions are vital to the patient's survival and recovery from injury. The paucity of adequate empirical studies on the management of patients with a raised ICP means there is currently insufficient evidence to provide strong recommendations for individual medical and nursing interventions.

Critical appraisal of a research paper

Perz-Barceno J, Llompart-Pou JA, Homar J, Abadal JM, Raunch JM, Frontera G, Brell M, Ibanez Javier, Ibanez Jordi (2008) Phenobarbitol versus thiopental in the treatment of refractory intracranial hypertension in patients with traumatic brain injury: A randomised controlled trial. *Critical Care* **12**(4), R112.

Reader activities

1. Read the research article written by Perez-Barcena et al. (2008)
2. Using the critical appraisal framework in Appendix, I consider the methodological quality of the paper
3. If relevant, reflect on this aspect of management within your clinical area and any implications for future practice this paper might raise

A commentary on this paper has been provided by the chapter author in Appendix XIII.

Recommended reading

Brain Trauma Foundation (BTF) American Association of Neurological Surgeons (2007) Guidelines *on Severe Traumatic Brain Injury*. Available online at: www.braintrauma.org. Recommended as they represent the most up to date and comprehensive set of guidelines currently available.

Maas AI, Dearden M, Teasdale GM, Braakman R, Cohadon F, Iannotti F, Karimi A, Lapierre F, Murray G, Ohman J, Persson L, Servadei F, Stocchetti N, Unterberg A (1997) EBIC guidelines for management of severe head injury in adults. *Acta Neurochirurgica* **139**(4), 286–294. These are the most recent European guidelines available but have probably been superceded by the BTF guidelines cited above.

National Institute of Health and Clinical Excellence (NICE) (2007) *CG56: Head Injury Triage, Assessment, Investigation and Early Management of Head Injury in infants, Children and Adults*. Available online at: www.nice.org.uk. Accessed 25 January 2010.

References

Arbour R (2004) Intracranial hypertension: monitoring and nursing assessment. *Critical Care Nurse* **24**(5), 19–32.

Available online at: www.medscape.com/viewarticle/542508?rss. Accessed 30 January 2010.

Azoulay E, Pochard F, Chevret S, Arich C, Brivet F, Brun F, Charles P-E, Desmettre T, Dubois D, Galliot R, Garrouste-Orgeas M, Goldgran-Toledano D, Herbecq P, Joly LM, Jourdain M, Kaidomar M, Lepape A, Letellier N, Marie O, Page B; Parrot A, Rodie-Talbere P, Sermet A, Tenaillon A, Thuong M, Tulasne P, Le Gall JR, Schlemmer B (2003) Family participation in care to the critically ill: opinions of families and staff. *Intensive Care Medicine* **29**, 1498–1504.

Brain Trauma Foundation (BTF), American Association of Neurological Surgeons (2007) *Guidelines on Severe Traumatic Brain Injury*. Available online at: www.braintrauma.org. Accessed 13 January 2010.

Clifton G, Miller E, Choi S, Levin H, McCauley S, Smith K, Muizelaar P, Wagner F, Marion D, Luerssen T, Chestnut R, Schwartz M (2001) Lack of effect of induction of hypothermia after acute brain injury. *New England Journal of Medicine* **344**(8), 556–563.

Clifton G (2004) Is keeping cool still hot? An update on hypothermia in brain injury. *Current Opinion in Critical Care* **10**: 116–119.

DH (2007) *Saving lives: reducing infection, delivering clean and safe care.* Department of Health. Available online at: http://www.clean-safe-care.nhs.uk/public/default.aspx?level=2&load=Tools&NodeID=181. Accessed 28 January 2010.

Eisenhart K (1994) New perspectives in the management of adults with severe head injury. *Critical Care Nurse Quarterly* **17**(2), 1–12.

Feldman Z, Kanter M, Robertson C (1992) Effects of head elevation on intracranial pressure, cerebral perfusion pressure, and cerebral blood flow in head injured patients. *Journal of Neurosurgery* **59**, 207–211.

Geraghty M (2005) Nursing the unconscious patient. *Nursing Standard* **20**(1), 54–60.

Gunnarsson T, Fehlings MG (2003) Acute neurosurgical management of traumatic brain injury and spinal cord injury. *Current Opinion in Neurology* **16**, 717–723.

Hlatky R, Valadka AB, Robertson CS (2003) Intracranial hypertension and cerebral ischaemia after severe traumatic brain injury. *Neurosurgical Focus* **14**(4), 1–4.

Ho AMH, Fung KY, Joynt GM, Karmakar MK, Peng Z (2002) Rigid cervical collar and intracranial pressure of patients with severe head injury. *Journal of Trauma* **53**, 1185–1188.

Hoffman WE, Charbel FT, Edelman G (1996) Brain tissue oxygen, carbon dioxide, and pH in neurosurgical patients at risk for ischaemia. *Anaesthesia and Analgesia* **82**, 582–586.

Huynh T, Messer M, Sing RF, Miles W, Jacobs DG, Thomason MH (2002) Positive end-expiratory pressure alters intracranial and cerebral perfusion pressure in severe traumatic brain injury. *Journal of Trauma* **53**, 488–492.

Iacono LA (2000) Exploring the guidelines for the management of severe head injury. *Journal of Neuroscience Nursing* **32**, 54–60.

Juul N, Morris GF, Marshall SB, Marshall LF (2000) Intracranial hypertension and cerebral perfusion pressure: influence on neurological deterioration and outcome in severe head injury. The Executive Committee of the International Selfotel Trial. *Journal of Neurosurgery* **92**, 1–6.

Kerr M, Crago EA. Nursing management: acute intracranial problems. In: O'Brien PG, Giddens JF, Bucher L, eds. *Medical-Surgical Assessment and Management of Clinical Problems.* St Louis, Mo: CV Mosby Inc; 2004: 1491–1524.

Ker K, Perel P, Blackhall K, Roberts I (2008) How effective are some common treatments for traumatic brain injury? *British Medical Journal* **337**, a865.

Kiening KL, Uterberg, AW, Bardt TF (1996) Monitoring of cerebral oxygenation in patients with severe head injuries: brain tissue PO_2 versus jugular vein oxygen saturation. *Journal of Neurosurgery* **85**, 751–757.

Lane PL, Skoretz TG, Doig G (2000) Intracranial pressure monitoring and outcomes after traumatic brain injury. In: Lettieri CJ (2006) Neurotrauma: management of acute head injuries. *Medscape Critical Care* **7**(2), 1–5. Available online at: www.medscape.com/viewarticle/542508?rss. Accessed 30 January 2010.

Layton AJ, Gabrielli A, Friedman WA (2004) *Textbook of Neurointensive Care*, Chap 25. WB Saunders, Philadelphia.

Lee ST (1989) Intracranial pressure changes during positioning of patients with severe head injury. *Heart and Lung* **18**, 411–414.

Lettieri CJ (2006) Neurotrauma: management of acute head injuries. *Medscape Critical Care* **7**(2), 1–5.

Liao J, So YT (2002) An approach to critically ill patients in coma. *Western Journal of Medicine* **176**(3), 184–187.

Lindsay K, Bone I, Callander R (2004) *Neurology and Neurosurgery Illustrated*. Churchill Livingstone, New York.

Maas AI, Dearden M, Teasdale GM, Braakman R, Cohadon F, Iannotti F, Karimi A, Lapierre F, Murray G, Ohman J, Persson L, Servadei F, Stocchetti N, Unterberg A (1997) EBIC guidelines for management of severe head injury in adults. *Acta Neurochirurgica* **139**(4), 286–294.

Mayer SA, Chong JI (2002) Critical care management of increased intracranial pressure. *Journal of Intensive Care Medicine* **17**, 55–67.

Menon DK (1999) Cerebral protection in severe brain injury: physiological determinants of outcome and their optimisation. *British Medical Bulletin* **55**(1), 226–258.

National Institute of Health and Clinical Excellence (NICE) (2007) *CG56: Head injury Triage, Assessment, Investigation and Early Management of Head Injury in Infants, Children and Adults*. Available online at: www.nice.org.uk. Accessed 26 January 2010.

Patterson J, Bloom SA, Coyle B, Mouradjian D, Maloney Wilensky E (2005) Successful outcome in severe traumatic brain injury: a case study. *Journal of Neuroscience Nursing* **37**(5), 263–242.

Perz-Barceno J, Llompart-Pou JA, Homar J, Abadal JM, Raunch JM, Frontera G, Brell M, Ibanez Javier, Ibanez Jordi (2008) Phenobarbitol versus thiopental in the treatment of refractory intracranial hypertension in patients with traumatic brain injury: a randomised controlled trial. *Critical Care* **12**(4), R112.

Ridley S, Smith G, Batchelor A (eds) (2003) *Core Cases in Critical Care*. Greenwich Medical Media Ltd., London.

Roundtable meeting (2002) Management of the agitated intensive care unit patient. *Critical Care Medicine (Supplement)* **30**(1), S97–S123.

Shepard S (2004) *Head Trauma*. Available online at: www.Emedicine.com. Accessed 21 August 2007.

Simmons BJ (1997) Management of intracranial haemodynamics in the adult: a research analysis of head positioning and recommendations for clinical practice and future research. *Journal of Neuroscience Nursing* **29**, 44–49.

Singh J, Stock A (2006) *Head Trauma*. Available online at: www.Emedicine.com. Accessed 14 January 2007.

Teasdale G, Jennett B (1976) Assessment and prognosis of coma after head injury. *Acta Neurochirurgica* **34**, 45–55.

Tortora GJ, Grabowski SJ (2000) *Principles of Anatomy and Physiology*. Wiley, New York.

Valadka AB, Gopinanth SP, Contant CF (1998) Relationship of brain tissue PO_2 to outcome after severe head injury. *Critical Care Medicine* **26**, 1576–1581.

Valadka AB, Yu F, Hlatky R, Robertson C (2000) Global and regional techniques for monitoring cerebral oxidative metabolism after severe traumatic brian injury. *Neurosurgical Focus* **9**(5). Available online at: www.medscape.com. Accessed 26 January 2010.

Vogelzang M, Nijboer JM, van der Horst I, Zijlstra F, ten Duis, Henk J, Nijsten MW (2006) Hyperglycaemia has a strong relation with outcome in trauma patients than in other critically ill patients. *Journal of Trauma* **60**, 873–877.

Yanko JR, Mitcho K (2001) Acute care management of severe traumatic brain injuries. *Critical Care Nursing Quarterly* **23**(4), 1–23.

Young JS, Blow O, Turrentine RN, Claridge JA, Schulman A (2003) Is there an upper limit of intracranial pressure in patients with severe head injury if cerebral perfusion pressure is maintained? *Neurosurgical Focus* **15**(6), 1–7.

Chapter 13

The patient with delirium

Deborah Slade and Kate Brown

Introduction

Delirium is a clinical syndrome characterised by disturbed consciousness, cognitive function or perception. It is a common but complex clinical syndrome associated with poor outcomes (National Institute for Health and Clinical Excellence (NICE) 2010). It occurs in up to 60–80% of patients in the intensive care unit (ICU), yet goes unrecognized by the managing physicians and nurses in 32–66% of cases (Pandharipande et al. 2005). Caring for patients with delirium (or confusion/agitation) presents significant challenges for critical care nurses. Delirium can have serious consequences for patients as it increases their length of critical care stay and places them at greater risk of hospital-acquired complications, such as infections, falls and pressure sores, and they are more likely to die (Morandi et al. 2009; NICE 2010). Ely and Truman (2005) noted that for many people who are in good physical condition but succumb to critical illness, cognitive decline poses the main threat to their ability to recover.

This chapter focuses on the assessment, diagnosis and management of a patient who has developed delirium following a period of admission to the ICU.

Patient scenario

Harry Faulkner is a 76-year-old man transferred from the ICU to a high-dependency unit (HDU). Harry has undergone abdominal surgery for a perforated bowel. Harry was in the ICU for ten days, as he required sedation and ventilation for a post-operative pneumonia. Harry has been successfully weaned from sedation and is now extubated. On arrival in the HDU, an assessment of Harry reveals the following information:

Airway/Breathing

Harry is self-ventilating on 40% oxygen.

Critical Care Nursing: Learning from Practice, 1st edition. Edited by Suzanne Bench and Kate Brown.
© 2011 Blackwell Publishing Ltd.

Circulation

Harry is haemodynamically stable and is afebrile.

Disability

Harry is confused, agitated and irritable. He is removing his oxygen mask and pulling at his lines. He frequently tries to get out of bed and is quite physically and verbally abusive.

Exposure/environment

Harry has an abdominal incision site, which is uncovered. He has a central-line and a naso-gastric tube for feeding. A penile sheath catheter attached to a urometer for hourly urine measurement. He is wearing knee-length thromboembolic stockings.

Reader activities

Having read this scenario, consider the following:

- Why has delirium become the recommended terminology for use in confusional states for hospitalised patients?
- What are some of the difficulties in obtaining universal definitions?
- What factors might have precipitated Harry's delirium?
- What is currently thought to be the pathophysiology of delirium?
- What non-pharmacological interventions might help to restore Harry's neurological status?
- What are the current opinions and guidance on the use of chemical and physical restraint in the UK? Do they differ from other countries, and what are your own views on their use in the critically ill patients?

Definitions of delirium

Delirium is the preferred term to explain confusion conditions in hospitalised patients without pre-existing dementia or psychosis (NICE 2010). It has replaced terms such as acute confusional state, ICU psychosis or acute brain dysfunction (Morandi et al. 2009). The prevalence of delirium amongst ICU patients is between 20% and 80% (Morandi et al. 2009), or may be as high as 60–80% (Pandharipande et al. 2005). Rates vary in relation to the severity of illness and the tools used to diagnose delirium (Ely et al. 2001). NICE (2010) defines delirium as a

clinical syndrome characterised by disturbed consciousness, cognitive function or perception (page 3)

NICE (2010) states that delirium is suspected by the presence of alterations in the following:

- Cognitive function: for example, worsened concentration, slow responses or confusion
- Perception: for example, visual or auditory hallucinations
- Physical function: for example, reduced mobility, reduced movement, restlessness, agitation, changes in appetite, sleep disturbance
- Social behaviour: for example, poor cooperation, withdrawal, or alterations in communication, mood and/or attitude.

Whatever diagnostic indicator is used, it is important that critical care nurses are aware of the patient risk factors for developing delirium and are able to assess and diagnose this condition. Best practice guidelines should be followed to treat delirium effectively and minimise the negative and sometimes serious sequelae for patients. Patients with any indicators of delirium should undergo assessment by a competent practitioner using a recognised diagnostic tool for this purpose (NICE 2010).

Patients may present with subtypes of delirium such as hyperactive, hypoactive or mixed activity delirium (Morandi et al. 2009). In hyperactive delirium, the patient is often agitated, mobile and verbal; in hypoactive delirium, the patient is often very quiet and lethargic, and in a mixed picture they may alternate unpredictably from one state to the other. Studies have generally revealed that hypoactive delirium is more prevalent in the ICU population (Pandharipande et al. 2007).

Harry would appear to fulfil the definition for hyperactive or mixed delirium using the criteria outlined above, as he has an acute onset of confusion, with agitation and cognitive dysfunction with attention deficit. At this time he is hyperactive but he should be monitored for episodes of hypoactivity. He will need to have a full assessment of delirium performed to confirm this diagnosis.

Diagnostics and assessment tools

There are a number of tools available for the assessment and diagnosis of acute confusion or delirium, but as yet there is no 'gold standard'. Most of these diagnostic tools were developed for use by psychiatrists and not devised to measure delirium in the non-verbal patient. They can be complex and time-consuming instruments that require the patient to be awake and verbalising (Ely et al. 2001). The confusion assessment method for ICU (CAM-ICU) (see Table 13.1) was developed purposefully to improve the assessment of delirium by non-psychiatrists and for patients who might be non-verbal (Ely et al. 2001). The aim of the CAM-ICU tool kit is to assist practitioners at the bedside to clinically assess patients, even whilst intubated, for compromised cognitive function with the aim of subsequently improving management outcomes within critical care. The CAM-ICU can be used on verbal or non-verbal patients to assess delirium (Ely et al. 2001).

Chevrolet and Jolliet (2007) caution that the CAM-ICU may have sacrificed a degree of sensitivity and specificity for speed and ease of use, but a number of studies have subsequently demonstrated that this tool has reasonable validity, with satisfactory sensitivity and specificity. It is relatively fast and easy to use and is also classed as reliable with good

Table 13.1 The confusion assessment method for the intensive care unit (CAM-ICU).

Delirium is diagnosed when both Features 1 and 2 are positive, along with either *Feature 3 or Feature 4*.

Feature 1. Acute Onset of Mental Status Changes or Fluctuating Course
- Is there evidence of an acute change in mental status from the baseline?
- Did the (abnormal) behaviour fluctuate during the past 24 hours, that is, tend to come and go or increase and decrease in severity?

Sources of information: Serial Glasgow Coma Scale or sedation score ratings over 24 hours, as well as readily available input from the patient's bedside critical care nurse or family.

Feature 2. Inattention
- Did the patient have difficulty focusing attention?
- Is there a reduced ability to maintain and shift attention?

Sources of information: Attention screening examinations by using either picture recognition or vigilance A random letter test (see Methods and Appendix 2 for description of attention screening examinations). Neither of these tests requires verbal response, and thus they are ideally suited for mechanically ventilated patients.

Feature 3. Disorganized Thinking
- Was the patient's thinking disorganised or incoherent, such as rambling or irrelevant conversation, unclear or illogical flow of ideas, or unpredictable switching from subject to subject?
- Was the patient able to follow questions and commands throughout the assessment?
1. 'Are you having any unclear thinking?'
2. 'Hold up this many fingers.' (Examiner holds two fingers in front of the patient.)
3. 'Now, do the same thing with the other hand.' (Not repeating the number of fingers)

Feature 4. Altered Level of Consciousness
- Any level of consciousness other than 'alert'.
- Alert – normal, spontaneously fully aware of environment and interacts appropriately
- Vigilant – hyperalert
- Lethargic – drowsy but easily aroused, unaware of some elements in the environment, or not spontaneously interacting appropriately with the interviewer; becomes fully aware and appropriately interactive when prodded minimally
- Stupor – difficult to arouse, unaware of some or all elements in the environment, or not spontaneously interacting with the interviewer; becomes incompletely aware and inappropriately interactive when prodded strongly
- Coma – unarousable, unaware of all elements in the environment, with no spontaneous interaction or awareness of the interviewer, so that the interview is difficult or impossible even with maximal prodding

inter-rater reliability (Ely et al. 2001). Despite the positive influence of the CAM-ICU tool, the presence of delirium is frequently missed as nurses often fail to diagnose it in their patients (Inouye et al. 2001). Nelson (2009) provides a useful and more detailed overview of the CAM-ICU tool and how to ensure it is used effectively.

Alternatively, the Intensive Care Delirium Screening Check List (ICDSC) devised by Bergeron et al. (2001) could be used to assess the ICU patient. This uses an 8-point score with each item scored as present or absent (0 or 1), a score of 4 or more defining delirium.

This tool is not, however, suitable for comatose or stuporous patients (Morandi et al. 2009).

The CAM-ICU is recommended for use by NICE (2010) and would be an appropriate assessment instrument for Harry.

Related pathophysiology

The precise mechanisms by which patients like Harry develop delirium are not clear, except where there is an obvious metabolic disorder such as hypoglycaemia (Chevrolet and Jolliet 2007). A number of theories have been postulated as to the cause of delirium and its possible long-term effects (Pandharipande et al. 2005; Morandi et al. 2009). Patients with delirium have abnormal brain scans, with evidence of hypoperfusion, and in some, cerebral atrophy is evident (Morandi et al. 2009). The brain abnormalities seen on neuroimaging of these patients points to a diffuse rather than a localised event, which is likely to be a result of global falls in cerebral blood flow. The cerebral hypoxia may be proportional to the severity of illness and be a consequence of responses to sepsis or other physiological insults (Chevrolet and Jolliet 2007; Morandi et al. 2009). The exact relationship between agitation, delirium and cerebral dysfunction remain poorly understood. It is not clear, for example, whether the brain is the passive victim of the physiological insult, along with many organs that dysfunction in critical illness, expressing its injury through agitation and delirium, or if it is the active player, participating and contributing to the extracerebral organ dysfunction (Chevrolet and Jolliet 2007).

Sepsis and the inflammatory and coagulation responses that ensue in this condition have a recognised association with the development of delirium, as the rates are much higher in these patients (Pandharipande et al. 2005; Morandi et al. 2009). The damage caused during sepsis may be related to the presence of large quantities of cytokines. Substances such as interleukin-1 and tumour necrosis factor cause endothelial damage and coagulopathy, and may alter the structure of the blood-brain barrier, resulting in a reduction of synaptic transmission and neuronal excitability (Morandi et al. 2009).

Delirium may also be related to imbalances in the synthesis, release and inactivation of neurotransmitters that are important in the regulation of cognitive function, behaviour and mood (Pandharipande et al. 2005). Three of the neurotransmitter systems involved in the pathophysiology of delirium are dopamine, g-aminobutyric acid (GABA) and acetylcholine. Dopamine increases the excitability of neurons, whereas GABA and acetylcholine decrease neuronal excitability. Imbalances in these neurotransmitters result in neuronal instability and unpredictable neurotransmission (Pandharipande et al. 2005). It is widely believed in delirium that there is an excess of dopamine and depletion of acetylcholine and this may be due to the effects of anticholinergic agents on brain function. Many drugs, likely to have been administered to Harry during his critical care stay, have anticholinergic properties, for example, antiarrhythmics and antibiotics, and these may cause an imbalance of dopaminergic and cholinergic neurotransmission.

A recent study by Pandharipande et al. (2008) examined the relationship between sedative drugs and GABA neurotransmission. GABA is an important inhibitory neurotransmitter but many of the sedative drugs, such as the benzodiazepines (lorazepam, midazolam) and propofol, commonly used in the ICU, have a high affinity for GABA receptors and may inhibit GABA neurotransmission leading to delirium. Pandharipande et al. (2008), in their study, found an association with both lorazepam and midazolam with delirium but not with propofol, fentanyl or morphine. This may have implications for the prescription and use of sedative agents (see Chapter 11 on care of the patient requiring sedation).

There does not appear to be, from the current data, a uniform or single causative agent for the development of delirium in the critically ill, or at least not one that is yet known. Further research is needed to establish stronger associations and provide evidence that might lead to effective prevention. It is likely, however, that delirium is multi-factorial in most patients. Many probably develop delirium from a combination of severe illness, sepsis, metabolic disturbances, coagulopathy, cerebral hypoxia or impaired neurotransmission as a result of drug or sedative therapy. Others may develop delirium from a single mechanism.

Risk factors

Risk factors for delirium can be divided into those that predispose the patient to delirium and those that may precipitate it (Arend and Christensen 2009; Morandi et al. 2009). Predisposing factors include older age (>65 years), lifestyle factors such as smoking and alcohol use and sensory impairments such as poor vision or hearing. There are a number of factors that may precipitate delirium: prolonged pain, the use of restraints, sedative drugs, sepsis, abnormal biochemistry and sleep deprivation (Chevrolet and Jolliet 2007; Pfister et al. 2008; Morandi et al. 2009) (see Table 13.2. for further factors causing distress in the critically ill).

Gustafson et al. (1991, cited in Webb et al. (2000) also identified hypoxia and a perioperative fall in blood pressure as major contributing factors in the surgical patient. Tune et al. and others have implicated not only obvious anticholinergic drugs but also many other commonly used drugs with anticholinergic side effects as causes of delirium (Tune et al. 1993, cited in Webb et al. 2000).

The ability to prevent delirium by recognition of predisposing factors and early structured interventions is yet to be established for the ICU patient (Morandi et al. 2009). Findings from studies on elderly patients, however, may provide useful evidence of preventative measures through controlling risk factors with structured interventions. Inouye et al. (1999) saw a reduction in delirium incidence from 15% to 9.9% with additional reduction in length of delirium in patients who were targeted for a protocol-based interventions targeted at six risk factors: cognitive impairment; sleep deprivation; immobilisation; psychoactive medications; visual or hearing impairment and dehydration. Many of these factors are common to patients like Harry and it would seem logical, therefore, that a similar approach might be effective in critically ill patients.

NICE (2010), in their guidance for managing delirium, highlight the importance of controlling risk factors and both NICE (2010) and Morandi et al. (2009) suggest using a multi-component intervention strategy aimed at achieving this. Morandi et al. (2009)

Table 13.2 Factors that contribute to critically ill patients developing physical and emotional distress.

Patient	Environment	People
• Age • Sex • Past medical history • Allergies • Alcohol and drug use • Previous drug reactions • Severity of illness	• Noise – equipment, radios, conversations, movement, pagers, telephones • Temperature • Lighting • Windows • Visiting times • Routine care times	• Family and friends • Nurses • Intensive care doctors • Other doctors • Physiotherapist • Radiologist • Pharmacist
Drugs • Sedatives • Analgesia • Muscle relaxants • Drug side effects • Drug–drug interactions	**Technology** Being attached to: • Ventilator • ECG monitor • Arterial line • Central venous line • Intravenous drug cannulae • Haemofilter/dialysis • Bispectral index (BIS) monitoring	**Miscellaneous** • Pain/discomfort • Sleep deprivation • Multi-profession rounds • Electrolyte imbalances • Nutrition • Scoring systems • Progress reports

Source: Data extracted from Roundtable Meeting (2002, Fig. 2).

suggest adapting a four-step nurse-led protocol originally developed for the acute setting by Bergmann et al. (2005), cited in Morandi et al. (2009):

1. Nursing detection of delirium with a validated instrument.
2. Evaluation of potential causes of delirium.
3. Preventative measures to manage common risk factors.
4. Creation of an therapeutic environment that promotes orientation.

Harry has a number of risk factors for delirium such as his age (76 years), significant sedative use whilst he was intubated and ventilated, infection and episodes of hypoxaemia, and he may well have various abnormal biochemistry results during his ICU admission. Nurses caring for Harry should have had a high suspicion and be alert to the possible development of delirium in this patient. They should also have taken a patient history to ascertain if Harry has any history of confusional episodes, the presence of any neurological or psychiatric conditions or any history of substance misuse, smoking and alcoholism (Webb et al. 2000; Chevrolet and Jolliet 2007).

Managing the patient with delirium

Interventions for Harry are discussed below and these should be aimed at limiting the current and potential risk of further episodes of delirium, limiting the negative physiological and emotional effects of delirium for Harry and reorientation to his environment (NICE 2010).

Airway/breathing

Harry's airway is currently patent but monitoring of his level of consciousness is ongoing to observe any potential airway compromise. Harry is self-ventilating and requires 40% oxygen. As he is agitated and picking at his lines, he may remove his mask and consequently be at risk of hypoxaemia, which could contribute to increased confusion and agitation and if sustained would prolong his delirium. Care should be taken to ensure that Harry receives adequate oxygen therapy and delivery via a nasal cannula might be more appropriate; although this will not guarantee a fixed oxygen percentage, Harry may be less inclined to remove this and may receive a more consistent gas delivery (O'Driscoll et al. 2008). His oxygen saturation should be monitored and oxygen titrated to maintain SpO_2 >94%.

Harry should be assisted to sit in an upright position and, if safe to do so, should be assisted to sit out in a chair for intervals during the day. This will improve basal oxygenation and improve alveolar gas diffusion, decreasing Harry's work of breathing and assisting in the prevention of hypoxaemia.

Circulation

Harry's heart is in normal sinus rhythm and his blood pressure is within acceptable limits. He should continue to have regular cardiovascular assessment to ensure maintenance of an adequate circulation. Any disturbances in cardiac rate or rhythm or a fall in blood pressure should be managed accordingly.

In relation to delirium, NICE (2010) and Morandi et al. (2009) both stress the importance of avoiding dehydration and electrolyte disturbances as these factors are significant predisposing factors for delirium. Oral fluid intake should be attempted and regular offers of preferred drinks for Harry are important in assisting him to normalise and begin activities of self-care. Assistance with oral intake can also be undertaken by family members and allows them an opportunity to perform care for their loved one. Harry should be carefully observed to avoid potentially harmful spillages of hot or cold liquids. It is unlikely at this time that Harry will maintain a sufficient oral intake and so may require additional intravenous fluid therapy; an appropriate crystalloid solution should be prescribed and delivered.

A daily blood test for urea and electrolytes should be performed and replacement of abnormal levels undertaken, as hyponatraemia, hypocalcaemia and hypomagnesaemia may influence delirium (Chevrolet and Jolliet 2007; Morandi et al. 2009). (Fluid therapy is discussed in more detail in Chapters 3 and 4.)

As infection is also a precipitating risk for delirium, Harry should have assessment of his temperature to detect early any new infectious episodes. Any evidence of clinically significant fever ($T \geq 38.3°C$) should prompt a septic screen (see Chapter 3) and treatment with antibiotic therapy (Department of Health (DH) 2007).

Disability of the central nervous system

Harry should have ongoing assessment of his neurological status using standard Glasgow Coma Score (GCS) assessment and delirium assessment with the CAM-ICU (NICE 2010).

Where possible, non-pharmacological management of Harry's delirium should be attempted (NICE 2010). A priority of care for Harry is in measures to assist him to orientate and engage in his surroundings (NICE 2010; Morandi et al. 2009). Harry should not be given large amounts of information at any one time but should be told appropriate information regarding his condition and treatment (Headway 2007). It would be advisable, at this stage, not to present Harry with too many alternatives to choose from and the use of closed questions to obtain essential information might be helpful (Pfaff 2006).

Harry, his family and friends should be kept apprised of his condition and his family should be encouraged to visit. They should be given information about delirium and offered reassurance that Harry's condition is not uncommon and that it can be treated (NICE 2010). They should also be advised to report to the staff any changes they note in Harry's behaviour. Family and friends may help by orientating the patient to place and time, and be always mindful that such prompting should not be excessive as this might exacerbate the patient's agitation (Pfaff 2006).

It is important that family, friends and staff do not take any physical or verbal abuse from Harry personally because he is reacting to his own perception of the environment, which includes those individuals present at that moment. If appropriate, the best approach might be to ignore abusive behaviour by walking away and returning when he appears less agitated, as reasoning or arguing with an agitated patient can be unproductive. If necessary it would be advisable to follow procedures for de-escalation and management of violence (NICE 2005).

Nurses should also ensure that Harry is provided with adequate sleep and rest. There is an association between sleep disruption delirium and systemic illnesses and mortality (Patel et al. 2008). Existing data demonstrate that sleep is commonly disrupted in critically ill patients, but data on the consequences of sleep disruption and deprivation on actual health outcomes are lacking (Bijwadia and Ejaz 2009). Sleep is thought to be an important precipitating factor in delirium (Morandi et al. 2009). Lack of sleep may cause activation of the stress response leading to raised blood glucose levels, and increased metabolic and oxygen requirements. It may increase the patient's risk of infection or lead to disordered thinking, confusion and agitation and is known to be a precipitating factor in the development of delirium.

The critical care environment is known to cause significant physiological and psychological discomforts for patients. The majority of patients, when asked, complain of lack of sleep with frequent disruptions and awakenings (Freise 2008; Patel et al. 2008; Bijwadia and Ejaz 2009). In fact many patients probably achieve average hours of sleep (7–9 hours) but this is mainly daytime sleep in short periods that does not allow for deeper, more satisfying REM sleep (Bijwadia and Ejaz 2009). Critical care areas are busy with activity occurring at any time of the day or night. Noise levels can be high due to alarms, staff conversations, equipment and general comings and goings (Richardson et al. 2007). Patients are also more anxious and may require frequent care activities that need to take place on a 24-hour basis, meaning that they are frequently awakened during the night (Freise 2008).

It is important to promote adequate sleep and rest for Harry as this may significantly decrease his agitation and confusion (NICE 2010). It may be advisable to place him in a side room, if this is available and without compromising any safety issues, remove noisy equipment and reduce the volume of alarms. Some studies have shown that ear plugs may be helpful for some patients but are not tolerated or liked by all (Scotto et al. 2009). For others, headphones with soft music may be appropriate to block more unpleasant sounds (De Niet et al. 2009). It is also important to reduce lighting whilst allowing continued safe observation of the patient; if lighting is a particular issue. The use of eye masks has been shown to improve sleep in some patients (Richardson et al.) but in Harry's confused state would unlikely to be safe, (Richardson et al. 2007). It is vital, however to ensure that Harry's safety is not compromised by Harry should have agreed additional rest periods during the day for additional sleep promotion. At these times visitors would be discouraged and nursing care activities kept to a minimum (Monsen and Edell-Gustafsson 2005). Clustering of nursing activities at night is recommended so that patients are disturbed less frequently and any non-essential care should be avoided if the patient is sleeping (Richardson et al. 2007).

Ensuring that Harry is able to see and hear adequately will also help to reduce confusion. Optimising sight and hearing would facilitate Harry in communicating and increase his ability to engage with his environment, increasing his familiarity with his surroundings, thus potentially reducing fear, anxiety and suspicions of harm that frequently accompany delirium. NICE (2010) and Morandi et al. (2009) highlight the importance of ensuring that any visual or hearing aids or devices normally used by the patient should be accessible to the patient and kept in good working order.

Chemical restraint

Wherever possible, pharmacological interventions involving sedatives should be avoided for patients with delirium as they may ultimately prolong critical care stay, contribute to confusion and have unwanted physiological effects for the patient (NICE 2010). If Harry has hyperactive delirium and is at risk of harming himself or others, it may be necessary to resort to drug management. This would involve the use of moderate sedation to protect necessary lines and infusions, allow for essential interventions and prevent harm to the patient (Webb et al. 2000).

In intensive care, obtaining the patient's consent to such chemical restraint is a challenge and so rarely sought (Van Norman and Palmer 2001). Braine (2005) emphasised that prescribing and administering medication is not in itself suggestive of abuse. However, overprescription, inappropriate use or failure to regularly review medication, whilst neglecting to consider other methods of management, might constitute abuse. Patients who receive pharmacological restraint should be prescribed medication with the least side effects, and once the drug is given, the patient should be regularly reviewed and monitored (Braine 2005). The fundamental consideration is that any drug used to sedate a patient should not be counterproductive by exposing the patient to side effects or potential for serious consequences.

Before a sedative is used, the presence of pain should be ascertained. Harry should undergo a pain assessment, as he may not be able to verbalise or explain his pain, whilst confused, physiological evidence of pain should also be assessed (see Chapter 10 for management of the patient in pain).

Haloperidol is the drug currently recommended for use in delirium and Harry would most likely be prescribed a 2 mg twice-daily dose of oral haloperidol with 5 mg bolus doses prescribed for serious episodes of agitation (Webb et al. 2000; Chevrolet and Jolliet 2007; Morandi et al. 2009, NICE 2010).

Benzodiazepines have traditionally been used in the management of anxiety associated with delirium (Chevrolet and Jolliet 2007) but have become less popular as long-term use may contribute to factors that might increase the risk of delirium, and their effects may be too sedative in some older patients. In the UK, NICE (2010) recommend that the antipsychotic/neuroleptic agent, haloperidol, is used for the management of delirium episodes that cannot be managed by non-pharmacological interventions. It has the advantage of a rapid onset of action and may additionally lower the epileptic threshold (subclinical epileptic seizures do occur in these patients) and may have a favourable effect on the outcome of patients with delirium (Webb et al. 2000; Chevrolet and Jolliet 2007; Morandi et al. 2009; NICE 2010). Due to the fact that benzodiazepines are thought to exacerbate or even cause delirium, their use cannot be justified. Other agents, such as dexmedetomidine, olanzapine and risperidone, are currently under review and may replace the use of haloperidol in the future. Although haloperidol is recommended at present, there is no clear evidence in establishing either its overall effectiveness in treating delirium or its long-term effects (Morandi et al. 2009; NICE 2010).

Exposure/environment

Other factors that would predispose Harry to continuance of his delirium or delay his recovery should also be addressed.

Harry should be protected against the risks of further infection. All staff should undertake appropriate hand-washing practices to avoid cross infection. An aseptic procedure should be used when handling or changing the dressing on his central venous catheter (DH 2007). A daily review of all invasive devices should take place with the multi-disciplinary team and unwanted lines; especially, indwelling urinary catheters should be removed. These devices increase the risk of infection and can be a source of irritation to patients, possibly contributing or exacerbating agitation in delirium (Harvey 1996; Webb et al. 2000; Roundtable Meeting 2002).

Harry's line sites and wounds should be observed for any clinical signs of infection. Swabs and specimens should be taken if indicated by clinical signs or suspicion of infection (DH 2007).

Harry should continue with regular nutritional assessments and his nutritional needs should be adequately maintained as poor nutrition may also be a precipitating factor in the development, or continuance, of delirium (follow NICE 2006) Clinical Guideline 32, for management of the adult with nutritional needs). Harry should begin oral nutrition as soon as he is able and should be encouraged to make his own food choices, as this will aid in restoring independence.

Harry should be assessed for his normal bowel function and for evidence of diarrhoea or constipation as these can lead to confusion and agitation. He should have regular toileting and bowel movements should be documented appropriately. An appropriate aperient should be prescribed and administered, if necessary, to maintain normal bowel function.

NICE (2010) also recommends that patients should be encouraged to mobilise as early as possible. Harry should be assisted to sit out in a chair for periods during the day and it may be prudent to time these to coincide with visitors as this will help to normalise him to his environment. Early mobilisation would also reduce his risk of thromboembolism and pressure sores (DH 2007).

The use of physical restraint

If Harry poses a danger to himself or others, it may also be necessary to consider the use of physical restraints (British Association of Critical Care Nurses (BACCN) 2004). Patients who are at risk of falling or removing invasive lines, drains or tubes that are essential in their care would fall into this category (BACCN 2004; Pfaff 2006). Many interventions in critical care compromise a patient's ability to take decisions, which impacts on our professional obligation to ensure patient freedom, dignity and respect for autonomy (BACCN 2004). The multi-professional team in critical care must maintain a moral obligation to do no harm – *non-maleficence* – and to support good practice – *beneficence* (Beauchamp and Childress 1994) – by considering the risks and benefits of any form of restraint and justifying all management decisions in the best interests of Harry and in compliance with the Mental Capacity Act (DH 2005).

There is a paucity of UK literature that explores the subject of restraint in critical care (BACCN 2004), and most data originate in the United States of America (USA) or Australia. Where all conceivable alternative approaches to managing a patient with agitation and confusion have been exhausted, it is seen as lawful, in the UK, to use reasonable force to restrain a patient when they are at risk of self- harm or physical injury; they are imposing an immediate risk of physical assault on staff; or to prevent dangerous, threatening or destructive behaviour (Dimond 2002). Ideally, a consensus should be reached between healthcare professionals, patient and relatives, if possible, to ensure any restraint is reasonable and proportionate to the circumstances and to preclude allegations of assault (DH 2001; Royal College of Nursing (RCN) 2004). The use of physical restraints may actually exacerbate Harry's agitation and can lead to injuries. A thorough documented assessment should be performed before taking a decision to use any form of physical restraint, and only devices manufactured for the purpose should be applied. Restraints should be taken off regularly to inspect the skin for any damage, and restraints should be removed as soon as Harry's condition permits.

Conclusion

Delirium is a common complication for patients in critical care and can have serious and potentially life-threatening consequences for the patient. Critical care practitioners should be aware of the risks factors that can predispose or precipitate delirium in the critically ill patient and follow multi-modal interventions aimed at prevention, detection and early interventions to minimise the negative sequelae that can ensue from this condition.

Key learning points from the scenario

- Critical care patients are at high risk for the development of delirium and a delirium screen should therefore be performed on all patients.
- Management of delirium should focus on limiting current and potential risk of further episodes of delirium, limiting the negative physiological and emotional effects of delirium and reorientation to the environment (NICE 2010).
- The use of any form of restraint (chemical or physical) should be reserved for cases where all other conceivable alternative approaches have been exhausted and/or where the patient presents a danger to themselves or others.

Critical appraisal of research paper

Ely EW, Margolin R, Francis J, May L, Truman B, Dittus R, Speroff T, Gautam S, Bernard GR, Inouye SK (2001) Evaluation of delirium in critically ill patients: validation of the Confusion Assessment Method for the Intensive Care Unit (CAM-ICU). *Critical Care Medicine* **29**(7), 1370–1379

Reader activities

1. Read the research article written by Ely et al. (2001).
2. Using the critical appraisal framework in Appendix I, consider the methodological quality of the paper.
3. Reflect on this aspect of your own practice and the implications for future practice management that this paper arises.

A commentary on this paper has been provided by the chapter author in Appendix XIV.

References

Arend E, Christensen M (2009) Delirium in the intensive care unit: a review. *Nursing in Critical Care* **14**(3), 145–154.

BACCN: British Association of Critical Care Nurses (2004) *Position Statement on the Use of Restraint in Adult Critical Care Units*. Available online at: www.baccn.org.uk. Accessed 28 January 2010.

Beauchamp TL, Childress JF (1994) *Principles of Biomedical Ethics*, 4th edn. Oxford University Press, New York.

Bergeron N, Dubois MJ, Dumont M, Dial S, Skrobik Y (2001) Intensive care delirium screening checklist: evaluation of a new screening tool. *Intensive Care Medicine* **27**, 859–864.

Bijwadia JS, Ejaz MS (2009) Sleep and critical care. *Current Opinion in Critical Care* **15**, 25–29.

Braine ME (2005) The managing of challenging behaviour and cognitive impairment. *British Journal of Neuroscience Nursing* **1**(2), 67–74.

Chevrolet J-C, Jolliet P (2007) Clinical review: Agitation and delirium in the critically ill – significance and management. *Critical Care* **11**, 214–219.

De Niet G, Tiemens B, Lendemeijer B, Hutschemaekers G (2009) Music-assisted relaxation to improve sleep quality: meta-analysis. *Journal of Advanced Nursing* **65**(7), 1356–1364.

Department of Health (DH) (2001) *Reference Guide to Consent for Examination or Treatment.* Available online at: www.doh.gov.uk/consent. Accessed 28 January 2010.

Department of Health (DH) (2005) *Mental Capacity Act 2005.* Available online at: http://www.dh.gov.uk. Accessed 1 February 2010.

Department of Health (DH) (2007) *Saving Lives: reducing infection, delivering clean and safe care.* Available online at: www.clean-safe-care.nhs.uk. Accessed 28 January 2010.

Dimond B (2002) *Legal Aspects of Nursing*, 3rd edn. Longman, London.

Ely EW, Margolin R, Francis J, May L, Truman B, Dittus R, Speroff T, Gautam S, Bernard GR, Inouye SK (2001) Evaluation of delirium in critically ill patients: Validation of the Confusion Assessment Method for the Intensive Care Unit (CAM-ICU). *Critical Care Medicine* **29**(7), 1370–1379.

Friese RS (2008) Good night, sleep tight: the time is ripe for critical care providers to wake up and focus on sleep. *Critical Care* **12**(3), 1–2.

Harvey M (1996) Managing agitation in critically ill patients. *American Journal of Critical Care* **5**, 7–15.

Headway, The Brain Injury Association (2007) Improving life after brain injury: *Post Traumatic Amnesia fact sheet.* Available online at: www.headway.org.uk Accessed 2 July 2007.

Inouye SK, Bogardus Jr ST, Charpentier PA, Leo-Summers L, Acampora D, Holford TR (1999) A multicomponent intervention to prevent delirium in hospitalized older patients. *New England Journal of Medicine* **340**, 669–676.

Inouye SK, Foreman MD, Mion LC, Katz KH, Cooney Jr LM (2001) Nurses' recognition of delirium and its symptoms. *Archives of Internal Medicine* **161**, 2467–2473.

Monsen MG, Edell-Gustafsson UM (2005) Noise and sleep disturbance factors before and after implementation of a behavioural modification programme. *Intensive and Critical Care Nursing* **21**, 208–219.

Morandi A, Jackson JC, Ely WE (2009) Delirium in the intensive care unit. *International Review of Psychiatry* **21**(1), 43–58.

Nelson LS (2009) Teaching staff nurses the CAM-ICU for delirium screening. *Critical Care Nursing Quarterly* **32**(2), 137–143.

National Institute for Health and Clinical Excellence (NICE) (2005) Violence: short-term management of disturbed/violence in inpatient psychiatric settings and Emergency Departments. *Clinical Guidelines 25*. NICE, London. Available online at: http://www.nice.org.uk/Guidance/CG25. Accessed 1 February 2010.

NICE and the National Collaborating Centre for Acute Care (2006) Nutrition support in adults: oral nutrition support, enteral tube feeding and parenteral nutrition. *Clinical Guideline 32*. NICE, London. Available online at: http://www.nice.org.uk/Guidance/CG32. Accessed 25 January 2010.

NICE (2010 CG 103) Delirium: diagnosis, prevention and management available online @ http://www. nice.org.uk/Guidance. Accessed 6 December 2010.

O'Driscoll BR, Howard LS, Davison AG on behalf of the British Thoracic Society (2008) BTS guideline for emergency oxygen use in adult patients. *Thorax* **63**(Suppl VI), 1029–47.

Pandharipande P, Jackson J, Ely EW (2005) Delirium: acute cognitive dysfunction in the critically ill. *Current Opinion in Critical Care* **11**, 360–368.

Pandharipande P, Cotton BA, Shintani A, Thompson J, Costabile S, Truman PB (2007) Motoric subtypes of delirium in mechanically ventilated surgical and trauma intensive care unit patients. *Intensive Care Medicine* **33**, 1726–1731.

Pandharipande P, Cotton BA, Shintani A, Thompson J, Pun BT, Morris Jr JA (2008) Prevalence and risk factors for development of delirium in surgical and trauma intensive care unit patients. *Journal of Trauma* **65**, 34–41.

Patel M, Chipman J, Carlin BW, Shade D (2008) Sleep in the Intensive Care Unit setting. *Critical Care Nursing Quarterly* **31**(4), 309–318.

Pfaff A (2006) *Post Traumatic Amnesia.* South Western Sydney Area Health Service. Available online: www.swsahs.nsw.gov.au. Accessed on 2 July 2007.

Pfister D, Siegemund M, Dell-Kuster S, Smielewski P, Rüegg S, Strebel SP, Marsch SC, Pargger H, Steiner LA (2008) Cerebral perfusion in sepsis-associated delirium. *Critical Care* **12**, R63.

Richardson A, Crow W Coghill E, Turnock C (2007) A comparison of sleep assessment tools by nurses and patients in critical care (2007). *Journal of Clinical Nursing* **16**, 1660–1668.

Roundtable Meeting (2002) Management of the agitated intensive care unit patient. *Critical Care Medicine (Supplement)* **30**(1), S97–S123.

Royal College of Nursing (RCN) (2004) Restraint revisited – rights, risk and responsibility. *Guidance for Nursing Staff.* Available online at: www.rcn.org.uk. Accessed 28 January 2010.

Scotto CJ, McClusky C, Spillan S, Kimmel J (2009) Earplugs improve patients' subjective experience of sleep in critical care. *Nursing in Critical Care* **14**(4), 180–184.

Van Norman G, Palmer S (2001) The ethical boundaries of persuasion: coercion and restraint of patients in clinical anaesthesia practice. *International Anaesthesiology Clinics* **39**(3), 131–143.

Webb JM, Carlton EF, Geehan DM (2000) Delirium in the Intensive Care Unit: are we helping the patient? *Critical Care Nursing Quarterly* **22**(4), 47–60.

Chapter 14

The patient with seizure activity

Clair Merriman

Introduction

A seizure is a single event that results in an altered state of brain function. Seizures can arise from a variety of clinical conditions and occur in a number of critically ill patients. A single seizure does not necessarily lead to the development of long-term seizure activity or epilepsy syndromes and often cease following resolution of the initial clinical disorder. Seizures may be difficult to detect in critically ill patients who are unconscious, heavily sedated or receiving neuromuscular blockade. Consequently, nurses in the ICU need to be vigilant for signs of altered neurological status as undetected seizure activity can lead to life-threatening status epilepticus (SE). This scenario focuses on the knowledge and skills necessary to manage a critically ill patient experiencing seizure activity.

Patient scenario

Simon is a 21-year-old man on the critical care unit. He was admitted two days ago with viral encephalitis. Simon is self-ventilating on room air, has a Glasgow Coma Score (GCS) of 15/15 and no neurological deficits. He has IV access via a peripherally inserted central catheter (PICC) line for IV antibiotics. An hour into your shift you witness Simon having a seizure, which commenced as a witnessed twitching of his entire right arm, progressing to impairment of his conscious level. The twitching lasted 45 seconds and stopped spontaneously. You undertake a physical assessment of Simon that reveals the following (see Table 14.1).

Reader activities

Having read the scenario, consider the following:

- What type of seizure has Simon experienced using current ILAE (International League Against Epilepsy) classification?

Critical Care Nursing: Learning from Practice, 1st edition. Edited by Suzanne Bench and Kate Brown.
© 2011 Blackwell Publishing Ltd.

Table 14.1   ABCDE assessment.

Airway	Maintaining own airway safely
Breathing	Respiratory rate: 14 bpm
Circulation	Heart rate: 100 bpm BP 140/80 mmHg Core temperature 37.5°C via tympanic thermometer
Disability	GCS 14/15, $E = 3$, $V = 5$, $M = 6$ Full power in both legs and arms Pupils equal and reacting to light (PEARL) BM 5.8 mmol/L
Exposure	No wounds or obvious traumatic injury

- Is the GCS a valid and reliable tool for assessing Simon's conscious level? Which other methods could be used and what are their possible advantages/disadvantages?
- What further assessments/investigations would be important for Simon in view of his seizure activity?

Related pathophysiology

An epileptic seizure is a transient occurrence of signs and/or symptoms due to abnormal, excessive or synchronous neuronal activity in the brain (Varelas and Spanaki 2006), causing an abrupt and temporary altered state of cerebral function (Hickey 2008; Fuller and Mansfold 2010; Barker 2008). The abnormal neuronal discharge results from an imbalance between excitation and inhibition within the central nervous system. Excessive excitation or inhibition can occur in focal areas of the cerebral cortex, causing focal seizures or throughout the cerebral cortex, causing generalised seizures (Hickey 2008; Barker 2008). The presentation of seizures depends on whether the seizure is focal (local) or generalised but both seizure types can cause alterations in sensation, behaviour, movement, perception or consciousness (Hickey 2008; Fuller and Mansfold 2010; Barker 2008).

Seizures may be caused by an acute insult, such as a head injury, or during an acute disorder of the central nervous system, such as encephalitis, as in Simon's case. Isolated seizures can also occur following drug toxicity, drug or alcohol withdrawal or metabolic disturbances (Barker 2008). In such cases, resolution of the underlying disorder usually leads to cessation of any further seizure activity; however, in some patients seizures may continue for no apparent reason. Simon is at risk of seizure activity due to his acute encephalitis. He has had an observed episode of 'twitching' in his right arm followed by a reduction in his conscious level and he will require further close observation as this event may not be an isolated one.

Seizure classification

The classification of seizures can be complex as it involves two interrelated classifications: the classification of seizure type and classification of epilepsy syndromes (Hickey 2008;

NICE 2004; Fuller and Mansfold 2010). It is recommended that confirmed epilepsy should be classified by epilepsy syndrome criteria (Barker 2008). Epilepsy is suspected following the occurrence of two confirmed seizures not arising from any other obvious, underlying cause (Fisher et al. 2005). As Simon has had a single seizure, most likely as a consequence of his encephalitis, he would not be diagnosed or treated for epilepsy at this time (NICE 2004). The risk of recurrence following a single seizure is variable but generally thought to be about 20–30%; however, recurrence may rise to 90% in patients with confirmed abnormal brain imaging or EEG results (Berg 1991; NICE 2004; Fuller and Mansfold 2010) and these patients may require treatment with anti-epileptic drugs (AEDs). Most neurologists would probably not recommend commencing anti-convulsants for Simon after a single seizure unless there was evidence of previous seizure activity, structural brain damage or a confirmed abnormal EEG recording (NICE 2004).

Classification of seizure type

Nurses need to be conversant with the classification of seizure type and the specific signs evident in a patient having a seizure (Mantri 2007). Seizures can manifest in a number of ways, such as involuntary changes in body movement or function, altered sensations, awareness or behaviour. The classification of seizures is currently undergoing review by the ILAE; consequently, some of the terminology cited in this chapter may be subject to imminent change. The most recent classifications are those issued by the ILAE in 2002 and NICE (2004) (see Table 14.2). The DH (2005) supports the use of this classification system in the UK.

Seizures are categorised as being either partial or generalised. Partial seizures (sometimes called focal or local) begin in a specific area of the brain with focal discharges. Partial seizures are additionally classed as being simple partial seizures, complex partial seizures or partial with secondary generalisation (Gambrell and Flynn 2004; Marthaler 2004). Simple partial seizures are those that do not cause the patient to lose consciousness and occur in a single hemisphere of the brain. The person will remain fully aware but may display behavioural and/or motor, sensory, experiential phenomena, clonic jerking of a body part, localised pain, auras or déjà vu (Marthaler 2004). Manifestations of simple partial seizures correspond to the area of the brain involved and the actions it controls. Seizures arising in the temporal lobe, for example, may cause alterations in memory and emotions or may lead to sensations of smells, tastes or sounds. Frontal lobe seizures commonly lead to uncontrolled movement of an extremity or changes in speech. The manifestations of these types of seizure may involve relatively subtle changes in behaviour or abnormal movements, which may be highly localised (e.g. eye twitching and involuntary movement of a finger or hand) and consequently overlooked or not regarded as significant. Nurses should therefore be vigilant in their observation of patients for any abnormal neurological activity, however slight.

The ictal phase (the seizure event) in simple partial seizures is frequently brief, making it difficult to confirm the diagnosis without continuous EEG monitoring. Simple partial seizures may sometimes progress to a complex partial seizure and it is, therefore, important for the nurse to observe the patients closely until they are fully recovered (Marthaler 2004).

Table 14.2 Classification of seizure type.

Partial (focal, local) seizures *Simple partial seizures* (consciousness not impaired) with any of the following symptoms: • With motor signs • With somatosensory or special-sensory symptoms such as simple hallucinations, e.g. tingling, light flashes, buzzing • With autonomic symptoms or signs such as epigastric sensation, pallor, sweating, flushing, piloerection and papillary dilatation • With psychic symptoms (disturbance of higher cerebral function) such as déjà vu, distortion of time sense, unprovoked fear or terrors, although these rarely occur without impairment of consciousness *Complex partial seizures* (with impairment of consciousness): • With simple partial onset followed by impairment of consciousness • With impairment of consciousness at onset *Partial seizures evolving to secondary generalized seizures* (generalized tonic–clonic, tonic or clonic): • Complex partial seizures evolving to generalized seizures • Simple partial seizures evolving to generalized seizures • Simple partial seizures evolving to complex partial seizures and then to generalized seizures **Generalized seizures (convulsive or non-convulsive)** • Absence seizures – impairment of consciousness alone or with mild clonic, atonic or tonic components, automatisms and/or autonomic symptoms or signs • Atypical absence • Myoclonic seizures • Clonic seizures • Tonic–clonic seizures • Atonic seizures **Unclassified seizures** • Includes all seizures that cannot be classified due to inadequate or incomplete data and some that defy classification

Source: Adapted from Commission on Classification and Terminology of the International League Against Epilepsy classification of seizure 1981.

Complex partial seizures impair consciousness and although the patients may appear to be awake, they will be unable to respond to commands and will not remember the event (Gambrell and Flynn 2004). This type of seizure originates mainly in the temporal lobe and common characteristics include automatisms (involuntary behaviours) such as chewing or picking or bizarre behaviours such as uncontrollable laughter, wanderings, hallucinations or unusual epigastric sensations (Gambrell and Flynn 2004). These seizures are often missed entirely as they are unobserved and the patient does not remember having them. They also have a minimal post-ictal phase and the person may return to normal behaviour rapidly. In addition, it is important to be aware that a partial seizure may sometimes develop into a generalised seizure, termed a partial seizure with secondary generalisation (Barker 2008).

Generalised seizures are classified as either non-convulsive or convulsive. Non-convulsive seizures include absence (originally termed petit mal) and myoclonic types. Absence seizures may manifest in staring, eye blinking or lip smacking and tend to occur with great frequency but are often undetected as they are short-lived events (Gambrell and Flynn 2004). Myoclonic seizures involve the jerking of a particular muscle group for a brief period. Non-convulsive seizures occur almost exclusively in children and adolescents; although they may sometimes happen in older patients, they are unlikely to be the type of seizures evident in Simon's case.

Convulsive generalised or tonic–clonic seizures cause the patient to lose consciousness, fall and have muscle spasms. Tonic spasms are characterised by contractions in which the arms flex and the legs extend. Clonic seizures lead to alternating contraction and relaxation of muscles. Tonic–clonic events often occur with little warning, and the patients will fall from standing, their breathing will be impaired during the event and they may lose bowel or bladder control or occasionally bite their tongue (Gambrell and Flynn 2004). There is a tonic phase in which the patients have violent convulsive muscular contractions and will appear pale, sweaty and tachycardic with an elevated blood pressure, sometimes becoming cyanotic during this period. As the seizure progresses, clonic muscle relaxations lengthen and gradually become more frequent as the seizure nears its end (Hickey 2008). A tonic–clonic seizure of more than five-minute duration is considered a serious event and requires a medical review of the patients, even if they are known to have seizures (NICE 2004). There is often a lengthy post-ictal phase following a tonic–clonic seizure, during which the patient lies still, is exhausted and may sleep for many hours. They will not remember the event and assessment for any traumatic injuries from the fall or convulsions should be undertaken (Gambrell and Flynn 2004).

A thorough understanding of the classification of seizures enables the nurse to identify the specific type of seizure their patient is experiencing and, consequently, promotes appropriate ongoing patient assessment and nursing management (Mirski and Varelas 2003). Witnessed seizures mean that nurses can document and report specific symptoms enabling confirmation of the type of seizure and its duration. The symptoms of Simon's seizure suggest that he has had a simple partial seizure that has progressed to a complex partial seizure. His seizure was initially partial (focal/local) as it did not involve a loss of consciousness and was manifested by clonic jerking of his right arm only, indicating that a single (the left) hemisphere of the brain was involved. Simon's seizure, however, progressed to a complex partial seizure in which his conscious level became impaired but the origin was still in a single hemisphere as only his right arm was involved.

Assessment tools/skills

Glasgow Coma Score and neurological assessment

The GCS is the most widely used neurological assessment tool worldwide. In critical care, it is also the cornerstone of many of the prognostic injury severity scoring systems forming a key part of the Trauma Score (TS), the Acute Physiology and Chronic Health Evaluation (APACHE) and the Trauma and Injury Severity Score (TISS) that are currently used to provide global assessment of critically ill patients in the ICU (Wayne et al. 1998).

Accurate GCS, neurological assessment and detection of seizure activity can be complex in many critically ill patients as they may be heavily sedated or receiving neuromuscular blockade (NMB), which will compromise their GCS score. Sedated and NMB patients cannot be assessed for eye opening, motor or verbal responses adequately, and ventilated patients who have endotracheal or tracheostomy tubes *in situ* will be unable to give verbal responses. Where it is important that accurate GCS scores are obtained, clinical studies have found that this can be achieved, in the absence of a verbal response in intubated patients, by calculating the verbal score from the motor and eye score using a specific mathematical formula (Wayne et al. 1998). Nurses should also bear in mind that pupil responses remain intact in the patient undergoing NMB and sedation, and consequently, regular observations of these are vital in the early detection of altered neurological status.

Electroencephalogram (EEG) and Continuous EEG (cEEG) monitoring

Continuous EEG (cEEG) technology utilises the placement of sensitive scalp electrodes to provide a detailed picture of brain activity. cEEG monitoring allows for the prompt detection and diagnosis of abnormal events, especially non-convulsive seizures (NCsz) that are impossible to detect by neurological assessments or observations (Arbour 2003). Non-convulsive seizures occur relatively frequently in the ICU patient and, if undetected, can lead to serious complications or the development of life-threatening SE (Hirsch 2004; Friedman et al. 2009). cEEG is recommended for patients who are heavily sedated, comatose or receiving NMB and those with severe traumatic brain injury (TBI), with CNS infection or with prior NCsz activity or non-convulsive status epilepticus (NCSE) (Hirsch 2004; Friedman et al. 2009). Simultaneous cEEG monitoring for a number of patients in a single ICU is now feasible as the large amounts of clinical data generated can be collated and analysed rapidly due to improved computer technologies (Friedman et al. 2009).

Simon does not fulfil a need for cEEG monitoring as he is awake and can be assessed by standard neurological assessment and GCS, but should he deteriorate and require sedation, his previous seizure activity might place him in need of cEEG monitoring.

Bispectral index monitoring (BIS)

The EEG-based BIS technology is increasingly being utilised in the ICU setting to monitor levels of sedation and arousal states in patients receiving NMB, bedside procedures or deep sedation during controlled ventilation and drug-induced coma, and would be indicated for a patient at risk of seizures who is sedated or on NMB (Arbour 2003). BIS is discussed more fully in Chapter 11 on managing pain and sedation.

Developing scenario

Three hours following his initial seizure, Simon has a generalised tonic–clonic seizure lasting two minutes. This is followed ten minutes later by a second tonic–clonic seizure of the same duration. During the seizure Simon appears pale, clammy and sweaty and he is incontinent of urine.

Nursing assessment and interventions

Airway/breathing

During a seizure it is not advisable to try and force anything into the mouth, such as airway adjuncts, as there is a high risk of damaging teeth or inducing gagging or choking. Simon should be given high-flow oxygen therapy during the seizure to relieve cerebral hypoxia as brain oxygen consumption may increase by 60% and cerebral blood flow by 250% during a seizure event (Hickey 2008).

On cessation of the seizure and during the post-ictal phase, Simon should be positioned on his side to ensure airway patency and facilitate drainage of secretions. Oral suctioning may be required if Simon has bitten his tongue or if he has hypersalivation and excess secretions (Gambrell and Flynn 2004). Monitoring of respiratory rate, depth and rhythm should commence. Most patients will return to an adequate spontaneous respiratory pattern following a seizure, provided airway patency is maintained, but oxygen therapy should be continued and titrated to achieve oxygen saturation (SpO_2) >94%. Should any patient not return to spontaneous breathing or become pulseless, cardiopulmonary resuscitation should commence without delay.

Circulation

A general assessment of Simon's circulatory system should be undertaken, although serious circulatory events are unlikely in seizures that do not progress to SE. Blood pressure and heart rate should be recorded and Simon's heart rhythm should be monitored. Seizures initiate sympathetic responses leading to vasoconstriction and an elevation in blood pressure, during the post-ictal phase; however, this ceases and Simon's blood pressure may dip, requiring re-assessment of his haemodynamic status and administration of appropriate fluid therapy. Simon is known to have encephalitis and monitoring of his temperature should continue two to four hourly for evidence of fever recurrence, as this would necessitate a review of his antibiotic therapy.

Disability of the central nervous system

During a convulsive seizure, the nurse needs to protect Simon from injury and must remain with him throughout the event (Hickey 2008). Eye glasses should be removed and restrictive clothing loosened, and if safe to do so, he should be placed on his side. It may also be possible to guide the movements of limbs to prevent injury but the nurse should not attempt to restrain Simon's movements.

As Simon has had repeated seizure activity, a benzodiazepine drug would normally be administered to instigate prompt termination of electrical seizure activity and prevent progression into SE (Varelas and Spinaki 2006; Barker 2008). Lorazepam 2–4 mg administered by intravenous push over 2 minutes or diazepam 10–20 mg similarly administered are used (Pena 2003). Both drugs have been shown to be effective in producing seizure cessation, although lorazepam may be more effective in preventing further seizures with fewer doses needed (Cock and Schapira 2002) and is the agent currently recommended for first-line use in the UK (NICE 2004). Benzodiazepine administration should bring about a rapid termination of seizure activity through depression of neuronal activity from gamma aminobyturic acid (GABA)-induced neurotransmission. Repeated doses of lorazepam may be given up to a maximum of 8 mg, should Simon have another seizure. It is important, however to be aware that lorazepam can cause apnoea and profound hypotension in excess doses.

Simon has now experienced multiple seizure activity and current guidelines recommend that he should be administered further AEDs in addition to further investigation of the underlying cause (NICE 2004) (see Table 14.3). In the critical care setting, phenytoin is the most commonly used AED for rapid therapeutic control of repeated seizures. It is given intravenously at a dose of 15–20 mg/kg. It should not be administered more rapidly than 50 mg/min as it can induce cardiac disturbances and is very irritant to veins (Pena 2003). Phenytoin can only be administered in normal saline and is highly protein bound, so blood levels may be difficult to ascertain in low albumin states (Valeras and Spanaki 2006). Phenytoin is absorbed well from the GI tract and, following intravenous loading, is given orally at 100 mg three times per day.

Table 14.3   Drug treatment by seizure type.

Seizure type	First line drug	Secondary drugs	Additional drugs that could be used	Drugs to be avoided (these could worsen seizures)
Generalised tonic–clonic	Carbamazepine Lamotrigine Sodium valproate Topiramate	Clobazam Levetiracetam Oxcarbazepine	Acetazolamide Clonazepam Phenobarbital Phenytoin Primidone	Tiagabine Vigabatrin
Absence	Ethosuximide Lamotrigine Sodium valproate	Clobazam Clonazepam Topiramate		Carbamazepine Gabapentin Oxcarbazepine Tiagabine Vigabatrin
Myoclonic	Sodium valproate (Topiramate)	Clobazam Clonazepam Lamotrigine Levetiracetam Piracetam Topiramate		Carbamazepine Gabapentin Oxcarbazepine Tiagabine Vigabatrin
Focal with/ without secondary generalisation	Carbamazepine Lamotrigine Oxcarbazepine Sodium valproate Topiramate	Clobazam Gabapentin Levetiracetam Phenytoin Tiagabine	Acetazolamide Clonazepam Phenobarbital Primidone	

Source: Adapted from NICE CG20 (2004).

Fosphenytoin can be given as an alternative to phenytoin. It is a newer water- soluble phenytoin prodrug that is activated by the body's metabolic processes (Pena 2003). This is prescribed at a dose of 15–20 mg/kg/PE (phenytoin equivalents) loading dose and intravenously 300–400 mg/day. Fosphenytoin cannot be given orally but can be administered

Table 14.4   Seizure documentation.

Information for documentation following a seizure
Document if patient remained conscious or had reduced or complete loss of consciousness.
Document the time seizure commenced and its duration. Seizures >5 minutes or repeated seizures require urgent review
Note time of cessation of ictal stage and beginning of post-ictal stage.
Document if the patient displayed any warning signs or auras (sense of doom, elation, déjà vu, smells, tastes or sounds).
Record abnormal movements and note which parts of the body were involved. Was the seizure simple partial (focal), complex partial or generalized?
Was there evidence of clonic or tonic–clonic activity?
Record any incontinence of urine or faeces.
Note any cognitive changes following the seizure.
Perform neurological observations note any pupil abnormalities, deviant gaze or motor weakness in any limbs and its duration.
Assess and document any injuries sustained during the seizure. Monitor the duration of sleep after the seizure.

Source: Adapted from Hickey (2008).

in 5% dextrose solution and infused at a more rapid rate than phenytoin as it causes fewer cardiac side effects. The goal of either drug is to achieve a therapeutic serum level of 10–20 µg/mL or free levels (not albumin bound) of 1–2 µg/mL but avoiding toxic levels. Patients who are intolerant to phenytoin should be given alternative AEDs such as intravenous or oral sodium valproate 600–3000 mg/day or oral carbamazepine 600–1200 mg/day.

Patients are often confused and agitated following a seizure and may become combative and aggressive. As Simon emerges from the seizure, it is important to remain with him and attempt to re-orient him to his surroundings, informing him of your nursing activities to reduce his anxiety (Marthaler 2004). It is important that the medical team is informed of Simon's recent seizures and detailed and accurate information documented concerning the specific nature and duration of the seizure activity (see Table 14.4). Simon should be investigated for possible contributing causes for this new onset of seizure activity. A blood glucose level should be obtained to rule out hypoglycaemia, as this can be a precipitating cause of seizure activity.

The post-ictal phase is the period following cessation of the seizure and lasts until the patient has recovered consciousness and orientation (or returned to his pre-seizure neurological status). During this time, Simon should be closely observed and, if necessary, GCS and neurological observations performed half- hourly (NICE 2004). It is important to distinguish alterations in Simon's neurological function arising from the seizure itself and those that might be due to new or extended neurological damage or function. Simon should return to his previous neurological function at the end of the post-ictal stage and, during this time, should be able to localise to painful stimuli. Medical review of the patient should be undertaken and further investigations considered if there is no return to his former state or any deterioration in neurological performance from the nursing assessment is detected.

As Simon has had repeated seizure activity, the medical team may request further investigations to determine if his encephalitis is worsening or to establish if he has developed an epilepsy syndrome. Diagnostic tests currently recommended by the NICE (2004) would be a computed tomography (CT) scan or magnetic resonance imaging (MRI) and EEG (or video EEG).

An EEG would be performed if a diagnosis of epilepsy was suggested by the developing clinical picture (NICE 2004). A CT or MRI scan of Simon would be indicated if there was suspicion that his encephalitis had worsened or if his seizure activity might be related to a new, undiagnosed condition or if Simon fails to return to his pre-ictal neurological status.

Accurate diagnosis of seizure type and epilepsy syndrome is key to the development of an appropriate treatment strategy as the selection of AEDs would largely be determined by these results (Hickey 2008; NICE 2004). Simon's longer term drug therapy would be reviewed by an epilepsy specialist prior to discharge as patient adherence to AED treatment is important in maintaining the patient seizure free. AED regimens should also be tailored according to seizure type, epilepsy syndrome, co-medication and the individual's lifestyle and preferences (NICE 2004).

Exposure/environment

Maintaining a safe environment for Simon can be difficult as seizures are unpredictable and can result in falls, traumatic injuries or disconnections from lines or tubes (Pena 2003). Simon will require close observation at all times whilst at risk of seizures and it may be prudent to lower his bed as near to the ground as possible in case of falls (Hickey 2008). In addition, padded cot sides may be required to protect limbs during a seizure. The nurse should also ensure that lines are anchored securely to prevent disconnections and ensure that during a seizure Simon does not become entangled in wires or tubing.

Simon may be incontinent of urine and/or faeces during convulsive seizures, and if he is not catheterised, this has implications for assessment of fluid balance, protection of his dignity and maintenance of hygiene and skin integrity. Following a seizure, Simon should be assessed for evidence of incontinence and appropriate hygiene measures undertaken as soon as feasible. In addition, he should be assessed for any signs of physical injury and this should be reported and carefully documented (Pena 2003; Hickey 2008).

Simon will also require appropriate nutritional assessment and maintenance of an adequate fluid and dietary intake. He should also have standard thromboembolic prophylaxis.

Conclusion

Seizures are fairly frequent events in the critically ill and can occur in a variety of critically ill patients. They arise from a number of clinical causes and are not necessarily the result of an existing epilepsy syndrome. Indeed, many seizures witnessed in the critically ill are sub-clinical and cease following resolution of the initial condition. Critical care nurses should be aware of the risks of seizure activity in their patients and be able to accurately assess seizure type using recognized classification criteria. In addition, nurses should be able to provide prompt and appropriate nursing management to maintain patient safety, terminate seizure activity using pharmacological measures and be conversant with standard AED treatments.

Key learning points from the scenario

- Pathophysiology of seizures
- Assessment, diagnosis and classification of seizures
- Evidence based management of seizure activity
- Understanding of the rationale for anti-convulsant drug therapy

Critical appraisal of a research paper

There is a paucity of quality, evidence-based and nursing-focused literature on the management of patients with seizures in the critical care environment, and further publication in this area is sorely needed.

Drislane FW, Lopez MR, Blum AS, Schjomer DLl (2008) Detection and treatment of refractory status epilepticus in the intensive care unit. *Journal of Clinical Neurophysiology* **25(4)**, 181–186.

The purpose of this US-based article was to research the underlying causes, prevalence and difficulties in identifying and treating SE in patients in a medical ICU. Undiagnosed SE is a significant problem in the ICU population as sub-clinical seizures may be undetectable in patients who are sedated or sedated and on NMB and where an altered mental state might arise from any number of causes. Sub-clinical seizures may be non-convulsive and difficult to observe in this patient population. Undiagnosed seizure activity may lead to SE with serious or life-threatening complications. Earlier diagnosis and prompt instigation of AED therapy may assist in the prevention of refractory SE and decrease mortality.

Reader activities

1. Read the research article written by Drislane et al. (2008).
2. Using the critical appraisal framework in Appendix I, consider the methodological quality of the paper.
3. Reflect on this aspect of your own practice and the implications for future practice management that this paper arises.

A commentary on this paper has been provided by the chapter author in Appendix XV.

References

Arbour R (2003) Continuous nervous system monitoring, EEG, the bispectral index, and neuro-muscular transmission. *AACN Clinical Issues* **14**(2), 185–207.

Barker E (2008) *Neuroscience Nursing: A Spectrum of Care*, 3rd edn. Mosby Elsevier, New York.

Berg AT, Shinnar S (1991) The risk of seizure recurrence following a first unprovoked seizure: a quantitative review. *Neurology* **41**, 965–72.

Cock HR, Shapira AH (2002) A comparison of lorazepam and diazepam as initial therapy in convulsive status epilepticus. *Quarterly Journal of Medicine* **95**, 225–231.

Department of Health (2005) *National Service Framework for Long Term Neurological Conditions*. DH, London.

Drislane FW, Lopez MR, Blum AS, Schjomer DLl (2008) Detection and treatment of refractory status epilepticus in the intensive care unit. *Journal of Clinical Neurophysiology* **25**(4), 181–186.

Fisher RS, van Emde W, Blume W, Elger C, Genton P, Lee P, Engel Jr J (2005) International League Against Epilepsy Special Article. Epileptic seizures and epilepsy: definitions proposed by the International League Against Epilepsy (ILAE) and the International Bureau for Epilepsy (IBE). *Epilepsia* **46**(4), 470–472.

Friedman D, Claassen J, Hirsch LJ (2009) Continuous electroencephalogram monitoring in the intensive care unit. *International Anesthesia Research Society* **109**(2), 506–523.

Fuller G, Mansfold M (2010) *Neurology: An Illustrated Colour Text*, 3rd edn. Churchill Livingstone, London.

Gambrell M, Flynn N (2004) Seizures 101. *Nursing* **34**(8), 36–41.

Hickey J (2008) *The Clinical Practice of Neurological and Neurosurgical Nursing*, 6th edn. Lippincott, Philadelphia.

Hirsch LJ (2004) Continuous EEG monitoring in the intensive care unit: an overview. *Journal of Clinical Neurophysiology* **21**(5), 332–340.

Commission on Classification and Terminology of the International League Against Epilepsy (ILAE) (1981) Proposal for revised clinical and ectroencephalographic classification of epileptic seizures. *Epilepsia* **22**, 489–501.

Mantri P (2007) Distinguishing between seizure types in adult epilepsy: a key role for nursing observations. *British Journal of Neuroscience Nursing* **3**(1), 560–567.

Marthaler MT (2004) Seizures revisited. *Nursing Management* **35**(4), 71–74.

Mirski MA, Varelas PN (2003) Diagnosis and treatment of seizures in the adult intensive care unit. *Contemporary Critical Care* **1**, 1–12.

National Institute for Health and Clinical Excellence (2004) *The Epilepsies: The Diagnosis and Management of the Epilepsies in Adults and Children in Primary and Secondary Care*. NICE, London.

Pena CG (2003) Seizure: a calm response and careful observation are crucial. *American Journal of Nursing* **103**(11), 73–81.

Varelas PN, Mirski MA (2001) Seizures in the adult intensive care unit. *Journal of Neurosurgical Anesthesiology* **13**, 163–175.

Varelas PN, Spanaki M (2006) Management of seizures in the critically ill. *The Neurologist* **12**(3), 127–139.

Wayne M, Rutledge R, Fakhry S, Emery S, Kromhout-Schiro S (1998) The conundrum of the Glasgow Coma Scale in intubated patients: a linear regression prediction of the Glasgow verbal score from the Glasgow eye and motor scores. *The Journal of Trauma, Injury, Infection and Critical Care* **44**(5), 839–845.

Chapter 15

The patient following poisoning

Sue Whaley

Introduction

3,4-Methylenedioxymethamphetamine (MDMA) is a designer drug, manufactured illic-
itly and sold in tablet (Figure 15.1) or liquid form for recreational use. Prevalent in the
dance and club scene, MDMA is a psychedelic amphetamine derivative and selective
neurotoxin known by various common names such as 'ecstasy', 'XTC' and 'love drug'.
This chapter focuses on a patient who has ingested ecstasy (MDMA) and explores the
common problems associated with its use necessitating an admission to critical care.

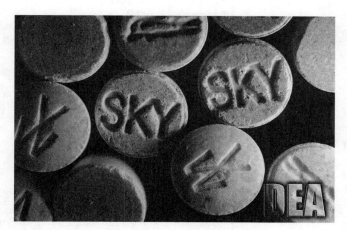

Figure 15.1   Ecstasy tablets. (Courtesy of Wikimedia Commons.)

Patient scenario

Femi is a 21-year-old female admitted to the emergency department in a collapsed state
following recreational ingestion of 2 'ecstasy' tablets over a 5-hour period. History from
the ambulance crew revealed that she was brought from a nightclub situated underground

Critical Care Nursing: Learning from Practice, 1st edition. Edited by Suzanne Bench and Kate Brown.
© 2011 Blackwell Publishing Ltd.

with high ambient temperatures and extremely poor ventilation. Friends at the scene reported that though witnessed to drink plenty of water, Femi had been dancing continuously prior to complaining of feeling unwell, vomiting and appearing disorientated. On arrival, she was self-ventilating, but drowsy and incoherent. Initial management included oxygen, cannulation, blood screen, urinalysis and fluid therapy. No antidote was given and initial treatment was based on symptom reduction.

Femi is fast-tracked to the high dependency unit (HDU) and, on arrival, is receiving 10 L of oxygen via a non-rebreathe mask. Peripheral access has been obtained and a 0.9% saline infusion is running. A urinary catheter has been inserted. Results from the initial assessment can be seen in Table 15.1.

Table 15.1   Initial assessment results.

Airway	Clear
Breathing	Self-ventilating
	Respiratory rate: 32 bpm
	Normal bilateral breath sounds on auscultation
	Arterial blood gases (ABG)
	pH 7.21
	PaO_2 13.7 mmHg (on high-flow oxygen)
	$PaCO_2$ 3.7 mmHg
	HCO_3^- 14 mmol/L
	Base excess −3.2
Circulation	Heart rate 132 bpm
	Blood pressure 126/84 mmHg
	Capillary refill time 4 seconds
	12-lead ECG shows sinus tachycardia.
Disability	Glasgow Coma Score 12/15
	Pupils equal, 6 mm, sluggish reaction to light bilaterally
	Blood glucose 4.4 mmol/L
Exposure	Temperature (tympanic) 38.5°C
Laboratory data	Hb 13.8 g/dL (normal)
	RBC 11.4×10^{12}/L
	WCC 9.3×10^9/L
	Platelets 294 (296×10^9/L)
	ESR 11 mm/h (0–16 mm/h)
	Coagulation screen is within normal range.
	Sodium (Na^+) 123 mmol/L (138–146 mmol/L)
	Potassium (K^+) 3.3 mmol/L (3.5–5 mmol/L)
	Urea 2.8 mol/L (2.5–6.4 mmol/L)
	Creatinine 114 mmol/L (70–120 mmol/L)
	Creatinine kinase 294 (5–150 U/L)
	Glucose 4.4 mmol/L (4.5–6 mmmol/L)
	Serum osmolality 262 (285–295 mOsm/kg)

Reader activities

Having read this scenario, consider the following:

• What are the physiological and toxicological effects of 'ecstasy'/MDMA?

- Why is Femi hyperthermic?
- What are the normal ranges of serum sodium and why might these be altered in the MDMA toxic patient?
- What are the priorities in the management of Femi?

Related pathophysiology

Ingesting MDMA would have resulted in the release of high levels of serotonin in Femi, stimulating serotonin, adrenergic and dopaminergic receptors. Onset of effects occurs within 30-60 minutes and users commonly report feeling euphoria, loss of inhibition, a distorted sense of time, mild visual distortions, reduced anxiety, greater insight, communicativeness and empathy, and increased sensuality. Femi might also have performed 'stacking', the intentional use of multiple staggered doses in order to enhance and prolong the effects of MDMA. 'Stacking' is a frequent behaviour amongst regular users (Ben-Abraham et al. 2003; Emde 2003; Galhinger 2004).

Femi may have also experienced other less-desired effects associated with the use of the drug, including diaphoresis (sweating), bruxism (teeth grinding), jaw clenching, dry mouth and blurred vision. MDMA also causes an enlargement in pupil size with the maximal change in pupil diameter usually occurring one to two hours post-ingestion. Larger doses can also produce significant oesophoria (tendency for the eyes to turn inwards) (de la Torre 2000; Hahn and Yew 2009).

Research into the cognitive performance of those under the effects of MDMA has further demonstrated memory deficits and a reduced ability to both concentrate and to process cognitive information (Parrott and Lasky 1998). Individuals such as Femi, who have taken the drug, may experience agitation, anxiety and toxic psychosis with symptoms of paranoia, as well as auditory and visual hallucinations. Related problems such as hyponatraemia can also cause confusion and disorientation.

Readily absorbed from the intestinal tract, MDMA is metabolised mainly in the liver by the enzyme cytochrome 450 oxidase – CYP2D6. Femi could be genetically deficient for this enzyme and thus more likely to develop liver damage and suffer exaggerated effects. Liver damage can also occur due to ischaemia resulting from both MDMA-induced hypotension and secondary to the hyperthermia. Thromboplastin released from injured myocytes can also cause clotting abnormalities.

Mechanisms of hyperthermia

The normal regulation of body temperature depends on both heat production and heat exchange with the surrounding environment. The relative magnitude of temperature elevation cannot be used to distinguish between the causes of hyperthermia, so consideration of event history, environmental factors and the drug behaviour of the individual are crucial to diagnosis (Bodenham and Mallick 1996). Following MDMA, intoxication hyperthermia is thought to be triggered by a failure of the thermoregulatory system due to interference with the serotonin pathway. This is in contrast to the controlled mechanism of fever induced by inflammation (see Chapter 3 for more information on fever).

Box 15.1   Causes of hyperthermia associated with MDMA.

Prolonged physical exertion
Warm environment

Amphetamine effects
Promotion of repetitive activity
Loss of sensation of thirst and tiredness

Mood-enhancing effects
Euphoria
Increased energy

Serotonin effects
Increased muscle tone
Heat production

Secondary effects of hyperthermia
Increased muscle tone
Further heat production

Source: Adapted from Hall and Henry (2006).

Femi's hyperthermia due to the MDMA toxicity may be caused by a number of co-related factors (see Box 15.1). Excessive diaphoresis due to the exertion of prolonged dancing will have resulted in a loss of water and electrolytes. This may have been compounded by a decreased sensorium, which in turn may have lessened any sensation of thirst or tiredness, leading to dehydration, electrolyte imbalance and additional physical exhaustion (Libiseller et al. 2005). It is likely that the high ambient temperatures and humidity at the nightclub, together with the vasoconstricting effects of MDMA, may have impaired Femi's normal heat loss by conduction and evaporation, thus limiting effective dissipation. Prolonged muscular contractions related to dancing will have added a further thermal burden leading to an increase in her core temperature.

Severe hyperthermia can result in neurological dysfunction. Delirium, seizures or coma associated with MDMA toxicity are reported as the most prevalent life-threatening complications (Kalant 2001). Susceptibility does not, however, appear to be related to ingested MDMA dose. Further potential complications of hyperthermia following MDMA ingestion include acute hepatic failure, rhabdomyolysis, disseminated intravascular coagulation (DIC) and non-cardiogenic pulmonary oedema.

Electrolyte disturbance

Femi is likely to have a range of electrolyte abnormalities including hyponatraemia, hyperkalaemia and hypoglycaemia.

Acute hyponatraemia is a serious complication of MDMA toxicity, linked to excessive sweating as a result of physical exertion, increased water intake and the abnormal release of vasopressin leading to excess levels of anti-diuretic hormone (ADH) secretion (Hartung et al. 2002; Devlin and Henry 2008).

Normal regulation of sodium levels in extracellular fluid is achieved through the actions of aldosterone and ADH. Plasma sodium and water concentration levels are continuously monitored by osmoreceptors situated in the hypothalamus. Any increase in the plasma concentration of sodium results in a corresponding increase in plasma osmolality. This triggers release of ADH from the posterior pituitary gland, resulting in greater permeability of renal tubular cells to water, increased water re-uptake, and subsequent expansion of plasma volume, reducing serum osmolality and concentrating the urine (Marieb 2006).

It is likely that Femi lost large amounts of sodium through profuse sweating in the hot and humid conditions of the nightclub. It is also probable that she drank excessive amounts of water (to avoid dehydration and over-heating), resulting in over-hydration. Alongside this, MDMA intoxication causes excess ADH production leading to a reduced renal response to water loading and subsequent dilutional hyponatraemia (Devlin and Henry 2008).

The consequences of hyponatraemia and increased water re-absorption are a fall in extracellular osmotic pressure, resulting in the passage of water from the blood into cells. Untreated, this leads ultimately to cerebral oedema causing obtundation, seizures and brainstem compression (Kalant 2001). Hyponatraemia should therefore be considered in all patients like Femi who present with suspected MDMA ingestion and neurological deficit, nausea and vomiting, headache, muscle cramps and weakness.

Rhabdomyolysis is a potentially fatal syndrome caused by the breakdown of skeletal muscle fibres. Characterized by the presence of myoglobin in the urine and raised creatinine kinase (CK) levels in excess of 3–5 times normal values (33–145 IU/L in women), rhabdomyolysis is associated with acute kidney injury and is a serious complication following MDMA ingestion.

Hyperkalaemia following ecstasy consumption (>5.0 mEq/L) has the potential to cause fatal cardiac arrhythmias. If rhabdomyolysis develops, raised levels of potassium ions are released from the cell into the extracellular fluid as a direct result of muscle cell degradation causing hyperkalaemia. This in turn causes hypoglycaemia due to the exchange of ions across the cell membrane.

Tests and investigations

Temperature assessment

Close monitoring of Femi's temperature is required during her critical care stay. A device which reflects core temperature should be used as peripheral temperature devices can be affected by a variety of other factors, which reduce reliability and validity. (see Chapter 3 for a critical review of the efficacy of different modes of temperature assessment).

Drug screening

As 50–70% of MDMA is excreted unchanged in the urine (Teter and Guthrie 2001), a spot urinalysis is the most feasible and appropriate method of screening for drugs of abuse. Tests available may simply identify amphetamines or specify MDMA. Femi's urine tested positive for amphetamine derivatives in the emergency department; however, this is of limited clinical value as there is little correlation between ingested dose and the subsequent severity of clinical symptoms (Dar and McBrien 1996). Sweat and saliva are also useful for the detection and analysis of recreational drugs, but use will be dependent on tests available in the department.

Blood screen

In order to identify fluid and electrolyte disturbances, Femi will require assessment of serum sodium, potassium and glucose concentration, and serum and urine osmolality. In addition, Femi's blood toxicity screen should include a full blood count, assessment of kidney and liver function, cardiac enzymes, CK, and clotting.

To monitor for rhabdomyolysis, serial monitoring of CK levels should be performed. The first 24 hours may reveal an initial increase in total CK until a peak level is determined (Cunningham 1997). Close monitoring of blood urea nitrogen and creatinine levels enables early detection of reduced kidney function. (see Chapter 9 for more information on acute kidney injury). Prothrombin time, activated partial thromboplastin time, and platelet count should be routinely tested in all patients with rhabdomyolysis.

If liver damage is evident, Femi may have jaundice, an enlarged liver, prolonged clotting times and raised plasma levels of liver enzymes (Kalant 2001; Brotto and Lee 2007).

Urinalysis

Femi's urinalysis is unremarkable except for a specific gravity of less than 1.005 (1.008–1.035) and osmolality of 253 mOsm/kg H_2O (275–295). The pH is 5. The rate of excretion of MDMA is thought to be linked to the pH of the urine; the greater the acidity, the faster the rate of excretion. As MDMA is highly toxic to the foetus in pregnancy, Femi's urine should also be tested for human chorionic gonadotropin (hCG).

Femi's high-urine osmolality despite a decreased serum osmolality and hyponatraemia is suggestive of syndrome of inappropriate anti-diuretic hormone (SIADH) found in MDMA toxicity. Laboratory tests determining raised levels of excreted sodium levels can confirm the diagnosis.

Analysis of Femi's urine must also include screening for haemoglobin and/or myoglobin in order to detect rhabdomyolysis.

12-lead ECG

Autonomic hyperactivity is commonly found in patients presenting with MDMA toxicity due to the amphetamine-induced surge of catecholamines causing tachycardias and dysrhythmias, which will be evident on a 12-lead ECG. The 12-lead ECG performed on Femi should also be examined for long QT syndrome and non-specific ST-T changes (Ben-Abraham et al. 2003) as individuals with pre-existing cardiac conditions are at an increased risk of fatal arrhythmias and cardiac collapse.

Box 15.2   Arterial blood gas.

pH	7.2
$PaCO_2$	5.5 mmHg
PaO_2	17 mmHg
HCO_3^-	19 mmol/L
Base excess	−3

Acid–base balance

Metabolic acidosis in MDMA toxicity is thought to occur as a complication of hyperthermia, rhabdomyolysis and seizures. Prolonged physical activity leads to increased lactic acid production, and in the presence of muscle cell breakdown, the resulting extracellular increase of potassium further acidifies the blood. Metabolic acidosis is linked to increased incidence of ventricular arrhythmias, and could predispose Femi to kidney injury if due to rhabdomyolysis. Regular arterial blood gases should therefore be undertaken in order to monitor Femi's acid–base status.

Developing scenario

One hour after admission, Femi suffers a tonic–clonic seizure lasting one minute during which intravenous (IV) diazepam (0.3 mg/kg) is administered. You reassess her and find the following: spontaneous ventilation, respiratory rate 10 breaths per minute, SpO_2 98% (on 10 L O_2 via a facemask), heart rate 114 beats per minute, blood pressure 98/75 mmHg, Glasgow Coma Score 11/15 and blood sugar 5.2 mmol/L.

You suspect either hyperthermia or hyponatraemia in the presence of MDMA as a possible cause for the seizure. Management of Femi's hyperthermia is ongoing with a cooling blanket *in situ* and reassessment reveals Femi's core temperature via a rectal probe is now 39.2°C. Hourly urine output is 20 mL and the urine appears concentrated. The decrease of urine output is significant and may be due to abnormally excessive production of ADH. Repeat blood tests reveal a serum sodium level of 121 mmol/L and serum osmolality of 259 mOsm/kg. Arterial blood gases show mild metabolic acidosis (see Box 15.2).

Evidenced-based discussion of interventions for MDMA toxicity

Airway/breathing

Femi should be placed in the recovery position whilst her conscious level is impaired in order to protect her airway (see Chapter 14 for more information on seizure management). Regular monitoring of her respiratory rate should be undertaken, and suction should be available due to the potential for Femi to vomit. Regular arterial blood gas analysis should also be performed to monitor the degree of metabolic acidosis. Femi's $PaCO_2$ may drop due to an increase in ventilation in an attempt to compensate for the metabolic acidosis as seen on initial presentation (Table 15.1). MDMA-induced metabolic acidosis may be corrected with sodium bicarbonate 50 mmol in 50 mL 8.4% solution. In this strength, it is an irritant to peripheral lines and thus should be administered centrally as extravasation causes skin necrosis. Rapid correction of significant acidosis in cases of a prolonged QT interval is vital in order to prevent onset of ventricular arrhythmias (NPIS 2009).

Circulation

Femi should remain attached to a cardiac monitor and have an arterial line inserted so that her cardiac rhythm and blood pressure can be continuously monitored. Although Femi remains tachycardic, such cardio-pulmonary manifestations of MDMA toxicity should only be treated if she becomes haemodynamically compromised (NPIS 2009). Pronounced hypotension may require the use of vasopressin. Conversely, if systolic pressures exceed 220 mmHg and diastolic exceed 140 mmHg in the absence of long-standing hypertension, NPIS (2009) guidelines recommend the use of IV diazepam 0.1–0.3 mg/kg and, if necessary, IV nitrates.

Management of hyponatraemia

Mild to moderate hyponatraemia in patients with normal kidney function may be treated conservatively with fluid restriction as serum sodium levels often correct spontaneously. In this case, repeat bloods indicate a serum sodium level of 124 mmol/L. To manage Femi's hyponatraemia and haemodilution, fluid intake is restricted to 60 mL/h infusion of 0.9% sodium chloride. Central venous pressure monitoring may be required to monitor intravascular fluid volume.

Serum sodium levels of below 120 mEq/L result in an increased risk of cerebral oedema and rapid serum sodium correction is required. Though controversial, in patients experiencing headaches, nausea and vomiting, seizures or coma, rapid correction may be achieved with hypertonic saline (3%) 1–2 mL/kg/h over 1–2 hours. Whilst treatment goals are to normalise serum sodium levels, once neurological symptoms improve, treatment must be halted to avoid over-correction (Decaux and Soupart 2003).

A complicating factor of fluid restriction in MDMA toxicity is a further decrease in urine output which, in conjunction with the potential for rhabdomyolysis, may predispose Femi to the development of kidney injury. Frequent monitoring of serum sodium levels, other electrolytes, kidney function and urine output is thus imperative during replacement therapy. Low-dose loop diuretics and mannitol may be used in order to rapidly diminish intracranial hypertension, although there is little evidence to support its use in MDMA toxicity (Hartung et al. 2002; Hall and Henry 2006). It is not recommended to acidify the urine as it may worsen the metabolic acidosis and increase myoglobin precipitation in renal tubules. Similarly, alkalinisation of the urine also is not indicated because it reduces the rate of MDMA excretion (Emde 2003). Of concern during sodium correction is the risk of osmotic demyelinating syndrome (ODS), a condition characterised by myelin sheath damage of nerves in the pons (brainstem) inhibiting nerve conduction (Decaux and

Soupart 2003). This is, however, less likely in Femi's case as the hyponatraemia is acute rather than chronic.

Decontamination

A principal aim for initial treatment of Femi is to ensure the maintenance of adequate hydration in order to promote elimination of the MDMA. Oral activated charcoal absorbs toxins on contact and may be used in order to reduce the amount of MDMA absorbed by Femi's gastrointestinal tract, thus decreasing the level of systemic toxicity. Although considered in cases of stacking, due to the rapid absorption of MDMA charcoal, it is only recommended for use within one hour of ingestion, where conscious level (and thus airway) is not compromised (National Poisons Information Service (NPIS) 2009). As Femi has been in the unit and has recently suffered a seizure, use of activated charcoal would not be recommended.

Disability of the central nervous system

Femi's conscious level should be regularly monitored and she should be closely observed for further seizure activity. Her blood glucose levels should also be closely monitored, and the critical care nurse should be aware that blood sugar will rise as serum potassium levels reduce. Due to the hyponatraemia, seizure activity and severe hyperthermia, communication with Femi and consent for procedures could be difficult. Femi's mental capacity may be temporarily impaired and judgements determining treatment must therefore be made in accordance with the Mental Capacity Act (DCA 2007).

Exposure/environment

Cooling measures

The relationship between the degree and duration of hyperthermia and increased mortality rates requires a prompt response to hyperthermia. As the hypothalamus is unable to control the core temperature, the use of anti-pyretics is contra-indicated in hyperthermia, and therapy should focus on the use of physical cooling. Mild hyperthermia can be treated with conventional cooling measures, such as the use of cooling blankets and jackets and cooled IV fluids. Invasive measures such as iced saline peritoneal, bladder and gastric lavage may also be utilised in order to achieve central cooling. However, as Femi's temperature is now above 39°C, more aggressive management is required which might include the use of sedation and Dantrolene (Eyer and Zilker 2007).

Established in the treatment of malignant hyperthermia, in MDMA intoxication Dantrolene is thought to bring about general reduction in heat production from muscle contraction and to attenuate neurotoxicity. NPIS (2009) guidelines recommend Dantrolene use if simple cooling measures are ineffective and temperature remains over 39°C. It is administered as a rapid IV bolus (1 mg/kg) and repeated as required to a cumulative dose of 10 mg/kg in 24 hours. In solution, Dantrolene has a pH of 9.5 and to avoid irritation and extravasation, and it must be administered in a large vein with a fast-running infusion (Krause et al. 2004) (see Chapter 3 for discussion of other cooling methods).

Psycho-social issues

Femi may be reluctant to share information with the healthcare team regarding her recreational drug use. This issue needs to be handled sensitively and Femi should be treated with respect and without judgement. Contacting Femi's next of kin, if this has not already been done, would be another priority. The information given to them would, however, need to be considered in light of Femi's wishes, if she is able to communicate these.

Conclusion

This chapter has discussed the management priorities and some of the challenges associated with the care of a patient following ingestion of ecstasy (MDMA). The condition affects many organ systems and a holistic approach to management is thus imperative.

Key learning points

- Identification of amphetamine/MDMA may be confirmed through urinalysis but is of limited clinical value as management is essentially supportive.
- Co-ingestion with other drugs complicates initial assessment and management. Other drugs commonly found in combination include cocaine, alcohol, and cannabinoids.
- Decontamination with active charcoal 50 g is effective only if administered within 1 hour of ingestion. In the hypovolaemic patient, hydration is paramount in order to promote diuresis and elimination.
- Holistic assessment should include cardiovascular status, core temperature, kidney and liver function, clotting profile and serum and urine electrolytes and osmolality.
- Rapid and aggressive cooling measures are necessary when core temperatures exceed 39°C. This may be achieved by use of invasive cooling methods, sedation and administration of Dantrolene.
- Mild to moderate hyponatraemia may be treated with fluid restriction. Severe hyponatraemia requires rapid but cautious correction with hypertonic saline.

Critical appraisal of research paper

Hartung TK, Schofield E, Short AI, Parr MJA, Henry JA (2002) Hyponatremic states following 3,4-methylenedioxymethamphetamine (MDMA, 'ecstasy') ingestion. *Quarterly Journal of Medicine* **95**, 431–437.

This paper reports a retrospective case series study that aimed to define clinical features of hyponatraemia following ingestion of MDMA.

Reader activities

1. Read the research article written by Hartung et al. (2002).
2. Using the critical appraisal framework in Appendix I, consider the methodological quality of the paper.
3. Reflect on this aspect of your own practice and the implications for future practice management that this paper arises.

A commentary on this paper has been provided by the chapter author in Appendix XVI.

Recommended further reading

Campbell GA, Rosner MH (2008) The agony of ecstasy: MDMA (3–4 methyldioxymethamphetamine) and the kidney. *Clinical Journal of the American Society of Nephrology* **3**(6), 1852–1869.

Patel MM, Belson MG, Longwater AB, Olson KR, Miller MA (2005) Methylenedioxynethamphetamine (Ecstasy)-related hyperthermia. *The Journal of Emergency Medicine* **29**(4), 451–454.

References

Ben-Abraham R, Szold O, Rudick V, Weinbroum AA (2003) 'Ecstasy' intoxication: life threatening manifestations and resuscitative measures in the intensive care setting. *European Journal of Emergency Medicine* **10**(4), 309–313.

Bodenham AR, Mallik A (1996) New dimensions in toxicology: hyperthermic syndrome following amphetamine derivatives. *Intensive Care Medicine* **22**, 622–624.

Brotto V, Lee G (2007) A literature review on the physiological effects of illicit substances on critically ill patients. *Intensive and Critical Care Nursing* **23**(2), 64–70.

Cunningham M, (1997) Ecstasy-induced rhabdomyolysis and its role in the development of acute renal failure. *Intensive and Critical Care Nursing* **13**, 216–223.

Dar KJ, McBrien ME (1996) MDMA-induced hyperthermia: report of a fatality and review of current therapy. *Intensive Care Medicine* **22**, 995–6.

DCA (2007) *Mental Capacity Act (2005)*. Department of Constitutional Affairs, TSO, London.

de la Torre R, Farré M, Ortuño J, Mas M, Brenneisen R, Roset P N, Segura J, Camí J (2000) Non-linear pharmacokinetics of MDMA ('ecstasy') in humans. *British Journal of Clinical Pharmacology* **49**(2), 104–109.

Decaux G, Soupart A (2003) Treatment of symptomatic hyponatraemia. *The American Journal of the Medical Sciences* **326**(1), 25–30.

Devlin RJ, Henry JA (2008) Clinical review: major consequences of illicit drug consumption. *Critical Care* **12**(1), 202.

Emde K (2003) MDMA (Ecstasy) in the Emergency Department. *Journal of Emergency Nursing* **29**(5), 440–443.

Eyer F, Zilker T (2007) Bench-to-bedside review: mechanisms and management of hyperthermia due to toxicity. *Critical Care* **11**(6), 236.

Galhinger PM (2004) Club drugs: MDMA, gamma-hydroxybutyrate (GHB), rohypnol, and ketamine. *American Family Physician.* **69**(11). Available online at: http://www.aafp.org/aafp/20040601/2619.html. Accessed 9 December 2009.

Hahn I, Yew D (2009) *Toxicity, MDMA*. Available online at: www.emedicine. com/emerg/ TOPIC927.htm. Accessed 17 March 2009.

Hall AP, Henry JA (2006) Acute effects of 'ecstasy' (MDMA) and related compounds: overview of pathophysiology and clinical management. *British Journal of Anaesthesia* **96**(6), 678–685.

Hartung TK, Schofield E, Short AI, Parr MJA, Henry JA (2002) Hyponatraemic states following 3,4-methylenedioxymethamphetamine (MDMA, 'ecstasy' ingestion. *QJM* **95**, 431–437.

Kalant H (2001) The pharmacology and toxicology of 'ecstasy' (MDMA) and related drugs. *CMAJ* **165**, 917–928.

Krause T, Gerbershagen MU, Fiege M, Weibhorn R, Wappler F (2004) Dantrolene – a review of its pharmacology, therapeutic use and new developments. *Anaesthesia* **59**, 364–373.

Libiseller K, Pavlic M, Grubwieser P, Rabl W (2005) Ecstasy – deadly risk even outside rave parties. *Forensic Science International* **153**(2–3), 227–230.

Marieb EN (2006) *Essential of Anatomy and Physiology*. Pearson Education Limited, London.

National Poisons Information Service (NPIS) (2009) *MDMA Guidelines*. Available online at: www.toxbase.org. Accessed 17 March 2009.

Parrott AC, Lasky J (1998) Ecstasy (MDMA) effects upon mood and cognition; before, during, and after a Saturday night dance. *Psychopharmacology* **139**, 261–268.

Teter CJ, Guthrie SK (2001) A comprehensive review of MDMA and GHB: two common club drugs. *Pharmacotherapy* **21**(12), 1486–1513.

Chapter 16

The patient with long-term needs

Ruth Cork

Introduction

More patients are now surviving critical care. Therefore, equal consideration should be given to both critical care rehabilitation and the more acute aspects of a patient's stay. This scenario focuses on a patient requiring a long-term stay within critical care, and explores how a multi-professional approach can improve both physiological and psychological recovery for both the patient and their family.

Patient scenario

Laura, a 19-year-old woman, was admitted to critical care three weeks ago. She remains ventilator dependent via a tracheostomy and frequently becomes tachypnoeic, hypertensive, sweaty and anxious after an hour on a spontaneous mode. Laura experiences pains in her legs, has obvious weight loss and muscle weakness. She is unwilling to get out of bed, partly because she hates the mechanical hoist and finds that the chair is uncomfortable.

Laura feels tired and appears anxious most of the time. Her anxiety is particularly acute at night, when she only sleeps for short periods, experiences nightmares and is hypervigilant and tearful when left alone. She appears emotionally attached to a few staff and apparently distrusts others. Laura can communicate using lip- reading but is too weak to write. She is able to swallow but takes only fluids like Coca Cola. She has no interest in food. She is receiving nasogastric feed 24 hours/day. Prior to her admission, Laura worked in a travel agency, went to a gym regularly and had a family and lots of friends who now visits frequently. She is nursed in an open area of a critical care unit.

Reader activities

- Identify the physiological problems Laura is experiencing/likely to experience as a result of her stay in critical care.
- Identify the psychological problems Laura appears to have and think about how they might have developed.

Critical Care Nursing: Learning from Practice, 1st edition. Edited by Suzanne Bench and Kate Brown.
© 2011 Blackwell Publishing Ltd.

- Discuss the critical care environment, staffing resources and workload patterns in terms of Laura's long-term recovery.

Discussion

Physiological

Laura's respiratory and other muscles have atrophied and weakened as a consequence of her prolonged ventilator dependency and immobility due to her critical illness (Deem 2006; Thirugnanam and Herridge 2007). Critical illness can lead to polyneuropathy, evidenced by Laura's general muscle weakness, leg pain and inability to write (Ricks 2007). Loss of muscle mass and changes in fat deposition have changed Laura's body shape and movement and may be contributing to her feeling uncomfortable in a standard hospital chair. She is at high risk of pressure area damage due to loss of fat deposits and poor nutrition (Plank et al. 1998). Laura is sleep deprived, which is both a physiological and psychological problem. The critical care environment and the effects of the sedative and analgesic drugs have contributed to sleep disturbance. Laura's loss of perception of a day and night cycle, combined with sensory monotony and overload, and high noise levels have disrupted her sleep pattern and quality. Drugs commonly used for critically ill patients affect the quality and duration of their natural sleep and can contribute to confusion and restlessness (Millbrandt and Angus 2006). Lack of sleep is affecting Laura's energy level during the daytime, therefore making her weaning progress slow.

The body's response to stressors is also both a physiological and psychological process. The physiological response to stress, which Laura is experiencing, includes increased adrenaline and cortisol levels, contributing to her tiredness, anxiety and immunocompetence. Pain, anxiety and sleep deprivation combined with a stress response are inhibiting her cognitive abilities causing memory loss, poor concentration and disturbing her emotional balance (Hopkins and Brett 2005).

Laura's tracheostomy may have changed her usual sensory awareness when she swallows. Nerves, muscles and reflexes may also have been affected by the presence of an artificial airway for such a long period. Laura is unable to experience the full flavours of fluid and food since she is not drinking and eating normally yet. Taste is also often affected (i.e. reduced taste or abnormal/unpleasant taste) by drugs. She is being tube fed continuously and obtaining adequate calories. Considering these factors, it is unsurprising that Laura is not experiencing an appetite.

Laura is also at high risk of developing a hospital-acquired infection due to suppressed immunity from septicaemia, antibiotic medication, intubation and other avenues for infection such as intravenous lines, the urinary catheter and nasogastric tube.

Psychological

Laura is at high risk of post-traumatic stress disorder (Cuthbertson et al. 2004; Hough and Curtis 2005; Hull and Cuthbertson 2007). Communication using lip reading is tiring and frustrating for patients and being unable to communicate isolates Laura from normal social interaction and autonomy (Hemsley et al. 2001). Laura's symptoms could also indicate that she is suffering from delirium (NICE 2009a), a commonly missed problem in critically ill patients (Morandi et al. 2009). Further information about delirium can be found at www.icudelirium.org and in Chapter 13.

Continuous, unpredictable intrusions into her personal space and her person, for example, suctioning, catheter care, her lack of visual and auditory privacy, inadequate and impersonal hospital gown clothing and few opportunities for choice or negotiation will also contribute to Laura's psychological difficulties. Laura has not been able to leave the unit to view the outside world, go to the gym, buy items from a shop or use the internet. These are all activities which Laura would normally do in her daily life, which provide mental stimulation and promote her sense of individuality, independence, choice and relationships with others.

Laura may consciously or subconsciously be aware of her dependency on nursing staff for every aspect of her current situation. Laura's motivation and ability to rationalise decisions is affected by these factors, for example, unwilling to eat or get out of bed. It is possible that she may start to withdraw mentally and become depressed, a common experience for long-stay critical care patients (Rattray and Hull 2008).

Environment, staffing resources, workload patterns

The critical care environment is predominantly a technical rather than homely place. Whilst it has the advantage of immediate access to life-sustaining equipment, drugs and a team of skilled staff 24 hours a day, for the recovering patient, there are some adverse effects. In an open area of a critical care unit, there is continuous exposure to unfamiliar, unpredictable sights, sounds (e.g. equipment alarms), sensory overload and monotony. There is also sensory deprivation of familiar input such as friendly human touch, daytime clothing, feeling hungry and lack of normal sources of mental stimulation. Noise and lighting levels are higher than in a normal hospital ward and night-time disturbance is common (Christensen 2007). Laura can see and hear other patients and may have been aware of other patients' (Hupcey 2000).

A cubicle could afford some visual and auditory privacy for Laura and protection from having to witness others' distress. They have the disadvantage, however, of possible social isolation and restricted scenery, depending on the provision of daylight, an outside view and facilities available to adapt the furniture content and position to suit individual needs, for example, re-positioning the bed to face an outside window. Critical care units within acute hospitals often lack equipment, facilities and the financial budget to purchase resources suited to rehabilitating long-stay critical care patients like Laura, for example, specialised chairs, laptop computers with voice-projection devices, patient toilets and bathrooms.

Staffing resources and workload patterns in most acute critical care units are focused on matching the expertise of staff with the illness/medical dependency of the patients in order to increase survival and maximise chances of recovery. Now that Laura is less dependent on medical equipment, she is likely to be nursed by less-experienced staff and also to share her nurse with another 'low-dependency' patient (Williams 2007).

Table 16.1   Factors affecting recovery for the long-term patient.

Physiological	Psychological
Reduced ability to communicate Muscle atrophy Critical care polyneuropathy Leg pains Decreased immunocompetence Effects of medication on levels of sleep, alertness and activity Decreased sense of taste Poor appetite Altered swallowing mechanism and sensation due to tracheostomy Effects of stress hormones on cognitive abilities, pain perception, blood glucose levels, cortisol levels	Reduced ability to communicate Post-traumatic stress disorder Sleep deprivation Sensory deprivation, overload, monotony Dreams/nightmares Potential flashbacks Anxiety Emotional imbalance and dependence Reduced autonomy Reduced privacy Reduced social interaction and role Reduced control over environment Delirium

These factors could delay her psychological recovery due to a lack of insight by health care staff an inability to meet her complex needs and the lack of time in which to do so (Scholes and Moore 1997; Williams 2003, 2007).

Table 16.1 summarises the common problems experienced by long-term patients in critical care.

Holistic assessment

A multi-professional and multi-system approach to assessing Laura is crucial, including what Laura recognises as her main problems. This is endorsed by NICE (2009b) in an important publication, which focuses on the early assessment of patients in critical care with regard to their rehabilitation needs.

Assessing Laura's progress in weaning from ventilation can be done using several different methods (see Chapter 2 for more information on weaning). Blood laboratory analysis should be performed twice weekly. Laura's phosphate and haemoglobin levels may require supplementing to optimise her weaning ability. A speaking valve can be used to check voice strength and provide an intermittent means of familiar verbal communication for Laura. A test can be done to assess Laura's ability to swallow oral fluids and food without aspiration risk. Weekly nutritional assessment, including a baseline weight and body mass index calculation can confirm whether Laura's nutritional intake is sufficient for her current metabolism in view of her needs for weaning and muscle building, for protection from infection and for relaying fat stores (Plank et al. 1998). Further, the physiotherapy team can comprehensively assess general muscle strength and the extent of any critical illness polyneuropathy and develop an exercise plan (Ricks 2007). Weekly microbiological screening of sputum, urine and skin swabs can confirm absence of infection and justify limiting antibiotics which would also reduce her resistance to bacterial and fungal infections.

Several scoring tools are available to aid assessment of pain (Gélinas et al. 2006), anxiety and depression (Zigmond and Snaith 1983), levels of sedation (Sessler et al. 2002) and delirium (Ely et al. 2001; NICE 2009a) (see Chapters 10, 11 and 13). Specialist nurses and therapists can aid baseline expert assessment and provide advice on Laura's needs, for example, a pain management nurse, clinical psychologist, specialist weaning nurse, speech and language specialist and occupational therapist. It is important, however, to select scoring or assessment methods which Laura finds useful and quick to use and to integrate them into evaluation so she can see her own progress. Too many visiting professionals may confuse and overwhelm Laura in her current emotional state and possibly reduce her trust in her primary team.

An environmental and social assessment, led as much as possible by Laura and her visitors, may lead to creative realistic adaptations which could promote her rehabilitation, sleep and social recovery (Hupcey 2000).

Scenario development

As Laura recovers, her family remain anxious and are viewed as 'demanding' by some of the nursing staff. For example, they frequently ask and repeat lots of questions about apparently minor, technical aspects of Laura's condition, for example, 'What's her oxygen saturation today?', and bring in information from the Internet to discuss and dispute some of her care, for example, 'These sleeping tablets are making her lack energy in the day', and 'You shouldn't be giving her Coke at all!'. They become angry and upset on days when they find that Laura had shared a nurse with another patient, even if Laura has received all the nursing care she requires and is, in her own words, 'having a good day'.

Reader activities

• Consider why Laura's family may have become 'demanding'.

Discussion

Laura's parents have witnessed her changing physical condition and experienced the stress of uncertainty regarding her survival/recovery, over a long period of time (Jones et al. 2004). Even though she is apparently not in danger of imminent death, they are probably still afraid that she may deteriorate and die. They have also experienced a loss of their natural parental role and opportunities to influence her survival/recovery, and have had to rely on the expertise of hospital staff to both help Laura and provide them with information (Leske 2000). This prolonged stress reduces physical and psychological coping mechanisms over time and may have affected their ability to think rationally and to build a trusting relationship with the clinical team (Johansson et al. 2005). Laura's parents may have recognised that their lack of technical and clinical knowledge limits their ability to identify key indicators of her recovery and understand how her clinical management is co-ordinated. They will be understandably utilising knowledge they have acquired through observing and talking to hospital staff and through familiar resources such as Internet sites, in order to try to gain an accurate perspective of Laura's current situation. It is possible that they now see an opportunity and view it as their responsibility to her to assert influence over her recovery by gaining knowledge and actively participating in decisions.

It is possible that the nurses have not recognised the complex emotional journey that Laura's relatives will be experiencing and therefore view her parents' questions and challenges negatively in terms of interfering with her care or as criticism of their efforts (Price 2004; Hughes et al. 2005; Latour 2005). Once their thought processes and emotions are understood through open conversation, Laura's family's mental focus and energy can be co-ordinated with the teams to help Laura's rehabilitation (Benner et al. 1999; Endacott and Berry 2007).

An evidence-based discussion of management

A multi-professional case conference should be organised to form a holistic management plan. This plan must be committed to by everyone who is involved, and clearly documented (NICE 2009b). Documentation and equipment should be kept at Laura's bed space at all times to ensure accessibility and consistency. Resources both within and outside of the hospital should be accessed for Laura. These might include a more comfortable and ergonomically suitable chair, occupational therapy and weaning advice.

An experienced nurse, physiotherapist and consultant should be the key co-ordinators, liaising with Laura and her family and ensuring that specific needs and care are met and that her progress is documented. The engagement and education of Laura's family requires sophisticated communication and relationship-building skills and prolonged commitment (Williams 2005; Endacott and Berry 2007). It is crucial that the nurse co-ordinator has insight and experience in meeting the challenges of rehabilitating a long-stay patient, since it is intensive work which includes building Laura's confidence and her family's involvement. One could argue that although Laura's acute medical needs are low, she is still highly nurse dependent and, therefore, would benefit from one-to-one nursing during her early rehabilitation. Conversely, it could be argued that Laura will gradually need to become more accustomed to less nursing attention as her independence increases, in readiness for her move towards ward care, and therefore sharing a nurse is appropriate. The role of the nurse co-ordinator and the reasons for either one-to-one or one-to-two nursing allocation must be explained diplomatically to Laura and her family.

Laura's rehabilitation and socialisation has to start within an acute environment, where limited facilities for privacy and occupational therapy are often evident. A daily and weekly plan will give Laura structure to her day and help her to recognise achievement of short-term goals such as getting dressed in her own clothes. Laura's plan should include general muscle building, short periods out of bed, rest periods and specific strengthening exercises with a mid-term aim of perhaps walking to the nearest window to see the view and a longer term aim of a hospital gym visit. Whilst Laura's muscles build up, a weaning plan can also be devised for her (Goodman 2006) (see Chapter 2). A speaking valve can be used for speaking during the day, with her tracheostomy cuff down, to enable verbal communication, thereby giving her more control over her activities and enhancing communication with the nurse caring for her. Critical care patients have often described feeling extremely anxious during the weaning phase of their recovery and its success has been shown to be positively influenced by their perception of the skill of their nurse.

Several aids are available to assist communication. These include picture and/or letter/word boards, which may be useful initially and at times when Laura is too tired to talk. However, using a pen and paper requires good dexterity, something which can be difficult for weaker patients.

Psychosocial and physical approaches can be combined to resolve some of Laura's problems. For example, her leg pain may be more tolerable with exercise, a more comfortable chair with leg rest and analgesia. She could be moved to a side room to promote sleep, privacy and independence. Laura could choose to use her head phones and iPOD for settling to sleep and her friends could provide evening 'pamper sessions' to reduce anxiety and aid relaxation (Urden et al. 2006). Laura should be encouraged to talk about her anxiety and nightmares and, if necessary, can take medication to aid sleep (Foa et al. 1999; NICE 2005). A call bell should always be close to Laura and answered promptly by the nearest nurse, to reassure her that she is safe.

Laura's parents can be involved in practical ways such as bringing in her computer/DVD player, post, clothes and home-made food snacks and by helping her to get dressed and to exercise (Endacott and Berry 2007). Laura's nasogastric feeding could be given only at night (via a new, fine-bore tube), and after passing a swallowing test, she can be encouraged to increase her oral diet gradually.

A patient diary may be useful to enable Laura to see her own progress over a period of days (Combe 2005; NICE 2009b). It could be completed by the nurses initially, then by Laura's parents and then jointly by Laura dictating to her parents. Laura and her family should be introduced to the critical care outreach nursing team, who may visit Laura on the ward when she is transferred from critical care, check on her progress and spend time listening and talking with her about her longer term recovery and eventual hospital discharge (Beard 2005).

Discharge from critical care to a general ward has been identified as a particularly stressful time for patients and relatives, with concerns about safety prominent (Chaboyer et al. 2005; Field et al. 2008; Bench and Day 2009), and common difficulties identified with cognitive function, sleep disturbances, eating and mobility (Jones et al. 2003; Robson 2003; Roberts and Chaboyer 2004; Hopkins and Brett 2005). Effective support and information at this time is paramount to ensure optimal rehabilitation continues (Bench and Day 2009). The introduction of critical care outreach services and follow-up clinics has helped to highlight some of these problems and enabled provision of ongoing support for patients and their families (NICE 2009b) before and after discharge from hospital.

Conclusion

The percentage of longer stay patients surviving critical care and experiencing difficulties following discharge is increasing. Therefore, critical care nurses must recognise the importance of critical care rehabilitation and follow-up, and this should be reflected in their clinical practice and in the education they receive. It also needs to be taken into account in managerial and budgetary allocation of resources.

Key learning points

- Patients and their families experience a complex array of physical and psychological challenges during critical illness.
- Rehabilitation needs should be assessed early for all critically ill patients.
- A multi-professional approach is key to effective rehabilitation.
- Longer term patients require identification and management of their specific needs.

Critical appraisal of a research paper

Jones et al. (2003) Rehabilitation after critical illness: a randomized, controlled trial. *Critical Care Medicine* **31**, 2456–2461.

This prospective, quantitative study evaluates the effects of adding a self-directed rehabilitation programme to routine follow-up care given to critical care patients.

Reader activities

1. Read the research article written by Jones et al. (2003).
2. Using the critical appraisal framework in Appendix I, consider the methodological quality of the paper.
3. Reflect on this aspect of your own practice and the implications for future practice management that this paper arises.

A commentary on this paper has been provided by the chapter author in Appendix XVII.

References

Beard H (2005) Does intermediate care minimize relocation stress for patients leaving the ICU?. *Nursing in Critical Care* **10**(6), 272–278.
Bench S, Day T (2010) The use experience of critical care discharge. *International journal of nursing studies*. **47:**487–499.
Benner P, Hooper-Kyriadkidis P, Stannard D (1999) *Clinical Wisdom and Interventions in Critical Care: A Thinking in Action Approach*. WB Saunders, Philadelphia.
Chaboyer W, Kendall E, Kendall M, Foster M (2005) Transfer out of intensive care: a qualitative exploration of patient and family perceptions. *Australian Critical Care* **18**(4), 138.
Christensen M (2007) Noise levels in a general intensive care unit: a descriptive study. *Nursing in Critical Care* **12**(4), 188–197.
Combe D (2005) The use of patient diaries in an intensive care unit. *Nursing in Critical Care* **10**(1), 31–34.

Cuthbertson B, Hull A, Strachan M, Scott J (2004) Post-traumatic psychopathology after critical illness requiring general intensive care. *Intensive Care Medicine* **30**, 450–455.

Deem S (2006) Intensive-care-acquired muscle weakness. *Respiratory Care* **9**(1), 1042–1053.

Ely EW, Inouye SK, Bernard GR, Gordon S, Francis J, May L, Truman B, Speroff T, Gautam S, Margolin R, Hart RP, Dittus R (2001) Delirium in mechanically ventilated patients: validity and reliability of the confusion assessment method for the intensive care unit (CAM-ICU). *Journal of the American Medical Association* **286**, 2703–2710.

Endacott R, Berry J (2007) Caring for relatives in intensive care – an exemplar of practice. *Nursing in Critical Care* **12**(1), 4–5.

Field K, Prinjha S, Rowan K (2008) 'One patient amongst many': a qualitative analysis of intensive care unit patients' experiences of transferring to the general ward. *Critical Care* **12**, R21.

Foa E, Davidson J, Frances A (1999) Treatment of post-traumatic stress disorder –the expert consensus guideline series. *Journal of Clinical Psychology* **60**, 1–75.

Gélinas C, Fillion L, Puntillo K, Viens C, Fortier M (2006) Validation of the Critical-Care Pain Observation Tool in adult patients. *American Journal of Critical Care* **15**(4), 420–427.

Goodman S (2006) Implementing a protocol for weaning patients. *Nursing in Critical Care* **11**(1), 23–32.

Hemsley B, Sigafoos J, Balandin S, Forbes R, Taylor C, Green V, Parmenter T (2001) Nursing the patient with severe communication impairment. *Issues and Innovations in Nursing Practice* **35**, 827–835.

Hopkins R, Brett S (2005) Chronic neurocognitive effects of critical illness. *Current Opinion in Critical Care* **11**, 369–375.

Hough C, Curtis J (2005) Long-term sequelae of critical illness: memories and health-related quality of life. *Critical Care* **9**, 145–146.

Hughes F, Bryan K, Robbins I (2005) Relatives' experiences of critical care. *Nursing in Critical Care* **10**(1), 23–30.

Hull A, Cuthbertson B (2007) Psychological consequences of critical; illness: aftercare or an afterthought? *British Journal of Hospital Medicine* **68**(9), 474–476.

Hupcey JE (2000) Feeling safe – the psychosocial needs of ICU patients. *Journal of Nursing Scholarship* **32**, 361–367.

Johansson I, Fridlund B, Hildingh C (2005) What is supportive when an adult next-of-kin is in critical care? *Nursing in Critical Care* **10**(6), 289–298.

Jones C, Skirrow P, Griffiths R, Humphris G, Ingleby S, Eddleston J, Waldman C, Gager M (2003) Rehabilitation after critical illness: A randomized, controlled trial. *Critical Care Medicine* **31**, 2456–2461.

Jones C, Skirrow P, Griffiths RD (2004) Post-traumatic stress disorder-related symptoms in relatives of patients following intensive care. *Intensive Care Medicine* **30**, 456–460.

Latour J (2005) Is family-centred care in critical care that difficult? A view from Europe. *Nursing in Critical Care* **10**(2), 51–53.

Leske JS (2000) Family stresses, strengths and outcomes after critical injury. *Critical Care Nursing Clinics of North America* **12**, 237–244.

Millbrandt E, Angus D (2006) Bench-to-bedside review: critical illness-associated cognitive dysfunction – mechanisms, markers, and emerging therapeutics. *Critical Care* **10**, 238–246.

Morandi A, Jackson, J, Ely EW (2009) Delirium in the intensive care unit. *International Review of Psychiatry* **21**(1), 43–58.

NICE (2005) *Post-traumatic Stress Disorder – The management of PTSD in Adults and Children in Primary and Secondary Care.* NHS National Institute for Health and Clinical Excellence (NICE), London. Available online at: www.nice.org.uk/pdf/CG026NICEguidelines. Accessed 15 October 2007.

NICE (2009a) *Delirium: Diagnosis, Prevention and Management (Draft Guideline)*. Institute for Health and Clinical Excellence (NICE), London. Available online at: www.nice.org.uk/CG83. Accessed 12 January 2010.

NICE (2009b) *Rehabilitation after critical illness*. NHS National Institute for Health and Clinical Excellence (NICE), London. Available online at: www.nice.org.uk/CG83. Accessed 9 October 2009.

Plank L, Connolly A, Hill G (1998) Sequential changes in the metabolic response in severely septic patients during the first 23 days after the onset of peritonitis. *Annals of Surgery* **228**, 146–158.

Price A (2004) Intensive care nurses' experiences of assessing and dealing with patients' psychological needs. *Nursing in Critical Care* **9**(3), 134–142.

Rattray JE, Hull AM (2008) Emotional outcomes after intensive care: literature review. *Journal of Advanced Nursing* **64**(1), 2–13.

Ricks E (2007) Critical illness polyneuropathy and myopathy: a review of evidence and the implications for weaning from mechanical ventilation and rehabilitation. *Physiotherapy* **93**(2), 151–156.

Roberts B, Chaboyer W (2004) Patients' dreams and unreal experiences following intensive care unit admission. *Nursing in Critical Care* **9**(4), 173–180.

Robson W (2003) The physiological after-effects of critical care. *Nursing in Critical Care* **8**(4), 165–171.

Scholes J, Moore M (1997) *Making a difference: the way in which the nurse interacts with the critical care environment and uses herself as a therapeutic tool*. Occasional Paper Series ITU NDU No 2. Brighton Centre for Nursing and Midwifery Research (Brighton Healthcare and University of Brighton), University of Brighton.

Sessler C, Gosnell M, Grap M, Brophy G, O'Neal P, Keane K, Tesoro E, Elswick R (2002) The Richmond Agitation–Sedation Scale: validity and reliability in adult Intensive Care Unit patients. *American Journal of Respiratory and Critical Care Medicine* **166**, 1338–1344.

Thirugnanam S, Herridge M (2007) Physical consequences of critical illness. *British Journal of Hospital Medicine* **68**(9), 477–481.

Urden L, Stacy K, Lough M (2006) *Thelan's Critical Care Nursing. Diagnosis and management*, 5th edn. Mosby Elsevier, Missouri.

Williams C (2003) *Nurse-patient Interaction in an Intensive Care Setting*. Unpublished PhD Thesis, University of Brighton, Brighton.

Williams C (2005) The identification of family members' contribution to patients' care in the intensive care unit: a naturalistic inquiry. *Nursing in Critical Care* **10**(1), 6–14.

Williams C (2007) Unpopular patients in the intensive care unit: is holistic care achievable? *Nursing in Critical Care* **12**(2), 59–60.

Zigmond A, Snaith R (1983) The Hospital Anxiety and Depression Scale. *Acta Psychological Scandanavia* **67**, 361–370.

Chapter 17

The patient requiring end-of-life care

Ruth Cork

Introduction

In critical care areas, most deaths are expected and follow a decision to withdraw or withhold treatment. Once it has been accepted that a patient is for end-of-life care, management shifts to the palliation of symptoms (BMA 2007) and the support of the family. The following scenario explores the complex array of skills and knowledge required to manage the process of treatment withdrawal, and to effectively support the patient and family during and after an end-of-life care decision has been made.

Scenario

Alan Smith, a 79-year-old gentleman, was admitted to the intensive care unit (ICU) with pneumonia complicated by severe sepsis and a myocardial infarction three weeks ago. He continues to require ventilation via a tracheostomy, and an echocardiogram demonstrates very poor left ventricular function despite increasing inotropic support. He also has methicillin-resistant *Staphylococcus aureus* (MRSA) in his sputum. Alan is semi-conscious. Although he appears to recognise his wife and son when they visit, he is otherwise passive and appears bewildered when awake. He is receiving naso-gastric Paracetamol to help him tolerate discomfort from his tracheostomy tube. The critical care consultant, in discussion with the team, decides to withdraw treatment and not to resuscitate him if he has a cardiac arrest.

The nurse caring for Mr Smith organises a meeting with the consultant and family, where this information is discussed with them. During this discussion, Mrs Smith appears passive and asks apparently unrelated questions such as 'Should I go and put some more money on the car parking ticket?', as if she has not heard the content of the information. Mr Smith's son, David, expresses anger directed towards the hospital staff for the fact that his father had acquired MRSA stating: 'If he hadn't got MRSA he would recover. You are obliged to continue treating him because it is your fault he is in the state he is in now.'

Critical Care Nursing: Learning from Practice, 1st edition. Edited by Suzanne Bench and Kate Brown.
© 2011 Blackwell Publishing Ltd.

Reader activities

- What factors should have been considered in reaching a decision to withdraw treatment from Alan?
- Who should the decision makers be? Discuss the role of Alan and his family.
- Explain the initial reactions of Alan's family to the bad news they had been given.

Discussion

Approximately 70–90% of deaths in the ICU follow a decision to withdraw treatment (Prendergast and Luce 1997; Winter and Cohen 1999). Medical treatment can legally and ethically be withdrawn when it is futile, and not in the patient's best interests to continue.

It is important to clarify the difference between judging an individual's previous quality of life, which is difficult and subjective, and making a clinical judgement about their inability to survive, despite treatment, which is more evidence based but no less complex. The reversible causes of Alan's current condition have been addressed. Further investigations are sometimes needed to confirm that the diagnosis and pathophysiology is non-reversible and that no other or further treatment will offer any clinical benefit to the patient at this stage in terms of survival and recovery (Twycross 2003). In Alan's case the echocardiogram indicated that his heart could not support his efforts to wean from the ventilator or the inotropes. Therefore, if Alan had a cardiac arrest, his chances of survival would be negligible. In addition, since he does not have the physical capacity to wean from the ventilator, continuing to treat him would be unjustifiable (Hall and Rocker 2000). The presence of MRSA in his sputum is much less clinically significant within the overall picture.

Medico-legally, the consultant is the decision maker since they are professionally accountable for the patient's management (GMC 2002; DCA 2005). Alan is semi/unconscious, unable to clearly express his thoughts and feelings and therefore unable to engage in a consent process with many aspects of his ongoing treatment. Involving Alan in a meaningful way in discussions regarding withdrawing treatment, although desirable in terms of his autonomy, is unrealistic (DCA 2005). Bearing this in mind, withdrawing treatment has obvious implications in terms of ethical principles (Gillon 1994) and the balance of power which families often perceive as existing wholly with the medical team (Jones et al. 1991; Wright 1999). Experienced nursing staff, familiar with the patient's condition, progress and the relatives' relationship with the patient, should be closely involved with the decision-making process. They should play a key role in promoting the relatives' trust in the whole team at this vulnerable time of starting to anticipate the death of their family member, when they often feel powerless to influence their survival.

The discussion should aim to achieve a consensus with the family (Curtis et al. 2001; Levy and Carlet 2001). The relatives do not have a clinical role in demanding either that treatment continue, as David attempted to do, or that it be discontinued. The Mental Capacity Act (DCA 2005), however, has introduced an opportunity for relatives to fulfil an advocacy role. Relatives can often accurately relay information about the patient's quality of life and any views which the patient may have expressed regarding life-saving treatment and the quality of their death, prior to the current hospital episode (Barnett 2002). Sometimes, relatives initiate a conversation suggesting that the patient 'would not want to carry on like this'. Caution must be used, however, when interpreting this information since the relatives' account may be influenced subconsciously by their own emotional stage of grieving and the actual rather than expressed quality of their relationship with the patient.

A request for a second opinion must be responded to honestly and realistically with time limits set for a final review of the patient's condition. It is crucial that relatives understand the clinical deterioration of the patient and that they are dying despite treatment (Fulbrook et al. 1999). It is also crucial that relatives do not perceive themselves as being responsible for 'switching off' the patient's 'life support' and thereby causing or allowing their death. It is helpful to state this fact to the relatives to prevent them from feelings of unjustified guilt in the future.

Unwanted, unexpected bad news triggers a normal stress response, including physical signs of stress, for example, pallor and/or shaking, and psychological signs for example, defensive/aggressive behaviour to protect the patient or themselves (Worden 1991). It is normal to expect that David and his mother would not be able to think rationally and realistically at this point.

Initially expressing denial or doubt is normal, as is seeking further clarification and confirmation that there is no longer any chance of survival. This is often both an intellectual process, which is understanding, and an emotional process, which is grieving. Mrs Smith's passive behaviour indicates that she has not yet absorbed the message being given. Her question regarding car parking is possibly a subconscious effort to divert away the bad news temporarily, until her mind starts to digest it (Wright 1999).

David expressed his distress as anger, blame and distrust directed at healthcare professionals. David's focus on Alan's hospital-acquired infection indicates that he is not only seeking information to try to understand the situation mentally but also diverting away from considering the less disputable facts of Alan's respiratory and cardiac insufficiency. His searching and bargaining behaviour ('you are obliged to carry on treating him') is normal and, if responded to with honest discussion, can help David to realise and accept that Alan is dying (Worden 1991).

Skills-based knowledge

Breaking bad news

Alan has been in the ICU for a few weeks, during which time the staff will have built a relationship with both him and his family. From the time of his admission, explanation of his condition and progress to Alan's family will have been an ongoing aspect of nursing care. It is likely that the question of Alan's survival has been raised either by his family or by the nursing and medical staff, and honest information given, so that his family will already be aware that his prognosis is poor. The ICU environment, however, is geared towards saving life and the transition to experiencing bereavement often appears sudden

Table 17.1   Stages of grief.

Stage	
Denial	Denial is usually only temporary. It is generally replaced with heightened awareness of situations and individuals that will be left behind after death
Anger	The individual recognises that denial cannot continue. They can be very difficult to care for due to misplaced feelings of rage and envy. Any individual that symbolises life or energy is subject to projected resentment and jealousy.
Bargaining	The third stage involves the hope that the individual can somehow postpone or delay death. Usually, the negotiation for an extended life is made with a higher power in exchange for a reformed lifestyle.
Depression	The individual begins to understand the certainty of death. Because of this, he or she may become silent and spend much of the time crying and grieving. It is an important time for grieving that must be processed.
Acceptance	This final stage comes with peace and understanding of the death that is approaching. Generally, the person in the fifth stage will want to be left alone. This stage has also been described as the end of the dying struggle.

Source: Data adapted from Kubler-Ross (1973).

for relatives, even for those who knew that the chances of recovery were slim (Seymour 2000). The conversation, involving breaking bad news to Alan's family, will therefore still have a massive impact on their understanding, emotional experience and memory of his death (Andrew 1998; Levy and Carlet 2001).

Preparing for and managing this conversation expertly is crucial (ICS 1998; Farrell 1999). Body language, giving clear facts in logical order using intelligent listening, non-technical language, timing of pauses, checking understanding, anticipating and responding to questions and reactions all require concentration, skill and uninterrupted time on the part of healthcare professionals. Both Mrs Smith's and David's initial responses were normal and they individually need assistance by the nurse to absorb this complex, emotionally difficult information over a period of time (Bolton 2000). Critical care staff need to have an understanding of the different stages of grief and how these might be expressed by both the patient and their family in order to effectively manage this aspect of care (Table 17.1).

Developing scenario

In accordance with the joint guidelines for best practice produced by the British Medical Association (BMA), the Resuscitation Council (UK) and the Royal College of Nursing (RCN) (2007), the consultant documents the discussion, Do Not Attempt Resuscitation decision and Alan's palliative care plan. The nurse disconnects and removes unnecessary monitoring and infusions and ensures Alan is clean and appears comfortable prior to his family returning to sit with him. An intravenous opiate infusion is commenced whilst his blood pressure is still high enough to circulate the opiate round his body, to prevent discomfort and facilitate a feeling of calm.

The nurse explains to Alan's family the provision of analgesia, sequence of stopping support and changes they can expect to see in Alan's breathing, skin colour and conscious level as he dies. She invites them to ask questions and to express their needs throughout this process. The nurse offers the services of the hospital chaplain, which are declined. Alan appears slightly aware but does not respond. The nurse then stops the inotropic drug infusion, reduces the oxygen delivery from the ventilator to 21% (i.e. room air) and reduces the ventilatory support that Alan is receiving.

His son, David, appears agitated, leaving the bedside and returning frequently. He asks some irrational questions, demands specific answers, expresses his distrust of hospital staff and seems unable to provide support to his mother. The nurse initiates conversation with Mrs Smith, asking about their life together. Mrs Smith talks freely and cries at times. David joins in with memories of family activities and gradually settles at the bedside, providing some physical comfort to his mother. Alan dies approximately six hours later, with both the nurse and his family present.

An evidence-based discussion of management

The care of Alan and that of his family are inextricably linked and need simultaneous management (Hall and Rocker 2000) (Figure 17.1).

Withdrawal of treatment plans and guidelines are increasingly used in critical care areas to aid accurate, unambiguous, thorough documentation and intra- and inter-professional collaboration, particularly when the withdrawal of treatment situation is especially complex (Marie Curie Palliative Care Institute Liverpool (MCPCIL) 2007). Plans should be flexible enough to adapt to the changing needs of the patient and family during the dying process. The Liverpool Care Pathway (LCP) (Ellershaw and Wilkinson 2003) is a multi-professional document that provides an evidence-based framework that can be used during the last hours and days of life. It is based on the standards of care delivery in the hospice environment. Its aim is to improve care of the dying in the last hours or days of

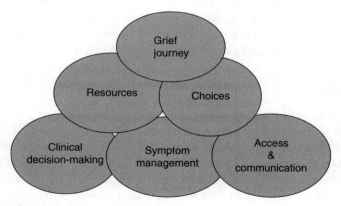

Figure 17.1   Nursing considerations in end of life care.

life, wherever the location, and to improve the knowledge related to the process of dying. The LCP is recommended as a template of best practice in UK national policy (DH 2008, 2009), and should guide the care of Alan and his family in the last hours or days of life. An example of the LCP template can be found at: http://www.mcpcil.org.uk/liverpool-care-pathway/pdfs/LCP-ICU-version11.pdf.

The dying process took several hours for Alan, providing an opportunity to utilise skills and creativity to influence the quality of his death and facilitate his family's natural grieving process.

Symptom management

Withdrawal of treatment does not equate to withdrawal of care. Every effort should be made to maintain the highest standard of care to the patient (Hunter et al. 2006). Pain relief should be given a high priority. An intravenous opiate infusion was provided for Alan to enhance comfort, not to accelerate the dying process (Truog et al. 2001; Twycross 2003). Titration of analgesia according to need is an important nursing role. All other infusions (apart from those for the control of unpleasant symptoms), and monitoring, should be discontinued (Cohen et al. 2003). In Alan's case, only cardiac monitoring was continued, at David's request, with the screen angled away from Mrs Smith's direct line of vision. This also enabled the nurse to monitor vital signs, such as tachycardia, that could indicate pain.

Truog et al. (2001) note that although guidelines suggest that any intervention that does not advance the patient's goals should be eliminated, this simple advice can be difficult to follow in reality. An example of this can be seen in Alan's care. Artificial nutrition and hydration are medical treatments and evidence from terminally ill cancer patients suggests that dying patients do not feel hunger or thirst in the later stages of death, and that their continuation can unnecessarily prolong death. However, Alan's naso-gastric feed was continued, since David expressed particular fear that his father would feel thirsty or hungry, depriving him of a basic human right.

Alan's ventilatory support was reduced to a minimum and his inotropic drugs discontinued. It would have been clinically appropriate to stop ventilation completely and just humidify the room air. Although he might have died more quickly, this may have increased his family's distress, bearing in mind that they needed time to communicate with him and with each other as part of the grieving process. Alan could also have been extubated, however, again this could have led to symptoms for example, gasping or gurgling sounds, that could have been construed as distressing for both Alan and his family.

Family needs

Box 17.1 outlines key aspects of family needs during end-of-life care.

Promoting access to the person and communication with them prior to death, at the moment of death and following death, is imperative (ICS 1998; Pattison 2006). The ICU environment lacks privacy, can be intimidating and often inhibits natural communication between family members. The provision of visual privacy, even if no side room is available, and the removal of unnecessary barriers to physical closeness between Alan and his family facilitate family communication and enable expression of emotional feelings. An

---

Box 17.1   Families' needs during end of life care

To be present
To assist in care for their loved one
To be informed about changes and decisions
To understand the care being delivered and its rationale
To be confident that their loved one is comfortable and cared for at all times
To be comforted and have opportunity to express their feelings
To feel confident that the correct decisions have been taken
To achieve an understanding of the death of their loved one
To have their own physical needs provided for

Source: Adapted from Truog et al. (2001).

---

expected death does not mean an emotionally accepted death. Therefore, time spent with the dying person is crucial to enable the reality of death to be emotionally and mentally acknowledged. The nurse deliberately provided a 'supportive presence' with Alan's family.

Providing choices and inviting requests and questions enable relatives to feel involved, make a contribution and acknowledge the reality of their loss. The nurse is the key coordinator and mobiliser of resources within the ICU and the hospital, and should initiate offering resources and services. Relatives may not realise that resources exist, for example, 24-hour religious support, the use of a private room to talk/take time away from the bedside and provision to make telephone calls (Cressey and Winbolt-Lewis 2000).

The stress of a crisis often disables coping abilities and routines and people require assistance to re-engage their personal resources. They often need repetition of the same information several times, or cannot remember things such as where they parked the car. After Alan's death, the nurse provided written information and the use of a telephone in a private room, enabling his family to cope with immediate practical tasks.

During and following Alan's death, David remained agitated, making unrealistic demands and asking some irrational questions. The nurse realised that it was not possible to resolve all David's concerns at this time of family crisis. Worden (1991) describes 'tasks' of grieving as part of a normal process, which some families need assistance with as they adjust to bereavement (Murray-Parkes 1998). An appointment with the Patient Advice and Liaison Services and with Alan's consultant could provide opportunities to talk through the clinical facts. Informing Alan's general practitioner of his death and encouraging Mrs Smith and David to contact him is another way of ensuring ongoing support (ICS 1998).

Relevant legislation and policy developments (e. g. Advanced Directives, the Human Rights Act, Organ Donor Registration (Branthwaite 2007)) also need to be incorporated into end-of-life care in order to meet the needs of patients and their families completely. Managing decisions making regarding end-of-life situations, progressing to holistic symptom management and achieving excellent communication with a patient's family are crucial aspects of modern critical care provision (Beckstrand and Kirchoff 2005).

Conclusion

End-of-life care is a therapeutic process. As such, it requires effective preparation and planning, with all individuals involved. Withdrawing treatment and care at the end of life is fraught with challenges. The process can be enhanced by the use of clear and unambiguous multi-professional guidelines, used to meet individual holistic needs of both the patient and their family.

Key learning points

- National guidelines should be used to guide clinicians in decisions related to the withdrawal or limitation of treatment.
- Withdrawal of treatment and subsequent end-of-life care will be individual to each patient and their family.
- Specific education should be provided for all clinical and non-clinical staff.
- National end-of-life care guidance (Liverpool Care Pathway) should be utilised to aid accurate, unambiguous, thorough documentation and effective inter-professional collaboration during treatment withdrawal and end-of-life care.

Critical appraisal of a research paper

Goodridge et al. (2008) Caring for critically ill patients with advanced COPD at the end of life: a qualitative study. *Intensive and Critical Care Nursing* **24**, 162–170.

Reader activities

1. Read the research article written by Goodridge et al. (2004).
2. Using the critical appraisal framework in Appendix I, consider the methodological quality of the paper.
3. Reflect on this aspect of your own practice and the implications for future practice management that this paper arises.

A commentary on this paper has been provided by the chapter author in Appendix XVIII.

References

Andrew CM (1998) Optimising the human experience: nursing the families of people who die in intensive care. *Intensive and Critical Care Nursing* **3**, 59–65.

Barnett MM (2002) Effect of breaking bad news on patient's perceptions of doctors. *Journal of the Royal Society of Medicine* **95**, 343–347.

Beckstrand RL, Kirchoff KT (2005) Providing end-of-life care to patients: critical care nurses' perceived obstacles and supportive behaviours. *American Journal of Critical Care* **14**, 395–403.

Bolton SC (2000) Who cares? Offering emotional work as a "gift" in the nursing labour process. *Journal of Advanced Nursing* **32**(93), 58–586.

Branthwaite MA (2007) The Introduction of a bill on assisted dying. *Care of the Critically Ill* **23**(5), 128–129.

British Medical Association (BMA) (2007) *Withholding or Withdrawing Life-Prolonging Treatment. Guidance for Decision Making*. BMA, London.

British Medical Association, Resuscitation Council (UK) and Royal College of Nursing (2007) *Decisions Relating to Cardiopulmonary Resuscitation*. Available online at: www.bma.org.uk. Accessed 12 January 2010.

Cohen SL, Bewley JS, Ridley S, Goldhill D (ICS Standards Committee) (2003) *Guidelines for Limitation of Treatment for Adults Requiring Intensive Care*. London, Intensive Care Society. Available online at: www.ics.ac.uk. Accessed 12 January 2010.

Cressey RW, Winbolt-Lewis M (2000) The forgotten heart of healthcare: a model of spiritual care in the National Health Service. *Accident and Emergency Nursing* **8**, 170–177.

Curtis JR, Patrick DL, Shannon SE, Treece PD, Engelberg RA, Rubenfeld GD (2001) The family conference as a focus to improve communication about end-of-life care in the intensive care unit: opportunities for improvement. *Critical Care Medicine* **29**(920), N26–N33.

Department of Health (2008) *End of Life Care Strategy – Promoting High Quality Care for All Adults at the End of Life*. DH, London.

Department of Health (2009) *End of Life Care Strategy: Quality Markers and Measures for End of Life Care*. DH, London.

Department for Constitutional Affairs (DCA) (2005) *The Mental Capacity Act*. Available online at: www.dca.gov.uk/capacity/index. Accessed 31 July 2009.

Ellershaw J, Wilkinson S (eds) (2003) *Care of the Dying: A Pathway to Excellence*. Oxford University Press, Oxford.

Farrell M (1999) The challenge of breaking bad news. *Intensive and Critical Care Nursing* **15**, 101–110.

Fulbrook P, Allan D, Carroll S, Dawson D (1999) On the receiving end: experiences of being a relative in critical care. *Nursing in Critical Care* **4**, 138–145.

General Medical Council (GMC) (2002) *Withholding and Withdrawing Life-Prolonging Treatments: Good Practice in Decision Making*. Available online at: www.gmc-uk.org. Accessed 31 July 2009.

Gillon R (1994) Medical ethics: four principles plus attention to scope. *British Medical Journal* **309**, 184–188.

Goodridge D, Duggleby W, Gjevre J, Rennie D (2008) Caring for critically ill patients with advanced COPD at the end of life: a qualitative study. *Intensive and Critical Care Nursing* **24**, 162–170.

Hall RI, Rocker GM (2000) End-of-life care in the ICU: treatment provided when end of life support was withdrawn. *Chest* **118**, 1424–1430.

Hunter J, Dean T, Gowan J (2006) Death with dignity: devising a withdrawal of treatment process. *British Journal of Nursing* **15**(3), 138–140.

Intensive Care Society (ICS) (1998) *Guidelines for Bereavement Care in Intensive Care Units*. ICS, London.

Jones C, Hussey RM, Griffiths RD (1991) Social support in the ICU? *British Journal of Intensive Care* **1**, 67–69.

Kubler-Ross E (1973) *On Death and Dying*. Routledge, London.

Levy MM, Carlet J (2001) Compassionate end-of-life care in the intensive care unit. Critical Care Medicine *29*, 2(supplement N1).

Marie Curie Palliative Care Institute Liverpool (MCPCIL) (2007) *The Liverpool Care Pathway – Non-Cancer Briefing Paper*. Available online at: www.mcil.org.uk. Accessed 31 July 2009.

Murray-Parkes CM (1998) Coping with loss: bereavement in adult life. *British Medical Journal* **14**(316), 7134.

Pattison N (2006) A critical discourse analysis of provision of end-of-life care in key UK critical care documents. *Nursing in Critical Care* **11**(4), 198–208.

Prendergast TJ, Luce JM (1997) Increasing incidence of withholding and withdrawal of life support from the critically ill. *American Journal of Respiratory Care Medicine* **155**, 15–20.

Seymour JE (2000) Negotiating a natural death in intensive care. *Social Science and Medicine* **51**, 1241–1252.

Truog RD, Cist AFM, Brackett SE, Burns JP, Curley MAQ, Danis M, DeVita MA, Rosenbaum SH, Rothenberg DM, Sprung CL, Webb SA, Wlody GS, Hurford WE (2001) Recommendations for end of life care in the intensive care unit: The Ethics Committee for the Society of Critical care Medicine. *Critical Care Medicine* **29**, 2332–2348.

Twycross R (2003) *Introducing Palliative Care*, 4th edn. Radcliffe Medical Press Ltd., Abingdon, UK.

Winter B, Cohen S (1999) ABC of intensive care: withdrawal of treatment. *British Medical Journal* **31**, 306–308.

Worden JW (1991) *Grief Counselling and Grief Therapy*, 2nd edn. Routledge, London.

Wright B (1999) Responding to autonomy and disempowerment at the time of sudden death. *Accident and Emergency Nursing* **7**, 154–157.

Appendices

Appendix I

Framework for critical appraisal of research studies

Based on Hamer S, Collinson G (2005) *Achieving Evidence-Based Practice*, 2nd edn. Bailliere Tindall, London.

Quantitative studies

- Was the aim/key question/hypothesis of this study clear? Do you think it warrants the research? Were the researchers credible?
- What type of study was it? Was this an appropriate design to answer the research question?
- Who comprise the sample? Is this appropriate? Was ethical approval sought?
- How were the subjects selected? Was this non-biased?
- What was the sample size? Consider the implications of this to the results.
- What (if any) interventions were used? Were all other factors kept static/controlled during this period? Why is this important?
- What measurement tools and data collection methods were used? Were the tools and data collection methods valid and reliable? Was there a systematic approach to data collection?
- What were the results? How were they collated and presented? Were any statistical tests done on any figures? Was this appropriate?
- What were the patient outcomes/conclusions and the researchers' interpretation of the results? Did the researchers' interpretation fit with the results? How do the findings fit with previous research in the area?
- What were the limitations of this study? Do the authors acknowledge these?
- Are the results generalisable? What limits their applicability to practice? What can you take away from the study?

Critical Care Nursing: Learning from Practice, 1st edition. Edited by Suzanne Bench and Kate Brown.
© 2011 Blackwell Publishing Ltd.

Qualitative studies

- Did the paper describe an important clinical problem addressed by a clearly formulated question?
- Was a qualitative approach appropriate?
- How were the setting and subjects selected?
- How does the researcher avoid researcher bias? What was the researcher's perspective, and has this been taken into account?
- What methods did the researcher use for collecting data and are these described in enough detail? Are the data collection processes transparent? Is there an audit trail?
- What methods were used to analyse the data, and what quality control measures were implemented? Were the transcribed and collated data returned to the participants to check accuracy?
- Are the results credible, and if so are they clinically important? Do the findings reflect the phenomena accurately?
- What conclusions were drawn and are they justified by the results?
- Are the findings of the study transferable to other clinical settings?

Appendix II

Chapter one article

Drakulovic et al. (1999) Supine body position as a risk factor for nosocomial pneumonia in mechanically ventilated patients: a randomised trial. *The Lancet* **354**(9133), 1851–1858.

Commentary

This paper by Drakulovic et al. (1999) is important as it is one of the research studies supporting the inclusion of head elevation in the ventilator care bundle, one of the high-impact interventions in the Saving Lives document produced by the Department of Health (DH 2007). Pneumonia is the most frequent nosocomial infection among intensive care unit (ICU) patients with the incidence of nosocomial pneumonia in medical and surgical ICUs having been reported to range from 12.8 to 17.6 per 1000 ventilator days. The American Centers for Disease Control and Prevention (CDC) have also emphasised the importance of preventing the development of VAP as the associated mortality ranges from 20% to 41% and it is the leading cause of death from nosocomial infections in hospital. Drakulovic et al. point out that although the semi-recumbent position has been strongly recommended by the CDC, its role in the prevention of nosocomial pneumonia has never been proven in a randomised clinical trial. They therefore investigated the frequency of nosocomial pneumonia in intubated and mechanically ventilated patients, randomly assigned to either supine or semi-recumbent body positions. The findings were so clear that the study was terminated at a scheduled interim analysis after only 86 patients had been recruited.

The strength of this study lies in the fact that it is a randomised controlled trial which allows the control of variables which could have an effect on the outcome. However, the study was conducted in only one hospital and in two ICUs which would have had a similar patient mix. Drakulovic et al. do not specify patients' presenting conditions in their paper. The question then arises as to how applicable the findings are to a general ICU population.

The patients allocated to be nursed in the supine position were more likely to have received ranitidine, to have a large-bore nasogastric tube in place and to have a higher APACHE II score than those in the semi-recumbent group. Although these differences between the groups did not reach statistical significance, all the *p*-values were less than 0.08. Combination of all these factors together may have led to a slight bias in the patients assigned to the supine group. More patients in the supine group also appear to have been ventilated for greater than seven days and there is no indication from the authors whether this difference is statistically significant or not. Drakulovic and colleagues, however, point out in their findings that ventilation for greater than seven days is a risk factor for development of nosocomial pneumonia. On the basis of the information presented, however, only six patients need to be treated in the semi-recumbent position to prevent one case of pneumonia.

This study highlights an interesting point regarding the pathogenesis of nosocomial pneumonia. The duration and the depth of sedation were associated with a significantly increased frequency of infection. There is now evidence that many of the sedatives commonly used in the ICU have immunosuppressive effects and, in fact, sedation is also addressed in the ventilator care bundle from the DH (2007).

During the study period patients in the semi-recumbent group were required to be nursed at an angle of 45 degrees. In practice this can be quite difficult to achieve and the authors do not make any comment how the angle was measured or what percentage of the time it was adhered to. This point has been further debated in later studies and, at present, it remains unclear as to the angle required to demonstrate a benefit. In fact the Saving Lives document suggests head elevation above 30 degrees as it is more realistic in practice (DH 2007).

There is no documented evidence of harm with the use of the semi-recumbent position and there is proof that that aspiration of gastric contents and associated nosocomial pneumonia are less likely when patients are nursed in the semi-recumbent position. Despite a few criticisms of this study by Drakulovic et al., it was stopped at the interim analysis as a result of the positive effects seen with the use of the semi-recumbent position, and this intervention is now recommended as part of the ventilator care bundle (DH 2007).

Reference

Department of Health (DH) (2007) *Saving Lives: Reducing Infection, Delivering Clean and Safe Care*. Crown copyright, London. Available online at: www.dh.gov.uk/. Accessed 6 August 2009.

Appendix III
Chapter article

Tonnelier et al. (2005) Impact of a nurse's protocol-directed weaning procedure on outcomes in patients undergoing mechanical ventilation for longer than 48 hours: a prospective cohort study with a matched historical control group. *Critical Care* **9**(2), 83–89.

Commentary

It is extremely difficult to compare the weaning of one patient with another even when the samples are matched as their trajectories can be so different. Studies like these tend to simplify weaning. However, this is a rather select group of patients in terms of the inclusion criteria and SBTs were conducted without PEEP.

A key difference between the retrospective sample and the prospective sample is that in the latter nurses used weaning protocols, whereas in the former, intensivists did not and, therefore, different intensivists would have different opinions, etc. The difficulty here is what made the difference: the nurse or the protocol? Using retrospective samples presents some methodological difficulties. Firstly, how can you ensure practices which will have an influence on the outcome have been controlled? For example, did sedation practices change over time? Even raising awareness of weaning will undoubtedly have some impact. Did the experience or expertise of the nurse have an impact? Jenny and Logan's work, for example, demonstrated that nursing expertise, knowing the patient and continuity of care were important features in accelerating weaning (Jenny and Logan 1992). The paper itself does consider the other methodological issues.

The emphasis was on screening for readiness for weaning with a SBT. The paper does not go on to explain what happened after a successful trial.

Reference

Jenny J, Logan J (1992) Knowing the patient: one aspect of clinical knowledge. *Image* **24**, 254–258.

Appendix IV

Chapter article

Giuliano KK et al. (1999) Temperature measurement in critically ill orally intubated adults: a comparison of pulmonary artery core, tympanic and oral methods. *Critical Care Medicine* **27**(10), 2188–2193.

Commentary

The paper is useful in that it attempts to add further evidence to establish the best method of non-invasive thermometry for the critically ill patient, which was by no means established at the time, or since. It is unlikely that more up–to-date studies will be able to replicate this type of research as so few PA catheters are now used and the study is, therefore, significant in its comparison of non-invasive devices compared to the 'gold standard'.

The sample size is reasonable at 102 and fairly distributed by sex and representative of a wide age range typical of the ICU population (35–95 years with average age 67.42). It would be reasonable to use convenience sampling in this instance as inserting a PA catheter solely for research purposes would not be permissible.

One of the strengths of the study is that the authors have attempted to account for influencing factors by controlling a number of variables. They have addressed interrater reliability by providing training of the operators, instruments were appropriately calibrated in the medical technology department and a number of patient factors such as pathology of the temperature taking site, clinical observations, ventilator circuit temperatures and ambient temperatures were accounted for. They did not, however, address other influencing factors, especially in the technique used in taking temperatures, for example, whether the tympanic thermometer lens was kept clean, whether both ears were used in obtaining data or whether an 'ear tug' technique was performed.

The inclusion of non-intubated control group would have improved this study, as it would have provided valuable information on the effect of intubation on oral temperatures. The study uses appropriate statistical methods of analysis for comparing instrument measurements, the Bland and Altman repeated measurement method. This is important as many researchers have fallen into the trap of using only correlational coefficients in analysing data from multiple measurements of different instruments, which invalidates their findings (see Bland and Altman (1986, 1995) for a full explanation of this statistical method).

The weaknesses in this study are the following: the authors use an inaccurate definition of the tympanic thermometer. A tympanic thermometer is a thermistor device that sits up against the tympanic membrane itself and measures conductive heat. This device is not suitable for clinical practice and the actual method used in this study was that of 'ear-based' thermometry using a device that measures temperature in the ear canal via infrared spectrometry. The point here is that one measures core temperature directly (tympanic) whereas the other thermometer estimates temperature. Another point of weakness in the study was in the comparison of the tympanic thermometer in the oral mode with the PA temperature as this accounted for the highest statistical degree of variability and inaccuracy. The thermometer in this mode would not equate to PA readings as it is specifically designed and preset to read the temperature as lower than core in this mode. It would have been better to compare this mode with the oral temperature readings.

The researchers also highlight a limitation of the study as a lack of hypo- and hyperthermic patients and so they could not assess the thermometers' performances over a broad range of temperatures.

The study does not provide conclusive evidence that oral temperature taking is more accurate than tympanic, but it does raise some interesting and important points. It is much more difficult than it appears to design studies that compare methods of clinical measurement as they are affected by so many variables, not all of which can be controlled. Tympanic temperatures should not necessarily be assumed to be effective in the critically ill. The study also highlights the poor training of staff in using instruments and how important this is in ensuring accurate temperature taking. It is also not at all easy to learn to take tympanic or ear-based temperatures properly.

Appendix V

Chapter article

Pronovost et al. (2006) An intervention to decrease catheter related bloodstream infections in the ICU. *The New England Journal of Medicine* **355**(26), 2725–2732.

Commentary

This is an important paper as it has been used by the DH in the UK as part of the evidence to support the central venous catheter care bundle, one of the high-impact interventions identified in the Saving Lives document (DH 2007). Additionally, it supports the guidelines produced by the American Centers for Disease Control (O'Grady et al. 2002). Both of these guideline sets recognise the huge impact that catheter-related bloodstream infection has on morbidity, mortality and cost, with data from the UK National Audit Office citing the added cost of bloodstream infection in England being £6209 per patient. Pronovost et al. (2006) in their paper also suggest that such infections could amount to an estimated 2.3 million dollars annually in the United States. Justification for studying the impact of interventions designed to reduce catheter-related bloodstream infection thus seems clear, although two multi-site studies had been previously conducted.

The strengths of this research lie in its prospective large sample multi-site approach, which included both general and specialist adult ICUs. This helped to ensure results were generalisable across a wide population. Intervention studies are traditionally conducted using randomised controlled trials which allow control of the many variables which could impact on the outcomes. This approach, however, would have required a control group who would have been denied interventions such as effective hand hygiene, known from previous studies to have a significant effect on reducing infection (DH 2007). This would have been ethically unsound.

The sample population consisted of those who volunteered following a request for participation from the research team. Those who chose not to participate were not followed up. This raises the question of what their characteristics were and whether they differed from those included within the sample.

At the same time as implementing the catheter-related interventions, three other sets of interventions were also introduced and monitored over a six-month period. This approach could have led to some contamination of the data sets retrieved, making it difficult to be sure that the results were entirely due to the implementation of the catheter-related interventions alone.

A common definition of catheter-related infection was agreed and distributed to all study sites, ensuring consistent diagnosis. However, it was not clear how frequently line sites were checked. The effects of individual components of the intervention set were also not examined, so it is difficult to know which aspects are more important, if any, than others. Other limitations of the methodology used were identified and discussed by the authors.

Significant reductions in catheter-related bloodstream infection were demonstrated using both p values, which were $< p = 0.002$, and narrow 95% confidence intervals. However, from examining the paper, it appears that 48 out of the 103 hospitals did not provide any baseline data for comparison and thus the comparisons between the two periods of time may not represent as significant a reduction as suggested by the authors. This does not detract from the startling fact that the median rate of infection 3 months after implementation was 0, and that this was then sustained for the remaining period of the study.

The implications of this study for current practice clear, and justify the results being used as evidence for practice within national UK and US guidelines (DH 2007; O'Grady et al. 2002).

References

Department of Health (DH) (2007) *Saving Lives: Reducing Infection, Delivering Clean and Safe Care*. Crown copyright, London. Available online at: www.dh.gov.uk/. Accessed 6 August 2009.
O'Grady N, Alexander M, Dellinger E, Gerberding J, Heard S, Maki D, Masur H, McCormick R, Mermel L, Pearson M, Raad I, Randolph A, Weinstein R (2002) *Guidelines for the Prevention of Intravascular Catheter-Related Infections*. Centers for Disease Control and Prevention. Morbidity and Mortality Weekly Report Recommendations and Reports 51(RR-10):10.

Appendix VI

Chapter article

De Laat E, Schoonhoven L, Grypdonck M, Verbeek A, de Graaf R, Pickkers P, van Achterberg T (2007) Early postoperative 30° lateral positioning after coronary artery surgery: influence on cardiac output. *Journal of Clinical Nursing* **16**, 654–661.

Commentary

This work is undertaken by a credible and comprehensive team of researchers (de Laat et al. 2007) with a wide range of expertise from the Netherlands. It is published in a respected, international, peer-reviewed journal with high impact factor.

Justification for the study is based on assertion by the research team that critically ill patients do not receive standard two hourly turns due to haemodynamic and oxygenation instability. Critical exploration of past studies are cited to offer support for this statement, but there is little reference to local/international clinical practices nor to normal physiological work in this area. A relevant hypothesis is posed.

The study appropriately cites itself as a clinical trial as there is some randomisation but not across the whole sample. The research method is well documented and extremely rigorous. There is a detailed sampling strategy for the 75 patients. The derivation of the four intervention groups is clearly outlined, but no detail is given as to how the size of this sample is determined: this would have been useful. The ethics process is well attended to in the paper. Only clinically stable patients were included. The use of the reference group is not entirely clear; a traditional control group may have strengthened this study.

The detailed interventions across the study groups are well presented; however, high-dose inotropic support is largely absent across the sample population, and whilst this is consistent with the sample inclusion criteria, it does raise questions as to study generalisability. There is full description of the equipment and procedures (calibration, etc.), with the primary outcome variable (cardiac output), collected with a pulmonary artery catheter. The data sampling process with five haemodynamic snapshots is clearly described.

The data analysis section is based on the premise of bioequivalence, and is supported by inferential statistical tests including one-sided and two-sided t-tests and chi-square tests. An assumption of normal distribution is made, which would appear reasonable, and a significance level of 0.05 used. The use of one- and two-sided t-tests with bioequivalence, and use of both parametric and non-parametric with normally distributed data, is not entirely clear. Greater justification would have been useful.

There are detailed results supporting the hypothesis, but this section lacks clarity. It is interesting to note that turning took place with two nurses and averaged 3.07 minutes; this is not entirely consistent with personal experience. The discussion section explores the team's findings with previous papers and appropriately cites limitations to other populations.

The finding of this study is that if a post-vein graft patient is haemodynamically stable, posturing should not cause cardiovascular problems. What is not known is what variables can be used to identify patients who will not tolerate posturing, and how pressure relief can be safely achieved in these patients. Whilst expert practitioners may have an instinct to the answers to these questions, this has not yet been confirmed by empirical study.

Appendix VII

Chapter article

Vincent JL, Sakr Y, Sprunh C (2008) Are blood transfusions associated with greater mortality rates? Results of the sepsis occurrence in acutely ill patients study. *Anesthesiology* **108**, 31–39.

Commentary

Patients were classified depending on whether they had received a blood transfusion at any time during their ICU stay. The study demonstrated that of the 3147 patients, 33% received a blood transfusion. It was noted, however, that these patients were marginally older (62 vs. 60 years, $P = 0.035$) and were more likely to have liver cirrhosis and hematologic cancer, to be a surgical admission and to have sepsis. The transfused patients had both a longer length of admission and a higher mortality rate but were more severely ill on admission (Simplified Acute Physiology Score II, 40.2 vs. 34.7; $P < 0.001$; Sequential Organ Failure Assessment score, 6.5 vs. 4.5; $P < 0.0016$).

However, in a multivariate analysis, blood transfusion was not associated with a higher mortality. Furthermore, findings from 821 matched pairs established that there was a higher 30-day survival in the blood transfusion group ($P = 0.004$).

Over the last two decades, practices relating to blood transfusions within critical care have altered with an increased knowledge of both the tolerance of lower haemoglobin thresholds and associated complications. However, this large European observational study does not support the view, and suggests that blood transfusions may not necessarily be associated with an increase in mortality in intensive care patients. These findings could perhaps be linked to the increased usage of leukodepleted blood throughout Europe. The researchers suggest that a large randomised controlled trial similar to that conducted by Hébert et al. (1999) is urgently needed to validate these findings.

Reference

Hébert P, Wells G, Martin C, Tweedale M, Marshall J, Blajchman M, Pagliarello G, Sandham D, Schweitzer I, Boiswert D, Calder L (1999) Variation in red cell transfusion practice in the intensive care unit: a multi centre study. *Critical Care* **3**, 57–63.

Appendix VIII

Chapter article

Aragon D (2006) Evaluation of nursing workload and perceptions about blood glucose testing and tight glucose control. *American Journal of Critical Care* **15**(4), 370–377.

Commentary

This study is one of very few nurse-led research studies looking into the practical aspects of tight glucose control. It uses a small sample of observations, finding a wide range of times taken to perform blood glucose monitoring. It makes no comment on the experience of the nurses undertaking this task and an increased number of observations need to be performed before a conclusion about the impact on nurses' workload can be made.

Aragon (2006) highlights the importance of nursing knowledge and understanding of the reasons for blood glucose monitoring and tight glucose control. As illustrated in Lily's case, a lack of knowledge about the effects of intensive insulin therapy and insufficient blood glucose measurements can have a catastrophic impact on the patient's morbidity and mortality. Some nurses in the study were found to favour point-of-care testing and capillary sampling over arterial sampling. This has an impact on the accuracy and the consistency of the blood glucose measurements obtained. This is an area which needs to be explored in further studies.

Appendix IX

Chapter article

Kimball E, Baragoshi G, Mone M, Hansen H, Adams D, Alder S, Jackson P, Cannon P, Horn J, Wolfe T (2009) A comparison of infusion volumes in the measurement of intra-abdominal pressure. *Journal of Intensive Care Medicine* **24**(4), 261–268.

Commentary

This recent study was justified by the current lack of agreement both in practice and within the literature about the optimal amount of infusion fluid to be used for IAP measurement, with the risks of over instillation cited as being bladder distension and a falsely elevated IAP (Kimball et al. 2009). The authors of the paper were credible and included Professor Wolfe, an expert in the management of intra-abdominal pressure management and a member of the World Society of the Abdominal Compartment Syndrome.

A small surgical population was chosen to study. This limitation is acknowledged by the authors. Data from these 18 patients in only one site is insufficient to draw firm conclusions. However, findings are supported by other studies quoted within the publication, adding credence to the results.

IAP measurements were undertaken using the AbVisor system. Authors do reinforce that this has been tested for validity and reliability, although they do not explicitly state whether this research was funded by the company who produces this system. Use of this single system also raises questions about whether data from this study defining appropriate instillation volumes are also applicable to other available systems.

A protocol developed by the investigators was used during the study. No information is provided, however, on how it was ensured that all users adhered to this or whether any training was provided during the study to ensure consistency of use. If IAP measurements were conducted exclusively by the research team, the impact of these problems would be limited. This is not, however, made clear in the publication, leading to speculation about the process.

Results were clearly displayed in table form, with adequate detail given of statistical analysis. Cited confidence intervals were moderate, indicating an acceptable spread of results, thus enhancing confidence in the clinical significance of the data.

Although only a few other studies have been conducted looking at this area of practice, the authors did attempt to discuss their results in light of these, again strengthening their overall findings. Useful recommendations were made for future clinical practice.

Appendix X

Chapter article

Rickard et al. (2004) Preventing hypothermia during continuous veno-venous haemodi-afiltration: a randomized controlled trial. *Journal of Advanced Nursing* **47**(4), 393–400.

Commentary

Although this study was a well-conducted RCT, the authors acknowledge that findings may have been different if the sample size had been larger or if the effect of individual differences had been controlled for. Additionally, authors note the important fact that these findings may only be relevant to use of CVVHD using the same equipment and blood flow rate as studied.

The scenario based on Elizabeth focuses on the use of CVVH, and these results may therefore not be applicable. What this paper does highlight, however, is the significant lack of nursing research evidence available to guide practice in this area, despite the incidence of hypothermia being 37–55% during RRT (Rickard et al. 2004), A search for more recent data to support or refute these findings was lacking, and limited nursing research was found on other aspects of nursing care relevant to Elizabeth.

Appendix XI

Chapter article

Clabo L (2008) An ethnography of pain assessment and the role of social context on two postoperative units. *Journal of Advanced Nursing* **16**(5), 531–539.

Commentary

Given that this research was carried out recently, it is suggested that the findings are applicable not only to UK practice but also to practice in critical care settings.

Although the framework used for this study, Bourdieu's theory of practice – an ethnographic approach – may not be familiar, the reader may find that it provided a cohesive framework which guided the ways in which data were collected and the subsequent analysis. Three phases of data collection were used, with multiple methods of data collection appropriate to each phase used, including participant observation and individual interviews,

The study found that all nurses used similar criteria in the assessment of pain. However, although nurses working on the same unit demonstrated remarkably similar approaches to pain assessment, the pattern of pain assessment was distinctly different in each of the units. In one unit, the nurses' knowledge gained from experience of particular surgical procedures appeared to be most important. In the second unit, the patients' individual experience seemed to be most important in pain assessment. This demonstrated, for the researcher, an example of a 'group think' approach, and the impact of the social context on pain assessment practice. The impact of the findings is important if considering how changes in practice can be sustained and shared across wide areas of nursing practice.

Shannon and Bucknall (2003) suggest that with much of the research in relation to barriers to pain assessment and management in critical care, some of the limitations of studies include a relatively small sample size and study population which limit the generalisability of the results. Although this study was not carried out in a critical care area, it was still relatively small, as it was limited to one teaching hospital in the United States of America. It could be argued that it is not relevant to critical care areas. It could also be argued that the size of the study is such that the findings could not be generalised. However, this does not mean that the research is not valuable – it can be used to provide a basis for further research.

Reference

Shannon K, Bucknall T (2003) Pain assessment in critical care: what have we learnt from research? *Intensive and Critical Care Nursing* **19**, 154–162.

Appendix XII

Chapter article

Egerod I (2002) Uncertain terms of sedation in ICU. How nurses and physicians manage and describe sedation for mechanically ventilated patients. *Journal of Clinical Nursing* **11**(6), 831–840.

Commentary

Although conducted in 2002, the findings are still supported by current observations, making these findings applicable to UK practice.

It is a descriptive/comparative study with a case study design, with data extracted from four adult ICUs in Denmark. Interestingly, most of the available research on sedation practices derives from Denmark and other neighbouring Scandinavian countries.

A tool was developed to measure the potential of nurses in relation to their knowledge of critical care, location of work and type of patients. Results indicated that the potential of the nurse is positively related to tacit knowledge. Experience was not defined by knowledge (theoretical) through certification but gained through experience.

Data were collected using semi-structured interviews. Themes were identified for the questions. Observation interviews comprised of on the spot questioning (in connection with direct observations). Notably, all sites had similar sedation practices and all were in agreement about the goal of sedation, namely, promoting comfort, breathing, safety through lighter sedation.

Themes that emerged from the data were:

Indications for sedation

Tube irritation
Ventilator dys-synchrony
Restlessness
Relieving the nurses

Interventions related to sedation

Choice of agent
Dosages
Administration of sedation

Outcome

Tube acceptance
Just below the surface (actual level of sedation)
Tube seeking (reaching for the tube)
Well sedated

Level of sedation was based on the subjective interpretation of the nurse caring for the patient. Sedative practices were further muddled by unclear physician orders as well as lack of documentation on the part of the nurses. Terminology used possibly also had an impact on the interpretation of the intervention. There was disagreement about the optimum choice of agent. Experienced nurses were more likely than those less experienced to consider changing ventilation settings instead of increasing sedation because they had accumulated more clinical knowledge.

This study demonstrates that the level of nursing skill may be inversely related to the level of sedation given, with more experienced nurses using less sedation and a wider range of options for optimum management. Results from this study suggest that sedation practices are inconsistent. Experienced nurses provided a better quality of sedation than less experienced nurses, which is ironic as it is often the less experienced nurses who are assigned to care for ventilated patients.

Appendix XIII

Chapter article

Perz-Barceno J, Llompart-Pou JA, Homar J, Abadal JM, Raunch JM, Frontera G, Brell M, Ibanez Javier, Ibanez Jordi (2008) Phenobarbitol versus thiopental in the treatment of refractory intracranial hypertension in patients with traumatic brain injury: A randomised controlled trial. *Critical Care* **12**(4), R112.

Commentary

This is a relevant paper because it focuses on an aspect of traumatic brain injury management for which there is a paucity of research data. The paper addresses an important consideration for patients with refractory intracranial hypertension and it complies with approaches outlined in the Brain Trauma Foundation (BTF) guidelines (BTF 2007). Perez-Barcena et al. (2008) and the BTF (2007) guidelines highlight the significance of deep sedation for patients with severe TBI and resultant refractory intracranial hypertension, which concurs with approaches to management that aim to balance restricting elevations in intracranial pressure with optimising cerebral perfusion. Owing to the paucity of research comparing the two agents, an important finding is the difference in neuroprotective potential that each agent has and how this may have some influence on therapeutic attempts to limit the impact of secondary brain injury, such as ischeamia and cerebral oedema formation.

The strengths of this research lie in the transparency of the inclusion and exclusion criteria, the robust invasive monitoring modalities used to generate patient data and the adherence to conventional approaches to patient management as outlined in the BTF guidelines as first-tier therapy. Unfortunately, the limiting factors of the research lie in the small sample group, which suggests that results must be interpreted with caution and cannot be generalised across a wide population. As with most intervention research, this study is a conventional randomised trial that accounts for multiple variables that might impact on the outcomes. The study does not use a 'control group' of patients, as it would be ethically unacceptable to deny patients either of the drugs because they are known to have potential benefits in the management of refractory intracranial hypertension (Lettieri 2006; Bader et al 2005). Ethical considerations can sometimes be the reason that underpins the paucity of primary research conducted in a particular aspect of management.

Perez-Barcena et al. (2008) highlight their inability to conduct the study 'blind' due to difficulties with concealing the distinct appearance of each agent. Interpretation of the daily electroencephalogram (EEG) recordings, however, was made by a neurologist who was blinded to the patients' treatment.

The randomisation technique generated disparate groups in terms of types of intracranial lesions shown on the CT results, which required Perez-Barcena et al. (2008) to adopt specific statistical analysis approaches to incorporate the dissimilar prognostic variable.

Effectiveness criterion, control of intracranial pressure, highlights the relevance of other interventions, such as surgical decompression, cerebrospinal fluid drainage and hyperosmolar treatments in providing a comprehensive approach to managing patients with refractory intracranial hypertension following traumatic brain injury. The data/findings are displayed in clear table format and it is easy to see comparisons and whether any components are statistically significant.

The significant finding of the paper is the neuroprotective potential associated with thiopental, but there is a need for more robust first level research to provide conclusive and generalisable findings. The reluctance to instigate barbiturate coma in many intensive care patients may be because it is associated with inducing hypotension and pupillary dilation which impede neurological assessment (Lettieri 2006). There is an accumulative effect when the drug is administered via continuous intravenous infusion, which requires the patient to be EEG monitored to optimise burst suppression but at the lowest dose. Following cessation of the infusion the accumulative effect can prolong the period over which the patient will waken to allow more accurate neurological assessment, or it may delay necessary testing of brain stem function.

The implications for current practice are not conclusive but the paper further supports approaches outlined in the BTF guidelines (2007) and justifies consideration of thiopental use in facilitating damage limitation in severely brain injured patients with refractory intracranial hypertension.

Appendix XIV

Chapter article

Ely EW, Margolin R, Francis J, May L, Truman B, Dittus R, Speroff T, Gautam S, Bernard GR, Inouye SK (2001) Evaluation of delirium in critically ill patients: Validation of the Confusion Assessment Method for the Intensive Care Unit (CAM-ICU). *Critical Care Medicine* **29**(7), 1370–1379.

Commentary

The focus of this paper is significant because it addresses the recognition of a disorder that is prevalent in intensive care patients. Agitation, anxiety and delirium are witnessed in intensive care patients and it is not known whether these mental states express different types of cerebral dysfunction or whether they represent a spectrum in the severity of cerebral damage (Chevrolet and Jolliet 2007). Sepsis-associated delirium is a disorder seen frequently in critically ill patients, who manifest not merely an unpleasant state of confusion, but a relevant and often severe organ dysfunction that is reflected by an increase in mortality (Pfister et al. 2008). Ely et al. (2001) acknowledge the need to be able to accurately assess patients at risk of delirium within the intensive care environment where a proportion of the patients would be non-verbal due to ventilatory support. The paper highlights that misnomers such as 'ICU psychosis' and 'intensive care syndrome' have been used too often to account for patients' agitation, anxiety or possible delirium, which has overshadowed the true incidence of delirium within intensive care.

The development of the confusion assessment method (CAM) enabled non-psychiatrist-trained practitioners to improve their assessment of patients at risk of delirium. The paper explores the adaptation of this method to accurately and reliably identify delirium in intensive care patients by employing both ventilated and non-ventilated adults in the study population. Much detail is given on how a target sample size was expected to ensure a statistically sound screening instrument. The prospective cohort study numbers, however, do appear quite small in comparison to intervention studies that utilise randomised controlled trials.

The validity of the study procedures assures that assessments were carried out in a blinded fashion with a mean time between assessments. For those readers not familiar with the CAM-ICU, the detail and illustrations of the method in the appendices are helpful and enable the reader to contextualise how they might implement the assessment format within their practice. Study variables were considered by gathering a broad range of patient data. Ely et al. (2001) analysed the performance, or reliability, of the method by also including a sub-group of patients in whom suspected dementia had already been identified. Whilst there was a 100% sensitivity and specificity in this sub-group, the authors highlight the need for further research on a much wider scale.

The strengths of this research were that at the time there was no validated method by which critical care practitioners could assess/monitor ventilated patients for delirium. It was suggested that the CAM-ICU could be completed in two to three minutes, and was proposed as easy to incorporate into a daily routine. The method offers practitioners the opportunity to identify patients with delirium, which can inform subsequent clinical management and potentially improve patient outcomes.

There could be more generalised acceptance and use of this approach to recognise critically ill patients with delirium if larger studies were conducted that included appropriately sized sample populations in a wide range of critical care environments. This paper highlights a very important aspect that is often the consequence of a person's experience of severe or acute illness whilst being cared for in the milieu of intensive care. There are so many factors that precipitate agitation, anxiety and delirium that more emphasis must be given to acknowledging and managing such manifestations of compromised cognitive function.

Appendix XV

Chapter article

Drislane FW, Lopez MR, Blum AS, Schjomer DLl (2008) Detection and treatment of refractory status epilepticus in the intensive care unit. *Journal of Clinical Neurophysiology* **25**(4), 181–186.

Commentary

The article presents an abstract and introduction outlining the purpose of the study and the significance of the problem of undiagnosed and untreated status epiliepticus (SE) in the ICU setting. The study aims to determine the causes, clinical features, difficulties in diagnosis and the effects of anti-epileptic drugs (AEDs) on the course of SE in ICU patients. The article does not state whether a literature search and review of the current body of evidence on this topic was undertaken, however, claims regarding the prevalence of SE and difficulties encountered in making this diagnosis in ICU patients are supported by references to relevant literature. The aims of the study are somewhat ambitious but not unattainable.

The study design is poorly described in the article and the authors do not make it clear precisely how the study was conducted. The study is quantitative in its methodology and appears to be a retrospective cohort study examining 20 years of medical records of patients who had a confirmed EEG (electroencephalograph) diagnosis of SE in the ICU departments of a single hospital in Boston, USA. The study does not make clear exactly how subjects were selected for inclusion but this appears to be based on a review by two EEG technologists of the initial EEG performed, and their confirmation that these patients had a correct diagnosis of SE. The reliability of the diagnosis of SE is strengthened by stating the professional expertise of the technologists and that their opinion was the sole determinant of inclusion in the study.

Other clinical data were collected from the medical notes to establish if the responsible physician believed that the patient was having seizures at the time of the EEG and an estimate from clinical data was made as to the time of onset of SE until a confirmed diagnosis of this. The notes were also reviewed to ascertain when AEDs were commenced and clinical observations reviewed to establish whether these had an effect on the neurological status. The clinical data confirming onset of seizure activity (witnessed seizure activity, altered mental or neurological status) appear to be appropriate but their reliability could be doubted as the data were reviewed retrospectively and are subject to possible interpretation inaccuracy or bias by the researchers. The article also does not state who undertook the review of the medical notes and makes no comment as to how reliability of data collection was achieved.

A satisfactory sample size of 91 patients was obtained, although the sample was selected from a diverse population of medical and surgical patients with a multitude of clinical conditions and this could have affected the results, for example, in ascertaining the degree of initial risk in developing SE or likely response to AEDs.

The main findings of the study provide evidence of the wide range of aetiologies and variety of seizure types that can give rise to SE in ICU patients. A poor diagnostic rate for seizure activity was evident with only 22% of patients diagnosed as having seizures prior to EEG confirmation and some patients were in SE for many hours or even days (up to 72 hours in some cases) before a diagnosis was made. This raises concerns that there may be insufficient clinical suspicion of the presence of seizure activity. Experienced clinicians also appeared to have great difficulty in identifying seizure activity in ICU patients. AED treatment appeared to improve neurological status in about 58% of patients with non-anoxic conditions but did not improve outcome in anoxic patients. The effect of AED treatment was marginal in those patients in the non-anoxic group who subsequently died but this could not be attributed to neurological events alone. Patients with partial seizure activity as opposed to generalized seizures improved more significantly to AED treatment.

In their discussion, the authors acknowledge some of the limitations of the study. The retrospective design casts some doubt over the finding of small or transient improvements following AED treatment, as improvements were subjectively determined by clinical signs in the medical records. The authors also highlight that anoxic patients have such a poor prognosis that inclusion of this patient population may not be helpful in determining outcomes of SE. The authors do maintain, however, that these patients were excluded from the findings of responsiveness to AEDs as these patients would be unlikely to show any improvement. Early AED treatment did appear to yield positive results in a significant number of non-anoxic patients. The study does provide evidence of significant underdiagnosis of seizures and SE in ICU patients and highlights the difficulty in recognizing seizures in unconscious and sedated patients. There is very limited analysis or discussion of the statistical data and this weakens the overall discussion of the study's findings.

Retrospective studies have inherent problems in data interpretation as they may be subject to bias or inaccuracy. The findings of this study should be viewed with some caution but it still provides valuable insights into the problems associated with seizure activity in ICU patients and the importance of diagnosis and treatment. The authors suggest that there should be a higher suspicion of the presence of seizures and that EEG should be used earlier and more frequently to assist diagnosis and early implementation of AED treatment.

Appendix XVI

Chapter article

Hartung TK, Schofield E, Short AI, Parr MJA, Henry JA (2002) Hyponatremic states following 3,4-methylenedioxymethamphetamine (MDMA, 'ecstasy') ingestion. *Quarterly
Journal of Medicine* **95**, 431–437.

Commentary

Seventeen patients (0.4%) were sampled through screening of all documented enquiries
to the London National Poisons Information Service (NPIS) involving MDMA or ecstasy.
All cases where MDMA use was complicated by hyponatremia (defined by a serum Na
of <130 mmol/L) were included for further scrutiny, and clinical details, blood and urine
biochemistry results were requested from the relevant hospitals. However, the exact time
frame for data collection is not made clear and though management advice was provided
by NPIS medical staff for cases identified after November 2009, the content or degree
of uniformity of clinical guidance is not stated nor is it made clear which cases received
this. Under-reporting by healthcare workers may also have led to an underestimation of
the frequency of MDMA toxicity-related events, though it is also possible that healthcare
referrals represented the more serious of cases, thereby leading to an overestimation of
the frequency of hyponatremia.

Results presented compare clinical course data from the 14 patients who made a complete recovery and one who survived but suffered further complications. Data from the
two fatalities are also compared and clearly presented in tabulated form. MDMA was not
confirmed by toxicological analysis in five cases, though history of MDMA ingestion was
obtained.

Findings reported highlight commonalities in the clinical course of events. Symptoms
of drowsiness, agitation, disorientation and muted state were observed, and in six patients hyponatremia, low serum osmolality and concentrated urine led to a diagnosis of
inappropriate ADH secretion. It is interesting to note that the two fatalities had both con-
sumed large amounts of fluid and developed cerebral oedema within five hours of MDMA
ingestion.

The study aims to simply define clinical features rather than determine causal associations and contributes to a small body of literature exploring possible associations between
MDMA toxicity, hyponatremia, inappropriate ADH secretion and excessive fluid ingestion. Discussion highlights controversy around the clinical need for hypertonic saline
versus fluid restriction to effectively correct hyponatremia; however, data regarding precise management of the cases presented is unfortunately limited.

Appendix XVII

Chapter article

Jones et al. (2003) Rehabilitation after critical illness: a randomized, controlled trial.
Critical Care Medicine **31**, 2456–2461.

Commentary

The aim of this research and its research approach are clear. It is relevant to the general population of recovering critical care patients in terms of harnessing their own motivation and their social support to accelerate and secure recovery, building on the follow-up care, which was already provided by the three hospital teams involved. The chosen intervention (rehabilitation programme) was justified by similar successful self-directed and exercise programmes used for comparable groups of recovering patients.

A transparent selection process was followed, with the participants and researchers double-blinded during the study and successful efforts made to restrict the patients from meeting each other. Ethical approval was given; consent and confidentiality were implied since all the patients were receiving follow-up and the usual professional commitments of confidentiality would have applied. The final sample size of 126 was smaller than that required for strong statistical significance to be reached. The researchers, however, acknowledged this in their analysis and accounted for 100% of their participants in their trial profile. A mixture of patients across three different hospitals were recruited, which strengthens the results and reduces opportunities for bias due to any particular professional's relationship with patients or the style of working. The fact that all three teams already followed a specific follow-up protocol, which continued during the study, also protected against bias.

The rehabilitation programme was a manual containing information on exercise, advice on aspects of recovery, and prompted the patients to use a diary and engage at least one supporter from their social network to help them. The fact that this intervention was actually a package of several approaches demonstrates clearly the multi-faceted approach to recovery that patients need and was justified during its pilot by patients.

Established measurement and data collection tools were used to examine a range of recovery indicators: physical, psychological and social. Standard analytical tests were completed to support the researchers' interpretations. Due to the moderate sample size, only a few of the results were statistically significant. Trends, however, indicated clinical significance. In particular, in the intervention group, physical recovery was accelerated, depression reduced, anxiety reduced (only towards the six-month stage) and indicators of post-traumatic stress disorder (PTSD) reduced. The researchers identified, however, the large percentage of patients across both groups (51%) who exhibited signs of PTSD at six-month follow-up, with a link to delusional memories, fitting with other studies and implying that more professional awareness and expert management is needed by patients.

In summary, the study provided insight into the difficulties patients experience during the part of their recovery journey which in-hospital professionals do not often witness. It indicates clearly that patients and relatives are able and willing to be further involved with their recovery and a specifically tailored rehabilitation programme can enhance their quality of life after critical illness.

Appendix XVIII

Chapter article

Goodridge et al. (2008) Caring for critically ill patients with advanced COPD at the end of life: a qualitative study. *Intensive and Critical Care Nursing* **24**, 162–170.

Commentary

This exploratory study had a clear purpose in aiming to examine nurses' and respiratory therapists' perceived obstacles to providing care of a high quality for patients with end-stage chronic obstructive pulmonary disease (COPD). The clinical and professional challenges and dilemmas inherent in caring for this group of patients are highlighted in the literature review and the qualitative focus group design justified by the lack of research identifying specific issues. The subjects were invited volunteers from three different ICUs within the same city, who were fully aware of the discussion topic and had consented to take part. The three groups were small and each group comprised of staff from the same ICU. The small size, homogeneity of the groups and the fact that they were recalling past experiences were limitations since there may have been a tendency for group members to agree with each other, depending on influential individuals and the established organizational culture within the group.

Researcher influence was avoided by the use of structured focus groups facilitated by three different moderators and the maintenance of a clear audit trail of original transcripts and audiovisual data. Relevant thematic analysis techniques were used by separate researchers to analyse the data and follow-up interviews were done to confirm themes, ensuring quality control. This data collection and their thorough analysis was a key strength in this study and gives credibility to the interesting and pertinent results. Three key themes emerged: 'managing difficult symptoms' (specifically dyspnoea and anxiety), 'questioning the appropriateness of life-sustaining care' and 'conflicting care priorities'. These themes were discussed in relation to the findings of other studies to provide wider insight into the issues surrounding caring for ICU patients who are dying.

In summary, this useful study reveals pertinent, current issues in providing life support to people who have probably reached the end of their chronic illness.

Index

Critical Care Nursing: Learning from Practice, 1st edition. Edited by Suzanne Bench and Kate Brown.
© 2011 Blackwell Publishing Ltd.